D1417235

Pediatric Chest Pain

Guest Editors

GUY D. ESLICK, PhD, MMedSc(Clin Epi), MMedStat
STEVEN M. SELBST, MD

PEDIATRIC CLINICS
OF NORTH AMERICA

www.pediatric.theclinics.com

December 2010 • Volume 57 • Number 6

SAUNDERS an imprint of ELSEVIER, Inc.

W.B. SAUNDERS COMPANY
A Division of Elsevier Inc.

1600 John F. Kennedy Boulevard • Suite 1800 • Philadelphia, Pennsylvania 19103-2899

http://www.theclinics.com

THE PEDIATRIC CLINICS OF NORTH AMERICA Volume 57, Number 6
December 2010 ISSN 0031-3955, ISBN-13: 978-1-4377-2478-3

Editor: Kerry Holland
Developmental Editor: Jessica Demetriou

The Pediatric Clinics of North America (ISSN 0031-3955) is published bimonthly by Elsevier Inc., 360 Park Avenue South, New York, NY 10010-1710. Months of issue are February, April, June, August, October, and December. Periodicals postage paid at New York, NY and additional mailing offices. Subscription prices are $179.00 per year (US individuals), $423.00 per year (US institutions), $243.00 per year (Canadian individuals), $563.00 per year (Canadian institutions), $289.00 per year (international individuals), $563.00 per year (international institutions), $87.00 per year (US students and residents), and $149.00 per year (international and Canadian residents and students). To receive students/resident rare, orders must be accompanied by name of affiliated institution, date of term, and the signature of program/residency coordinator on institution letterhead. Orders will be billed at individual rate until proof of status is received. Foreign air speed delivery is included in all *Clinics* subscription prices. All prices are subject to change without notice. **POSTMASTER:** Send address changes to *The Pediatric Clinics of North America*, Elsevier Health Sciences Division, Subscription Customer Service, 3251 Riverport Lane, Maryland Heights, MO 63043. **Customer Service: 1-800-654-2452 (US and Canada). From outside of the US and Canada: 1-314-447-8871. Fax: 1-314-447-8029. For print support, E-mail: JournalsCustomerService-usa@elsevier.com. For online support, E-mail: JournalsOnlineSupport-usa@elsevier.com.**

Reprints. For copies of 100 or more, of articles in this publication, please contact the Commercial Reprints Department, Elsevier Inc., 360 Park Avenue South, New York, NY 10010-1710. Tel.: 212-633-3812; Fax: 212-462-1935; E-mail: reprints@elsevier.com.

The Pediatric Clinics of North America is also published in Spanish by McGraw-Hill Inter-americana Editores S.A., Mexico City, Mexico; in Portuguese by Riechmann and Affonso Editores, Rua Comandante Coelho 1085, CEP 21250, Rio de Janeiro, Brazil; and in Greek by Althayia SA, Athens, Greece.

The Pediatric Clinics of North America is covered in *MEDLINE/PubMed (Index Medicus), Excerpta Medica, Current Contents, Current Contents/Clinical Medicine, Science Citation Index, ASCA, ISI/BIOMED*, and *BIOSIS*.

Printed in the United States of America.

Contributors

GUEST EDITORS

GUY D. ESLICK, PhD, MMedSc(Clin Epi), MMedStat
Associate Professor, Discipline of Surgery, The Whiteley-Martin Research Centre, Sydney Medical School, The University of Sydney, Nepean Hospital, Penrith, New South Wales, Australia

STEVEN M. SELBST, MD
Professor of Pediatrics, Vice-Chair for Education, Pediatric Residency Program Director, Attending Physician, Division of Pediatric Emergency Medicine, Jefferson Medical College, Nemours/A.I. duPont Hospital for Children, Wilmington, Delaware

AUTHORS

BRETT R. ANDERSON, MD, MBA
Fellow, Division of Pediatric Cardiology, Morgan Stanley Children's Hospital of New York-Presbyterian, Columbia University Medical Center, New York, New York

ZULFIQAR A. BHUTTA, MBBS, FRCP, FRCPCH, FCPS, PhD
Division of Women and Child Health, Aga Khan University, Karachi, Pakistan

LORIN R. BROWNE, DO
Assistant Professor, Department of Pediatrics, Children's Corporate Center, Medical College of Wisconsin, Milwaukee, Wisconsin

STEPHEN JOHN CICO, MD
Assistant Professor, Attending Physician, Division of Emergency Medicine, Department of Pediatrics, Seattle Children's Hospital, University of Washington, Seattle, Washington

YAMINI DURANI, MD
Assistant Professor of Pediatrics, Department of Pediatrics, Thomas Jefferson University, Jefferson Medical College, Philadelphia, Pennsylvania; Attending Physician, Division of Emergency Medicine, Alfred I. duPont Hospital for Children, Wilmington, Delaware

ERIN E. ENDOM, MD
Assistant Professor, Section of Emergency Medicine, Department of Pediatrics, Baylor College of Medicine, Texas Children's Hospital, Houston, Texas

GUY D. ESLICK, PhD, MMedSc(Clin Epi), MMedStat
Associate Professor, Discipline of Surgery, The Whiteley-Martin Research Centre, Sydney Medical School, The University of Sydney, Nepean Hospital, Penrith, New South Wales, Australia

JOSE M. GARZA, MD
Assistant Professor of Pediatrics, Division of Gastroenterology, Hepatology and Nutrition, Cincinnati Children's Hospital Medical Center, Cincinnati, Ohio

KATIE GIORDANO, DO
Pediatric Emergency Medicine Fellow, Division of Emergency Medicine, Alfred I. duPont Hospital for Children, Wilmington, Delaware

MARC H. GORELICK, MD, MSCE
Professor and Chief, Pediatric Emergency Medicine; Jon E. Vice Chair in Emergency Medicine, Children's Hospital of Wisconsin, Medical College of Wisconsin, Milwaukee, Wisconsin

BRETT W. GOUDIE, MD
Clinical Instructor, Division of Cardiology, Department of Pediatrics, The Nemours Cardiac Center, Alfred I. duPont Hospital for Children, Wilmington, Delaware

NAKIA N. JOHNSON, MD
Fellow, Section of Emergency Medicine, Department of Pediatrics, Baylor College of Medicine, Texas Children's Hospital, Houston, Texas

AJAY KAUL, MD
Associate Professor of Pediatrics, Division of Gastroenterology, Hepatology and Nutrition, Cincinnati Children's Hospital Medical Center, Cincinnati, Ohio

YASIR KHAN, MD
Division of Women and Child Health, Aga Khan University, Karachi, Pakistan

CASSANDRA J. MCDONNELL, MA
Doctoral Candidate, Department of Psychology, University of Missouri-St Louis, St Louis, Missouri

CAROLYN A. PARIS, MD, MPH
Assistant Professor, Attending Physician, Division of Emergency Medicine, Department of Pediatrics, Seattle Children's Hospital, University of Washington, Seattle, Washington

STEVEN M. SELBST, MD
Professor of Pediatrics, Vice-Chair for Education, Pediatric Residency Program Director, Attending Physician, Division of Pediatric Emergency Medicine, Jefferson Medical College, Nemours/A.I. duPont Hospital for Children, Wilmington, Delaware

MARY BETH F. SON, MD
Instructor in Pediatrics, Division of Immunology, Harvard Medical School, Children's Hospital Boston, Boston, Massachusetts

ROBERT P. SUNDEL, MD
Associate Professor of Pediatrics, Division of Immunology, Harvard Medical School, Children's Hospital Boston, Boston, Massachusetts

MASATO TAKAHASHI, MD
Professor of Pediatrics Emeritus, Children's Hospital Los Angeles, University of Southern California Keck School of Medicine, Los Angeles, California

ALEXANDER TOLEDO, DO, PharmD
Fellow, Section of Emergency Medicine, Department of Pediatrics, Baylor College of Medicine, Texas Children's Hospital, Houston, Texas

VICTORIA L. VETTER, MD, MPH, MSHP
Professor of Pediatrics, Division of Pediatric Cardiology, The Children's Hospital of Philadelphia, University of Pennsylvania School of Medicine, Philadelphia, Pennsylvania

KAMILA S. WHITE, PhD
Assistant Professor, Department of Psychology, University of Missouri-St Louis, St Louis, Missouri

GEORGE A. WOODWARD, MD, MBA
Professor and Chief, Division of Emergency Medicine, Department of Pediatrics, Seattle Children's Hospital, University of Washington, Seattle, Washington

Contents

> The epidemiology and associated risk factors of pediatric chest pain are not well described. Several studies report the prevalence of chest pain types among children and adolescents; however, detailed prospective studies that aim to determine continued morbidity, mortality, health-care seeking behaviors, continued medication use, and quality of life are lacking. A greater understanding of pediatric chest pain epidemiology and risk factors is required.

> Children frequently present to a pediatric office or emergency department with the complaint of chest pain. Between 0.3% and 0.6% of visits to a pediatric emergency department are for chest pain. Unlike adult patients with chest pain, most studies have shown that children with chest pain rarely have serious organic pathology. Infrequently, a child with chest pain will present with significant distress and require immediate resuscitation. Most children with chest pain are not in extremis, and for many, the pain is not acute in nature.

> Chest pain is regularly encountered in pediatric medical settings and may be associated with many organic diagnoses that vary widely in morbidity and mortality. Patients with chest pain with and without organic disease may also suffer from comorbid, exacerbating, or causal psychopathology. This article provides practical general guidelines for psychological diagnosis and alleviation of emotional and behavioral difficulties. Specific medical conditions that may benefit from psychological consultation are highlighted. Pediatric chest pain, including an analysis of medically unexplained chest pain, is examined from a psychological perspective that includes a critical review of relevant literature and suggestions for the clinical management of this condition.

> Cardiac ischemia in children is usually not an isolated disease in an otherwise normally formed coronary artery but is part of more complex

congenital or acquired diseases. Although cardiac ischemia is not a frequent occurrence, it must be recognized as a serious, life-threatening event. This article lists and characterizes major causes of cardiac ischemia in children, describes signs and symptoms of each, and provides therapeutic considerations.

Myocarditis and pericarditis are rare but important causes of pediatric chest pain. The diagnositic criteria, clinical course, causes, and treatment of myocarditis is reviewed. There is particular attention to the relationship of myocarditis with dilated cardiomyopathy. Supportive therapy remains the standard of care for pump dysfunction. The identification and treatment of pericarditis with associated large pericardial effusion can be life-saving. This article reviews the important clinical features that might lead the clinician to diagnose either myocarditis or pericarditis and thus separate the few patients with either of these conditions from the legions of children with noncardiac chest pain.

Although cardiac causes of chest pain in children are infrequent, arrhythmias are implicated in most cardiac related cases. The most common arrhythmias associated with chest pain are supraventricular tachycardias, but more ominous rhythms, such as ventricular tachycardia or bradycardias, can manifest as chest pain. Investigation of all children with chest pain suspected of arrhythmia should include detailed history and physical examination and a 12- or 15-lead electrocardiogram. In some cases echocardiogram, 24-hour Holter monitoring, exercise stress testing, or other cardiac evaluations may be indicated. Children with a history of cardiac disease or cardiac surgery are particularly at risk for arrhythmias and may experience chest pain in association with their arrhythmias.

Even though chest pain in children is a common complaint, an underlying gastrointestinal cause is rare. The four common gastrointestinal conditions that present with chest pain include eosinophilic esophagitis, gastroesophageal reflux disease, esophageal dysmotility, and foreign body ingestion. Other than ingestion of certain foreign bodies, most of these conditions are not life-threatening. Associated symptoms and history may be helpful in distinguishing these disorders, but further evaluation is often indicated to identify the precise cause.

Chest pain remains a common complaint among children seeking care in the United States. Asthma and lower respiratory tract infections such as pneumonia can be significant causes of chest pain. Children with chest pain caused by either of these pulmonary etiologies generally present with associated respiratory symptoms, including cough, wheezing, tachypnea, respiratory distress, and/or fever. Although analgesic medications can improve chest pain associated with pulmonary pathologies, the mainstay of therapy is to treat the underling etiology; this includes bronchodilator and/or steroid medications in children with asthma and appropriate antibacterial administration in children with suspicions of bacterial pneumonia. The chest pain generally resolves along with the resolution of other respiratory symptoms.

This article discusses pneumothorax, pneumomediastinum, and pulmonary embolism in pediatric practice. Although children appear to have better outcomes than adults, the risk factors are substantial. Topics covered include the pathophysiology incidence, presentation, diagnosis, and management of these diseases.

Musculoskeletal chest pain is the most common identifiable cause of chest pain in children and adolescents. A lesion or irritation of any layer of the anterior chest wall may lead to pain. Causes range from the common, such as costochondritis, to the rare, such as chronic recurrent multifocal osteomyelitis. Regardless of the cause, chest pain raises concern of cardiac abnormalities, and may rapidly lead to significant anxiety and lifestyle alterations. Thus, efficient and accurate identification of the cause of pediatric chest pain by a thorough history and physical examination is important to minimize the disruption it may cause.

This article describes some of the miscellaneous etiologies of pediatric chest pain that are important to recognize early and diagnose. Up to 45% of pediatric chest pain cases may elude definitive diagnosis. Serious morbidity or mortality is infrequent. Accurate diagnosis of more obscure causes may help to avoid unnecessary emergency department evaluation and cardiology referral, while also alleviating the concern and stress families and patients experience when dealing with chest pain.

Several contributory factors such as poverty, lack of purchasing power, household food insecurity, and limited general knowledge about appropriate nutritional practices increase the risk of undernutrition in developing countries. The synergistic interaction between inadequate dietary intake and disease burden leads to a vicious cycle that accounts for much of the high morbidity and mortality in these countries. Three groups of underlying factors contribute to inadequate dietary intake and infectious disease: inadequate maternal and child care, household food insecurity, and poor health services in an unhealthy environment.

THE CLINICS ARE NOW AVAILABLE ONLINE!

Access your subscription at:
www.theclinics.com

GOAL STATEMENT

The goal of the *Pediatric Clinics of North America* is to keep practicing physicians and residents up to date with current clinical practice in pediatrics by providing timely articles reviewing the state-of-the-art in patient care.

ACCREDITATION

The *Pediatric Clinics of North America* is planned and implemented in accordance with the Essential Areas and Policies of the Accreditation Council for Continuing Medical Education (ACCME) through the joint sponsorship of the University Of Virginia School Of Medicine and Elsevier. The University Of Virginia School of Medicine is accredited by the ACCME to provide continuing medical education for physicians.

The University of Virginia School of Medicine designates this educational activity for a maximum of 15 *AMA PRA Category 1 Credits*™ for each issue, 90 credits per year. Physicians should only claim credit commensurate with the extent of their participation in the activity.

The American Medical Association has determined that physicians not licensed in the US who participate in this CME activity are eligible for a maximum of 15 *AMA PRA Category 1 Credits*™ for each issue, 90 credits per year.

Credit can be earned by reading the text material, taking the CME examination online at http://www.theclinics.com/home/cme, and completing the evaluation. After taking the test, you will be required to review any and all incorrect answers. Following completion of the test and evaluation, your credit will be awarded and you may print your certificate.

FACULTY DISCLOSURE/CONFLICT OF INTEREST

The University of Virginia School of Medicine, as an ACCME accredited provider, endorses and strives to comply with the Accreditation Council for Continuing Medical Education (ACCME) Standards of Commercial Support, Commonwealth of Virginia statutes, University of Virginia policies and procedures, and associated federal and private regulations and guidelines on the need for disclosure and monitoring of proprietary and financial interests that may affect the scientific integrity and balance of content delivered in continuing medical education activities under our auspices.

The University of Virginia School of Medicine requires that all CME activities accredited through this institution be developed independently and be scientifically rigorous, balanced and objective in the presentation/discussion of its content, theories and practices.

All authors/editors participating in an accredited CME activity are expected to disclose to the readers relevant financial relationships with commercial entities occurring within the past 12 months (such as grants or research support, employee, consultant, stock holder, member of speakers bureau, etc.). The University of Virginia School of Medicine will employ appropriate mechanisms to resolve potential conflicts of interest to maintain the standards of fair and balanced education to the reader. Questions about specific strategies can be directed to the Office of Continuing Medical Education, University of Virginia School of Medicine, Charlottesville, Virginia.

The faculty and staff of the University of Virginia Office of Continuing Medical Education have no financial affiliations to disclose.

The authors/editors listed below have identified no financial or professional relationships for themselves or their spouse/partner:
Brett R. Anderson, MD, MBA; Zulfiqar A. Bhutta, MBBS, FRCP, FRCPCH, FCPS, PhD; Lorin R. Browne, DO; Stephen John Cico, MD; Yamini Durani, MD; Guy D. Eslick, PhD, MMedSc(Clin Epi), MMedStat (Guest Editor); Erin E. Endom, MD; Jose M. Garza, MD; Katie Giordano, DO; Marc H. Gorelick, MD, MSCE; Brett W. Goudie, MD; Carla Holloway, (Acquisitions Editor); Nakia N. Johnson, MD; Ajay Kaul, MD; Yasir Khan, MD; Cassandra J. McDonnell, MA; Carolyn A. Paris, MD, MPH; Karen Rheuban, MD (Test Author); Steven M. Selbst, MD (Guest Editor); Mary Beth F. Son, MD; Robert P. Sundel, MD; Masato Takahashi, MD; Alexander Toldeo, DO, PharmD; Victoria L. Vetter, MD, MPH, MSHP; and Kamila S. White, PhD.

The authors/editors listed below identified the following professional or financial affiliations for themselves or their spouse/partner:
George A. Woodward, MD, MBA is a consultant for the Joint Commission Resources, and is an intermittent consultant for the Joint Commission International.

Disclosure of Discussion of Non-FDA Approved Uses for Pharmaceutical Products and/or Medical Devices
The University of Virginia School of Medicine, as an ACCME provider, requires that all faculty presenters identify and disclose any off-label uses for pharmaceutical and medical device products. The University of Virginia School of Medicine recommends that each physician fully review all the available data on new products or procedures prior to clinical use.

TO ENROLL

To enroll in the Pediatric Clinics of North America Continuing Medical Education program, call customer service at 1-800-654-2452 or visit us online at www.theclinics.com/home/cme. The CME program is available to subscribers for an additional fee of $223.00

Preface

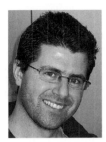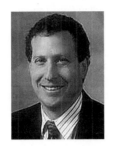

Guy D. Eslick, PhD,   Steven M. Selbst, MD
MMedSc(Clin Epi), MMedStat
Guest Editors

It is with immense pleasure that we welcome you to this issue of *Pediatric Clinics of North America*, which is devoted to one of the most common reasons for children and adolescents to present to a physician, that is, "chest pain." Chest pain is an alarming symptom and the importance of careful evaluation cannot be understated. Determining a "cause" for pediatric chest pain can be very challenging as it is a complex symptom with a myriad of potential pathologies. Clinicians are rightfully concerned about some serious causes of chest pain in children, but there is also concern about ordering expensive studies to make a diagnosis when this may not be necessary. There are several prospective studies and case reports to guide clinicians, but many questions about chest pain remain. Investigation/management is often dictated by the emotional concerns of the family and physicians.

Evaluating a child with chest pain can be a frustrating experience for the clinician, the patient, and the family. Despite careful evaluation, in almost half of all pediatric chest pain cases, the cause is unknown, which adds stress to the parents of sick children and the concern that they may have a potentially fatal form of chest pain. Often the pain disturbs the child's daily routine. Many children with this complaint are awakened from sleep by the pain, while many others miss school because of chest pain. The clinical picture of chest pain for children is different than that of adults along with the causes and associated conditions, with risk factors such as obesity, an essentially unassessed problem.

In this issue of *Pediatric Clinics of North America*, we aim to produce a diverse yet practical collection of topics that will be of use not only to general pediatricians but also for specialists in cardiology, emergency medicine, gastroenterology, and other areas of medicine.

In preparing this issue we selected authorities in medicine, including cardiology, gastroenterology, respiratory medicine, rheumatology, psychological medicine, internal medicine, and pediatrics. Most importantly, we would like to thank all the authors who contributed their expertise and precious time in developing these useful articles.

Pediatr Clin N Am 57 (2010) xiii–xiv
doi:10.1016/j.pcl.2010.09.015
0031-3955/10/$ – see front matter © 2010 Elsevier Inc. All rights reserved.

pediatric.theclinics.com

We believe these articles are educational and practical and we hope they will be of use to clinicians and researchers around the world. We would also like to thank Carla Holloway, the Editor of *Pediatric Clinics of North America*, for providing excellent guidance and keeping us on track during the production of this issue. Dr Eslick would like to give special thanks to Enid, Marielle, and Isacc for their love and continued support. Dr Selbst would like to thank his wife Andrea and children Lonn and Eric for their tremendous support and encouragement.

We hope this issue of *Pediatric Clinics of North America* will be an excellent resource for all who play a role in the diagnosis and treatment of pediatric patients with chest pain.

Guy D. Eslick, PhD, MMedSc(Clin Epi), MMedStat
The Whiteley-Martin Research Centre
Discipline of Surgery
Sydney Medical School
The University of Sydney
Nepean Hospital, Level 5
South Block, PO Box 63
Penrith, Sydney, New South Wales 2751
Australia

Steven M. Selbst, MD
Division of Pediatric Emergency Medicine
Jefferson Medical College
Nemours/A.I. duPont Hospital for Children
1600 Rockland Road
Wilmington, DE 19803–3607, USA

E-mail addresses:
eslickg@med.usyd.edu.au (G.D. Eslick)
sselbst@nemours.org (S.M. Selbst)

Dedication

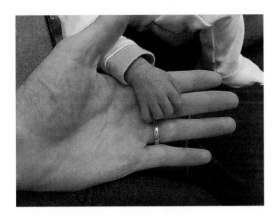

I would like to dedicate this issue of the *Pediatric Clinics of North America* to my newborn son, Isaac-Guillaume Eslick, who was born six weeks early on the 24th of March at 12:08 AM. Once again I have been blessed by God.

The Lord says, "Do not be afraid! I am with you—do not be afraid! Do not let your troubles overwhelm you, I hold you in the palm of My hand. I love you! I sustain you; I give you strength; I lead and guide you. Trust in Me! Trust in Me!! Isaiah 43:1-7."

Guy D. Eslick

Pediatr Clin N Am 57 (2010) xv
doi:10.1016/j.pcl.2010.09.014
0031-3955/10/$ — see front matter © 2010 Elsevier Inc. All rights reserved.

pediatric.theclinics.com

Epidemiology and Risk Factors of Pediatric Chest Pain: A Systematic Review

Guy D. Eslick, PhD, MMedSc(Clin Epi), MMedStat

KEYWORDS

• Chest pain • Pediatric chest pain • Risk factors • Epidemiology
• Prevalence

Chest pain among children and adolescents is common[1–4]; however, knowledge of the epidemiology of pediatric chest pain and risk factors associated with it is scant. An understanding of the epidemiology of chest pain among children is important, because it provides information about changes that may occur in behavior, culture, and environment, not to mention risk factors and causes of chest pain. Chest pain is an important alarm symptom. In adults, the presence of chest pain conjures up the possibility of a potentially fatal cardiac event. Fear of a serious life-threatening condition also exists for parents of children with acute chest pain, but the literature suggests that pediatric chest pain is generally a benign condition.[5–7] However, at present, there are very little mortality data related to chest pain as the primary presenting symptom, and further studies are required to validate these claims. The literature is scattered in prevalence studies and other reports on risk factors; this article aims to consolidate this literature and provide an overview of all studies assessing the epidemiology and risk factors of pediatric chest pain.

SYSTEMATIC REVIEW

The search strategy for this review included the following major electronic databases: MEDLINE, EMBASE, and Current Contents (1950–September 2010). The search strategy used combinations of the keywords (1) chest pain, (2) pediatric, (3) children, (4) adolescents, (5) epidemiology, and (6) risk factors. Additional manual searches were made using the reference lists from all published papers. No language restriction was placed on any of the literature searches. The search revealed 219 potential studies. The abstracts of all potential studies were read to determine if they were epidemiologic in nature or on risk factors. There were 69 epidemiologic studies and

The Whiteley-Martin Research Centre, Discipline of Surgery, Sydney Medical School, The University of Sydney, Nepean Hospital, Level 5, South Block, PO Box 63, Penrith, New South Wales 2751, Australia
E-mail address: eslickg@med.usyd.edu.au

Pediatr Clin N Am 57 (2010) 1211–1219
doi:10.1016/j.pcl.2010.09.013
0031-3955/10/$ – see front matter Crown Copyright © 2010 Published by Elsevier Inc. All rights reserved.

Table 1
Characteristics of chest pain studies conducted on pediatric populations

Study	Year	N	M/F	Age (Mean)	Cardiac (%)	Gastrointestinal (%)	Psychological (%)	Musculoskeletal (%)	Respiratory (%)	Idiopathic (%)
Driscoll et al[5]	1976	40	22/18	12–19 (12.35)				22.5	12.5	45
Asnes et al[14]	1981	123	41/82	4–13			29			
Kashani et al[15]	1982	100					13			
Pantell and Goodman[12]	1983	100						45		
Fyfe[30]	1984	67	40/27	8–19	6	1		1	2	85
Selbst[34]	1985	267								
Rowland and Richards[11]	1986	31	23/8	8–18			26			
Nudel et al[16]	1987	180	112/68	5–22					18	
Selbst et al[35]	1988	407	180/227	2–19	4	4	9	15	21	21
Berezin et al[36]	1988	51		8–20		6		41		53
Selbst et al[9]	1990	149	69/80	(11.34)	4	3	11	11	20	34
Rowe et al[37]	1990	336	159/166	2–18			5	28	19	12
Woolf et al[38]	1991	17		(14.00)		59				
Zavaras-Angelidou et al[39]	1992	134	74/60	1.2–19	19	7		16	12	20
Glassman et al[18]	1992	83	42/39	1–20		48				56.6

Study	Year	N	F/M	Age						
Wiens et al[40]	1992	88	47/41	4–20			74			92
Tunaoglu et al[41]	1995	100	46/54	2.5–16						
Gunther et al[33]	1999	456		4–17						
Silva et al[32]	2000	104	59/45	4–16	10.6		13.5	22.1	7.6	46.2
Evangelista et al[10]	2000	50	33/17	5–21		8	4	76	12	
Lam and Tobias[42]	2001	55	28/27	6–20	12	15	4	32	4	30
Sabri et al[31]	2003	132	21/23	(12.10)	33.1	36.1				
Gastesi Larranaga et al[43]	2003	161								
Yildirim et al[50]	2004	300	172/128	3–17	8	4.7	18.7	1.6	3	63.4
Massin et al[44]	2004	168	133/104	3–15	5	4	9	64	13	
Wojcicka-Urbanska et al[51]	2004	60		(13.00)	23		10	4	11	52
Sadurska et al[49]	2005	132			22.7	11.4	25.8	1.5	6.8	46.2
Lipsitz et al[45]	2005	27	15/12	8–17			59			
Cagdas and Pac[46]	2009	120	66/54	5–16	42.5					
Danduran et al[47]	2008	263	141/122	5–22						
Lin et al[48]	2008	103	64/39	4–17	2	5.8	2	6.7	24.3	59.2
Hambrook et al[8]	2010	818	368/450	0–18	2.8	6.4	2.2	12.8	9.4	36.4
Total		5,222			13.5	14.63	20.30	22.00	11.84	44.35

Abbreviations: F, female; N, number; M, male.

27 on risk factors for pediatric chest pain. In the final review, only 36 epidemiologic studies were used. Full versions of these studies were read and the data used in this systematic review.

EPIDEMIOLOGY

The first published study to determine the epidemiology of chest pain amongst children and adolescents was published more than 30 years ago.[5] It was a prospective study of 43 children with a mean age of 12 years. The major categories of chest pain reported from this study were idiopathic chest pain (45%), costochondritis (22.5%), chest pain secondary to bronchitis (12.5%), miscellaneous (10%), chest pain secondary to muscle pain (5%), and chest pain secondary to trauma (5%). The average duration of chest pain varied considerably: idiopathic, approximately 2 years; miscellaneous, around 8 months; costochondritis, 3 months; trauma, just over a week; bronchitis, just under a week; and muscle strain, 1 day. The conclusions reached from this study were that chest pain in children was not as ominous as in adults and that cardiac disease represented a very small proportion of presentations.

Since then, there have been almost 40 studies on the prevalence of chest pain amongst children and adolescents. The study by Driscoll and colleagues[5] was the only one published in the 1970s; however, in the 1980s, there were 11 additional studies and in the 1990s, slightly fewer, with 8 studies published; in the first decade of the twenty-first century, there have been 16 studies. These studies have included 5222 patients from numerous countries around the world (**Table 1**).

The most recent study,[8] which is also the largest one published (N = 818), was drawn from the 2002–2006 National Hospital Ambulatory Medical Care Survey (NHAMCS) in the United States. This included all emergency department visits with a main complaint of chest pain for individual's aged less than 19 years. Chest pain was classified into 9 different groups (**Fig. 1**). Chest pain not otherwise specified made up the majority (36.8%) of presentations, followed by infectious (21.1%), trauma-musculoskeletal (12.8%), respiratory (9.4%), other (8.2%), gastrointestinal (6.4%), cardiovascular (2.8%), psychiatric (2.2%), and hematologic (0.3%) presentations. This suggests that chest pain related to cardiovascular disease represents a very small proportion of all chest pain presentations to emergency departments.

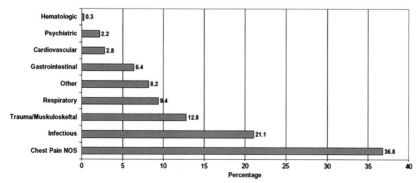

Fig. 1. Emergency department discharge diagnosis from the largest study in pediatric chest pain. (NOS, not otherwise specified). (*From* Hambook JT, Kimball TR, Khoury P, et al. Disparities exist in the emergency department evaluation of pediatric chest pain. Congenit Heart Dis 2010;5:285–91; with permission.)

However, if all studies conducted on pediatric chest pain are analyzed, there seems to be a significantly greater proportion of chest pain presentations associated with a cardiac cause (9.57%). The difference may be explained by some of these studies being taken from pediatric cardiology departments in which a diagnosis of cardiovascular disease is more likely to be found than in an emergency department setting. But if these data are taken as a whole, then it suggests that cardiac causes are more common than previously thought, relative to other types of chest pain. Moreover, the groupings of these chest pain types could also be an important factor, for example, with groups like *other* and *chest pain not otherwise specified*, a substantial proportion of patients have no known cause for their chest pain, at least in initial diagnostic workup in an emergency setting. It would seem worthwhile to follow up these patients over long periods to determine what subsequent diagnosis is applied to these cases and determine important clinical outcomes (eg, mortality, morbidity, repeat presentations).

A limited number of prospective studies have been conducted among pediatric patients,[4,9–12] seeming to have similar problems to adult studies in terms of very small sample sizes, low follow-up rates, and short follow-up periods (3 years maximum).[13] The largest of these studies consisted of 407 children at baseline, of whom, 149 were followed up for 6 months or more and 51 patients were followed up for 2 years of more.[9] Patients had 3 repeat visits in the follow-up period, during which time, the initial diagnoses changed in just over a third of patients (34%), sometimes more than once (5%). Almost half the patients (43%) continued to experience intermittent or persistent chest pain.

The analysis of the studies in this systematic review based on the type of chest pain reported has generally consisted of 6 different groups, usually based on organ systems. These data suggest that idiopathic chest pain was most prevalent (35.62%), followed by musculoskeletal (19.75%), then psychological (16.31%), gastrointestinal (10.36%), cardiac (9.57%), and respiratory (8.39%) conditions as the primary cause of presentation (**Fig. 2**).

RISK FACTORS

There is very little information on the risk factors associated with chest pain in children and adolescents (**Box 1**). Risk factors in adults and children with chest pain differ significantly, with overlap for certain types of chest pain. Some of these risk factors are discussed in greater detail in other articles. The author only gives a brief overview of what currently exists in the literature. Currently, all published reports on pediatric chest pain are case reports or case series.[14–29] As yet, no studies have been published reporting on the risk factors in relation to chest pain frequency and severity within a pediatric population experiencing chest pain. It would seem that a study assessing the type and magnitude of risk factors is warranted.

Some of these risk factors occur in both adult and pediatric groups; for example, certain beverages like coffee and carbonated drinks. Other risk factors, such as aspirin use, NSAID use, smoking, and alcohol use are more of an issue in an adult group; however, this does not exclude the possibility of them being of importance in some pediatric presentations for chest pain. A risk factor of increasing importance among pediatric populations is obesity, the impact of which has not been determined in a clinical or community sample. Obesity may be important on its own or in combination with other conditions, such as gastroesophageal reflux disease.

Also, future studies should assess the role of illness behavior between adult family members and their children, which could represent a substantial proportion of patients

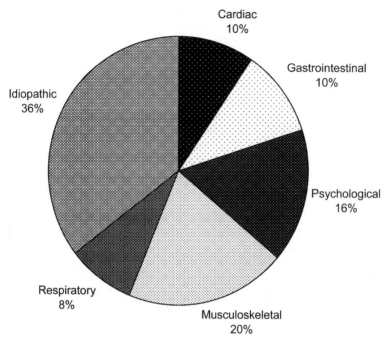

Fig. 2. Summary of the classification of chest pain types from all studies.

Box 1
Published risk factors for children with chest pain

- 5-Aminosalicylic acid
- Infections (*Mycoplasma pneumoniae*, mycobacterial disease)
- Tetracycline
- Cocaine
- Marijuana
- Ephedrine
- Psychological disorders (panic disorder, anxiety, depression)
- Dipyridamole
- Methacholine inhalation
- Exercise-induced asthma
- Spinal arteriovenous malformation
- Kawasaki disease
- Esophageal disorders
- Caffeinated beverages (ie, coffee)
- Carbonated beverages

with chest pain who are currently classified as suffering from either idiopathic or noncardiac chest pain.

SUMMARY

Currently, the epidemiology of chest pain among children and adolescents is poorly understood, with little data on risk factors or the epidemiology of pediatric chest pain in the general population. Further, large, long-term prospective studies are required.

ACKNOWLEDGMENTS

The author thanks Dr Brigitte Nanan for translation of the German paper, Beatriz Belmar for translation of the Spanish paper, and Ms Maree Yabsley for assistance with the table.

REFERENCES

1. Kocis KC. Chest pain in pediatrics. Pediatr Clin North Am 1999;46:189–203.
2. Brenner JI, Ringel RE, Berman MA. Cardiologic perspectives of chest pain in childhood: a referral problem? To whom? Pediatr Clin North Am 1984;31:1241–58.
3. Balfour IC, Syamasudar Rao P. Chest pain in children. Indian J Pediatr 1998;65: 21–6.
4. Eslick GD. Classification, natural history, epidemiology, and risk factors of noncardiac chest pain. Dis Mon 2008;54:593–603.
5. Driscoll DJ, Glicklich LB, Gallen WJ. Chest pain in children: a prospective study. Pediatrics 1976;57:648–51.
6. Thull-Freedman J. Evaluation of chest pain in the pediatric patient. Med Clin North Am 2010;94:327–47.
7. Gokhale J, Selbst SM. Chest pain and chest wall deformity. Pediatr Clin North Am 2009;56:49–65.
8. Hambrook JT, Kimball TR, Khoury P, et al. Disparities exist in the Emergency Department evaluation of pediatric chest pain. Congenit Heart Dis 2010;5: 285–91.
9. Selbst SM, Ruddy RM, Clark BJ. Chest pain in children follow-up of patients previously reported. Clin Pediatr (Phila) 1990;297:374–7.
10. Evangelista JA, Parsons M, Renneberg AK. Chest pain in children: diagnosis through history and physical examination. J Pediatr Health Care 2000;14:3–8.
11. Rowland TW, Richards MM. The natural history of idiopathic chest pain in children. A follow-up study. Clin Pediatr (Phila) 1986;25:612–4.
12. Pantell RH, Goodman BW. Adolescent chest pain: a prospective study. Pediatrics 1983;716:881–7.
13. Eslick GD, Talley NJ. Natural history and predictors of outcome for non-cardiac chest pain: a prospective cohort study. Neurogastroenterol Motil 2008;20:989–97.
14. Asnes RS, Santulli R, Bemporad JR. Psychogenic chest pain in children. Clin Pediatr (Phila) 1981;20:788–91.
15. Kashani JH, Lababidi Z, Jones RS. Depression in children and adolescents with cardiovascular symptomatology: the significance of chest pain. J Am Acad Child Psychiatry 1982;21:187–9.
16. Nudel DB, Diamant S, Brady T, et al. Chest pain, dyspnea on exertion, and exercise induced asthma in children and adolescents. Clin Pediatr (Phila) 1987;26: 388–92.

17. Woodward GA, Selbst SM. Chest pain secondary to cocaine use. Pediatr Emerg Care 1987;3:153–4.
18. Glassman MS, Medow MS, Berezin S, et al. Spectrum of esophageal disorders in children with chest pain. Dig Dis Sci 1992;37:663–6.
19. Izumi N, Haneda N, Mori C. Methacholine inhalation challenge in children with idiopathic chest pain. Acta Paediatr Jpn 1992;34:441–6.
20. Tomita H, Ikeda K, Nagata N, et al. Dipyridamole-provoked chest pain implies severe coronary artery disease in children. Acta Paediatr Jpn 1993;35:289–93.
21. Chen CC, Wang CM, Chu NK, et al. Spinal cord arteriovenous malformation presenting as chest pain in a child. Spinal Cord 2008;46:456–8.
22. Madhok AB, Boxer R, Green S. An adolescent with chest pain-sequela of Kawasaki disease. Pediatr Emerg Care 2004;20:765–8.
23. Kundra M, Yousaf S, Maqbool S, et al. Boerhaave syndrome–unusual cause of chest pain. Pediatr Emerg Care 2007;23:489–91.
24. Gilleland J, Blount RL, Campbell RM, et al. Psychosocial factors and pediatric noncardiac chest pain. J Pediatr Psychol 2009;34:1170–4.
25. Milov DE, Cynamon HA, Andres JM. Chest pain and dysphagia in adolescents caused by diffuse esophageal spasm. J Pediatr Gastroenterol Nutr 1989;9: 450–3.
26. James LP, Farrar HC, Komoroski EM, et al. Sympathomimetic drug use in adolescents presenting to a pediatric emergency department with chest pain. J Toxicol Clin Toxicol 1998;36:321–8.
27. Hascelik S, Ozer S, Taner Y, et al. Panic disorder in a child with recurrent chest pain. Turk J Pediatr 2007;49:105–8.
28. Atay O, Radhakrishnan K, Arruda J, et al. Severe chest pain in a pediatric ulcerative colitis patient after 5-aminosalicylic acid therapy. World J Gastroenterol 2008;14:4400–2.
29. Cohen M, Kelly K, Shaw KN. Chest pain and cardiomegaly without pulmonary involvement: An atypical presentation of pediatric mycobacterial disease. Pediatr Emerg Care 1995;11:35–6.
30. Fyfe MD. Chest pain in pediatric patients presenting to a cardiac clinic. Clin Pediatr (Phila) 1984;23:321–40.
31. Sabri MR, Ghavanimi AA, Haghighat M, et al. Chest pain in children and adolescents: epigastric tenderness as a guide to reduce unnecessary work-up. Pediatr Cardiol 2003;24:3–5.
32. Silva A, Aires Pereira S, Alvares S. Chest pain - retrospective study. Nascer E Crescer 2000;9:171–6.
33. Gunther A, Kapke C, Stern K, et al. Etiology and symptomatology of chest pain in children referred to a cardiology practice. Monatsschr Kinderheilkd 1999;147: 339–45.
34. Selbst SM. Chest pain in children. Pediatrics 1985;75:1068–70.
35. Selbst SM, Ruddy RM, Clark BJ, et al. Pediatric chest pain: a prospective study. Pediatrics 1988;82:319–23.
36. Berezin S, Medow MS, Glassman MS, et al. Chest pain of gastrointestinal origin. Arch Dis Child 1988;63:1457–60.
37. Rowe BH, Dulberg CS, Peterson RG, et al. Characteristics of children presenting with chest pain to a pediatric Emergency Department. CMAJ 1990;143:388–94.
38. Woolf PK, Gewitz MH, Berezin S, et al. Noncardiac chest pain in adolescents and children with mitral valve prolapse. J Adolesc Health 1991;12:247–50.
39. Zavaras-Angelidou KA, Weinhouse E, Nelson DB. Review of 180 episodes of chest pain in 134 children. Pediatr Emerg Care 1992;8:189–93.

40. Wiens L, Sabath R, Ewing L, et al. Chest pain in otherwise healthy children and adolescents is frequently caused by exercise-induced asthma. Pediatrics 1992; 90:350–3.
41. Tunaoglu FS, Olgunturk R, Akcabay S, et al. Chest pain in children referred to a cardiology clinic. Pediatr Cardiol 1995;16:69–72.
42. Lam JC, Tobias JD. Follow-up survey of children and adolescents with chest pain. South Med J 2001;94:921–4.
43. Gastesi Larranaga M, Fernandez Landaluce A, Mintegi Raso S, et al. [Chest pain in pediatric emergency departments: a usually benign process]. An Pediatr (Barc) 2003;59:234–8 [in Spanish].
44. Massin MM, Bourguignont A, Coremans C, et al. Chest pain in pediatric patients presenting to an Emergency Department or to a cardiac clinic. Clin Pediatr (Phila) 2004;43:231–8.
45. Lipsitz JD, Masia C, Apfel H, et al. Noncardiac chest pain and psychopathology in children and adolescents. J Psychosom Res 2005;59:185–8.
46. Cagdas DN, Pac FA. Cardiac chest pain in children. Anadolu Kardiyol Derg 2009; 9:401–6.
47. Danduran MJ, Earing MG, Sheridan DC, et al. Chest pain: characteristics of children/adolescents. Pediatr Cardiol 2008;29:775–81.
48. Lin CH, Lin WC, Ho YJ, et al. Children with chest pain visiting the Emergency Department. Pediatr Neonatol 2008;49:26–9.
49. Sadurska E, Kosciesza A, Jawniak R, et al. The causes of chest pain in children and adolescents with special focus on cardiac problems in our experiences. Pediatr Pol 2005;80:169–74.
50. Yildirim A, Karakurt C, Karademir S, et al. Chest pain in children. Int Pediatr 2004; 19:175–9.
51. Wojcicka-Urbanska B, Kotowska A, Wroblewska-Kaluzewska M. Chest pain in children. Pediatr Pol 2004;79:433–7.

Approach to the Child with Chest Pain

Steven M. Selbst, MD

KEYWORDS

• Child • Pediatric chest pain • Treatment • Diagnosis

Children frequently present to a pediatric office or emergency department (ED) with the complaint of chest pain. Between 0.3% and 0.6% of visits to a pediatric emergency department are for chest pain.[1,2] Unlike adult patients with chest pain, most studies have shown that children with chest pain rarely have serious organic pathology.[1–4] Infrequently, a child with chest pain will present with significant distress and require immediately resuscitation. Most children with chest pain are not in extremis and for many the pain is not acute in nature.[1]

Treat the complaint of chest pain seriously, because underlying heart disease or other serious pathology can sometimes exist. Many patients and their families associate chest pain with heart disease.[4,5] Dramatic media accounts of sudden deaths in young athletes have focused attention on chest pain as a sign of serious heart disease. Also, young people are aware of risk factors for cardiac disease because the medical community has emphasized the prevalence of hypertension and atherosclerotic cardiovascular disease in adults. Although serious, fatal heart disease is extremely rare in the pediatric population, families seek reassurance when they bring their child to the pediatric office or ED with the complaint of chest pain.[5]

Furthermore, treat this complaint seriously because the symptom of chest pain often disturbs a child's daily routine. About one-third of children with this complaint are awakened from sleep by the pain and one-third miss school because of the pain.[1] In one study, 16% of children with chest pain made more than 1 visit to an ED with this same complaint.[6] Chest pain often becomes a chronic problem, lasting more than 6 months in 7% to 45% of children.[1,3] About 8% of children have chest pain for more than 1 year.[1,6]

Because there are occasional children with serious pathology related to chest pain, the pediatrician and ED physician must carefully contemplate an extensive differential diagnosis when evaluating a child with chest pain (**Box 1**).

Age is a factor in the etiology of pediatric chest pain. Young children are more likely to have a cardiorespiratory cause for their pain, such as cough, asthma, pneumonia, or

Division of Pediatric Emergency Medicine Jefferson Medical College Nemours/A.I. duPont Hospital for Children, 1600 Rockland Road, Wilmington, DE 19803–3607, USA
E-mail address: sselbst@nemours.org

Pediatr Clin N Am 57 (2010) 1221–1234
doi:10.1016/j.pcl.2010.09.003
0031-3955/10/$ – see front matter
pediatric.theclinics.com

Box 1
Differential diagnosis of chest pain in children

Cardiac-related causes

    Coronary artery disease-ischemia/infarction

        Anomalous coronary arteries

        Kawasaki disease (coronary arteritis)

        Diabetes mellitus (long standing)

    Arrhythmia

        Supraventricular tachycardia

        Ventricular tachycardia

    Structural abnormalities of the heart

        Hypertrophic cardiomyopathy

        Severe pulmonic stenosis

        Aortic valve stenosis

    Infection

        Pericarditis

        Myocarditis

Noncardiac-related causes

    Musculoskeletal disorders

        Chest wall strain

        Direct trauma/contusion

        Rib fracture

        Costochondritis

    Respiratory disorders

        Severe cough

        Asthma

        Pneumonia

        Pneumothorax/pneumomediastinum

        Pulmonary embolism

    Psychological disorders

        Stress-related pain

    Gastrointestinal disorders

        Reflux esophagitis

        Pill-induced esophagitis

        Esophageal foreign body

    Miscellaneous disorders

        Sickle cell crises

        Abdominal aortic aneurysm (Marfan syndrome)

        Pleural effusion (collagen vascular disease)

        Shingles

Pleurodynia (coxsackievirus)

Breast tenderness (pregnancy, physiologic)

Tietze syndrome

Texidor's twinge/precordial catch syndrome

Chest mass

Idiopathic

heart disease; whereas, adolescents are more likely to have pain associated with stress or a psychogenic disturbance.[1]

DIFFERENTIAL DIAGNOSIS

There are numerous causes of chest pain in children (see **Box 1**). The following articles in this issue of *Pediatric Clinics of North America* will address these etiologies in detail. Keep a broad differential diagnosis in mind while assessing the child with chest pain. *Cardiac Disease* that was previously undiagnosed is a rare cause of chest pain in children.[1–4] Some children may have an underlying medical condition that results in a higher likelihood of angina or myocardial infarction. For instance, children who have long-standing diabetes mellitus, past history of Kawasaki disease, chronic anemia, or use of cocaine are at risk for cardiac pathology.[5,7–9] In many cases, exercise induces the chest pain with these disorders because coronary blood flow is limited. Pain with exertion should therefore be given careful consideration. Syncope may also be associated.[10,11]

In addition, some children may have an arrhythmia that causes symptoms, such as palpitations or an abnormal cardiac examination.[2] Supraventricular tachycardia is the most common of these arrhythmias, but ventricular tachycardia can also lead to brief, sharp, chest pain.

Consider a structural cardiac abnormality, such as hypertrophic obstructive cardiomyopathy, when evaluating a child with chest pain.[11,12] There may be a family history of this condition, as it has an autosomal dominant pattern of inheritance. Children with this disorder have a murmur heard best when patients are standing or performing a Valsalva maneuver. These patients are at risk for ischemic chest pain, especially when exercising.[5] Most other structural disorders of the heart rarely cause chest pain, however, severe pulmonic stenosis with associated cyanosis, coarctation of the aorta, and aortic valve stenosis can lead to ischemia.[5,13] The pain in these conditions may be described as squeezing, choking, or as a pressure sensation in the sternal area. Finally, mitral valve prolapse (MVP) may cause chest pain by papillary muscle or left ventricular endocardial ischemia. With MVP, a midsystolic click and late systolic murmur are often found. MVP is not a frequent cause of pediatric chest pain and it is no more common in children with chest pain than in the general population.[1,12]

Cardiac infections are important, although uncommon, causes of pediatric chest pain. For instance, pericarditis produces sharp stabbing pain that improves when patients sit up and lean forward. The child with this infection is usually febrile, in respiratory distress, has a friction rub, distant heart sounds, neck vein distention, and pulsus paradoxus.[14] Myocarditis is a more common infection and is often difficult to diagnose because it presents as many other viral infections. Children with myocarditis may have pain for several days, albeit mild and not disruptive. After a few days of fever and other systemic symptoms, such as vomiting and lightheadedness, patients may develop chest pain with exertion and shortness of breath. Examination may reveal muffled heart sounds, fever, a gallop rhythm, tachycardia or tachypnea that is out of proportion to the degree of fever present.[15–17] Patients also may have orthostatic changes in pulse or blood pressure. This is often misinterpreted as volume depletion because children with this infection may not be taking oral fluids well and may indeed have mild dehydration. However, when orthostatic changes do not improve after fluid resuscitation, cardiogenic causes, such as myocarditis, should be suspected. A chest radiograph usually shows cardiomegaly in both of these infections and an electrocardiogram will be abnormal, prompting a further evaluation, such as an echocardiogram (see the article by Durani and colleagues elsewhere in this issue for further exploration of this topic).

Musculoskeletal disorders are perhaps the most common causes of chest pain in children.[1,2] Active children frequently strain chest wall muscles while wrestling, carrying heavy books, or exercising.[11,12] Some children complain of chest pain after direct trauma to the chest, resulting in a mild contusion of the chest wall or, with more significant force, a rib fracture, hemithorax, or pneumothorax. In most cases, there is a straightforward history of trauma and the diagnosis is clear. Careful physical examination reveals chest wall tenderness or pain with movement of the torso or upper extremities.

Costochondritis is a common musculoskeletal disorder in children. Pain related to this condition is generally sharp, may be bilateral, and is exaggerated by physical activity or breathing. The diagnosis is made by eliciting tenderness over the costochondral junctions with palpation. Pain from costochondritis may persist for several months (see the article by Son and Sundel elsewhere in this issue for further exploration of this topic).[5,12]

Respiratory Conditions frequently lead to chest pain. For instance, children with a severe, persistent cough; asthma; or pneumonia may complain of chest pain caused by overuse of chest wall muscles. Diagnosis of one of these conditions is made by history or the presence of rales, wheezes, tachypnea, or decreased breath sounds on physical examination. Some children who complain of chest pain with exercise will be found to have exercise-induced asthma, which can be determined with a treadmill test. Consider a spontaneous pneumothorax or pneumomediastinum in children with sudden chest pain, especially if they have respiratory distress. Children at high risk for these conditions are those with asthma, cystic fibrosis, and Marfan syndrome.[18,19] Also, previously healthy children may develop a pneumothorax by rupture of an unrecognized subpleural bleb with minimal precipitating factors, such as cough or stretching. Examination often reveals respiratory distress, decreased breath sounds on the affected side (if the pneumothorax is significant), and possibly palpable subcutaneous air. Adolescents who snort cocaine are also at risk for barotrauma and may complain of severe, sudden chest pain with associated anxiety, hypertension, and tachycardia.[9,20] Finally, consider pulmonary embolism (PE) as a cause of chest pain. This condition is rare in pediatric patients, but is occasionally diagnosed in teenage girls using birth control pills or after recent surgery/abortion, or young males with recent leg trauma. Patients with PE will experience dyspnea, fever, pleuritic pain, cough, and hemoptysis (see the article by Johnson and colleagues elsewhere in this issue for further exploration of this topic).[21–23]

Psychogenic Disturbances cause chest pain in both boys and girls at equal rates.[1,2] Consider this etiology if the child has had a recent major stressful event, such as separation from friends, divorce in the family, or school failure that correlates temporally with the onset of the chest pain, Often the anxiety or stress that results in somatic complaints is not easily apparent; hyperventilation or an anxious appearance are not always present (see the article by McDonnell and White elsewhere in this issue for further exploration of this topic).[12]

Gastrointestinal disorders, such as reflux esophagitis, frequently cause chest pain in young children and adolescents.[1,2] The pain is classically described as burning, substernal in location, and worsened by reclining or eating spicy foods. This condition is diagnosed by history or with a therapeutic trial of antacids.[22] In addition, some adolescent patients may take medications, such as doxycycline, with little water and then lie down. They may develop severe pill esophagitis as the undissolved pill lodges in the esophagus.[24]

Also, consider the ingestion of a coin, button battery, or other foreign body that is lodged in the esophagus when a young child presents with sudden severe chest pain, perhaps with drooling or difficulty swallowing. Usually, the child or parent gives a clear history that a foreign body was recently ingested and a simple radiograph can confirm the diagnosis (see the article by Garza and Kaul elsewhere in this issue for further exploration of this topic).[22]

Miscellaneous causes of chest pain include pain related to underlying diseases. For instance, patients with sickle cell disease may have pain related to vasoocclusive crises or acute chest syndrome.[25] Marfan syndrome may cause chest pain because of a dissection of an abdominal aortic aneurysm.[26] Collagen vascular disorders may lead to pleural effusions. Varicella zoster infection may cause shingles, resulting in severe chest pain that can precede the classic rash or occur simultaneously. Coxsackie virus infection may cause pleurodynia with paroxysms of sharp pain in the chest or abdomen. Children may also complain of chest pain with breast tenderness from physiologic changes of puberty or early changes of pregnancy (see the article by Cico and colleagues elsewhere in this issue for further exploration of this topic). Tietze syndrome is a rare condition that causes sternal chest pain. Suspect this condition when physical examination reveals tender, spindle-shaped swelling at the sternochondral junctions. Etiology of Tietze syndrome is unknown and it can last for months. Finally, Texidor's Twinge is a syndrome of left- sided chest pain that is brief (<5 minutes duration) and sporadic. This pain may recur frequently for a few hours in some individuals and then remain absent for several months. The pain seems to be associated with a slouched posture or bending, and is not related to exercise. It is usually relieved when the individual takes a few shallow breaths, or one deep breath, and assumes a straightened posture. This pain syndrome is also referred to as *precordial catch* or *stitch in the side*. The etiology remains unclear.[27,28]

Idiopathic chest pain is a label given to children when no clear etiology can be found. In 20% to 45% of cases of pediatric chest pain, no diagnosis can be determined with certainty.[1,4]

IMMEDIATE APPROACH TO CHILDREN WITH CHEST PAIN

It is rare for a child with chest pain to present in extremis. However, conditions, such as pneumothorax, trauma, cocaine toxicity, or an arrhythmia, can lead to cardiovascular compromise. Before going on with a detailed evaluation, determine if patients need immediate support. If patients have tachypnea, dyspnea, shortness of breath, or poor color attach a monitor and support the patients' airway and breathing. Measure the patients' oxygen saturation and give oxygen supplementation if needed.

Next, evaluate the patients' cardiac rate and rhythm and support the patients' circulation. Consider an intravenous (IV) line and IV fluids to restore intravascular volume. Give an IV bolus of normal saline, 20 mL/kg, if patients have signs of shock, dizziness with standing, orthostatic changes in vital signs, or if they have not been drinking well.

GENERAL APPROACH TO CHILDREN WITH CHEST PAIN

Most children with chest pain do not need immediate management. Take a thorough history and perform a careful physical examination. These practices will guide the physician to determine when laboratory studies, specific treatments, and referral to a specialist for further evaluation are necessary.[5,12]

History

A thorough history will reveal the etiology of chest pain in most cases (**Box 2**). First, determine when the pain began. Children with acute onset of pain (within 48 hours of presentation) are more likely to have an organic etiology for the pain. The etiology is not always serious, but pneumonia, asthma, trauma, pneumothorax, and arrhythmia are more likely if the pain is recent.[1] In a young child with sudden onset of pain, consider a foreign body (coin or button battery) in the esophagus or injury. Those with chronic pain who have gone for extended periods without a diagnosis are much more likely to be idiopathic or have a psychogenic etiology.[1,11]

Next, determine what *precipitates the pain*. Chest pain precipitated by running or exercise is concerning because this may relate to cardiac disease or, more commonly, exercise-induced asthma.[29,30] Inquire about trauma, rough play, or recent overuse of chest wall muscles. Major trauma and direct chest injury are easily recalled; however, patients often overlook minor trauma and muscle overuse. History of wrestling, playing football, doing multiple pushups, lifting weights, or participating in gymnastics may suggest muscle strain as the cause of the chest pain. Discover if the child recalls choking on a foreign body or swallowing a coin. Determine if the child has recently eaten spicy foods or is taking any medications, such as tetracycline. In an older child or teenager, inquire about the use of cocaine, oral contraceptives, or if there was recent leg trauma.[12]

Ask about *associated complaints*. Chest pain that is associated with syncope or palpitations is more significant and may relate to arrhythmia or other cardiac disease. Dizziness with standing in association with chest pain suggests dehydration, but could also be related to cardiac insufficiency. Associated fever is concerning for an infection, such as pneumonia, myocarditis, or pericarditis. Joint pain or rash in association with chest pain may indicate a collagen vascular disease. Psychogenic chest pain is often associated with other somatic complaints. Inquire about school phobias, sleep disturbances, family turmoil, or recent significant stress (eg, move, death of loved one, serious illness.) Children with chest pain often experience increased levels of psychological symptoms.[31] Assess the severity of the patients' pain and how often patients

---

Box 2
Value of history in the differential diagnosis of chest pain

1. Consider thoracic trauma if patients recall a specific incident.

2. Consider stress or emotional upset as the cause of pain, if an important life event is temporally correlated.

3. Consider esophageal foreign body (coin or button battery ingestion) in a young toddler with acute onset of chest pain.

4. Consider pneumonia or viral myocarditis if the child has fever.

5. Consider cardiac disease if the pain is associated with exertion, syncope, and dizziness.

6. Consider serious associated conditions, such as asthma, lupus, sickle cell disease, and Marfan's syndrome.

have chest pain. Determine if the pain is so severe that the child is missing school or work. Serious etiology is not well correlated with frequency or severity of pain. However, constant, frequent severe pain is more likely to be distressing and interrupts daily activity. Children who wake from sleep because of the pain are more likely to have an organic etiology, though not necessarily serious.[1,12]

Ask patients to *describe the pain*. The location and quality of the pain sometimes points to an etiology for the pain. This history is less helpful in young children because they are imprecise in language and description. Many cannot localize the pain sensation. However, if patients describe burning pain in the sternal area, esophagitis may be suspected. If a febrile child describes sharp pain that is relieved by sitting up and leaning forward, suspect pericarditis.

Review the patients' *past medical history*. History of asthma places patients at risk for more serious causes for chest pain, such as pneumonia or pneumothorax. Previous heart disease or conditions like long-standing insulin-dependent diabetes mellitus (hyperlipidemia) or Kawasaki disease (coronary artery aneurysms) may increase the risk for cardiac pathology.[7,8] Consider serious cardiac or pulmonary complications or life-threatening acute chest syndrome in children with a history of sickle cell disease. Patients with Marfan syndrome have increased risk for aortic dissection and pneumothorax. Children with chest pain who have an underlying collagen vascular disease have an increased risk for pleural effusion or pericarditis. Ask about previously diagnosed heart disease, although most underlying structural cardiac lesions rarely produce chest pain.

Family history may be helpful because some cardiac disorders are familial. Consider hypertrophic cardiomyopathy in families with this condition or those with a history of sudden death.[10] Negative family history goes against this condition, but does not rule out this possibility. In children with a family history of heart disease or chest pain, the parents may be unusually concerned about the symptom, yet the child often has a nonorganic etiology.[1]

Finally, allow patients and families to express their fears and concerns about the symptom, which may help direct the therapeutic approach. Determine which medications have been given to treat the pain and what management has been instituted by the family. Pain that resolves with parental attention may imply an emotional etiology.[5,12] See **Box 3** for important history questions to ask for children with chest pain.

Box 3
Important history in a child with chest pain

When did the pain begin?

How severe is the pain?

How often does the pain occur?

What is the pain like?

How long does the pain last?

What makes the pain better or worse?

Are there associated symptoms (dizziness, syncope)?

What triggers the pain (exercise)?

What is the past medical history?

Is there a family history of heart disease, sudden death, or other conditions?

What treatments have been tried?

Physical Examination

A careful physical examination is likely to point to the cause of pain. To avoid overlooking an important clue to the etiology, *it is wise not to focus exclusively on the chest* (**Box 4**). With a quick general assessment, differentiate patients in severe distress who need immediate treatment for life-threatening conditions, such as pneumothorax. Distinguish hyperventilation from respiratory distress. The absence of cyanosis or nasal flaring, and the presence of carpopedal spasm and acral paresthesias, suggests hyperventilation. Measure the *vital signs*. Orthostatic changes suggest depleted intravascular volume (dehydration), but could relate to cardiac insufficiency (pump failure). Fever is notable and serves as a branch point in narrowing the differential diagnosis. Fever associated with chest pain points to an infectious process, most commonly pneumonia.[1,2] Consider other less common infections, such as myocarditis and pericarditis. Osteomyelitis of the rib is another rare infection that could cause chest pain.[32] Children with fever are far less likely to have muscle strain, conversion disorder or gastrointestinal pathology.

Next, look for *signs of chronic disease*, such as pallor, poor growth, and a sallow appearance. These signs suggest the chest pain is a symptom of a more complex problem, such as Hodgkin's lymphoma or a collagen vascular disease, such as lupus. Consider Marfan syndrome if patients are tall and thin with an upper extremity span that exceeds their height. Note any signs of anxiety that could indicate the presence of emotional stress.[5,12]

Examine the *skin* for rashes, bruises, or other lesions. A rash may suggest a systemic illness, such as a collagen vascular disease. Bruises on the chest or elsewhere may indicate unrecognized trauma to the chest.

Carefully examine the *abdomen*. Abdominal tenderness or mass may indicate a source of pain that is referred to the chest. Examine the *joints* to determine the presence of arthritis in consideration of a collagen vascular disease.

Perform a complete *chest examination* (**Box 5**). Inspect the chest for an abnormal breathing pattern, signs of trauma, or asymmetry caused by cardiomegaly, scoliosis, or breast enlargement. Auscultate for rales, wheezes, or decreased breath sounds. Listen to the heart for a murmur, rub, muffled sounds, or arrhythmia.[5,12] Absence of such findings does not rule out cardiac disease. A murmur that intensifies with a Valsalva maneuver and the standing position is the hallmark of hypertrophic cardiomyopathy. Examine the heart in the upright, supine, and standing positions.

Next, *palpate the chest wall* assessing for tenderness over major muscle groups, including the pectoral muscles. Musculoskeletal chest pain is usually reproducible by palpation or by moving the arms and chest through a variety of positions. Tenderness of the sternum at the costochondral junctions suggests costochondritis. If subcutaneous air is palpable, consider a pneumothorax or pneumomediastinum.[12,19]

Box 4
Approach to the general physical examination in children with chest pain. Look for:

Acute distress, abnormal vital signs

Chronically ill appearance

Skin rash or bruising

Abdominal pathology

Arthritis

Anxiety

Box 5
Approach to the physical examination of the chest in children with chest pain

Inspect for signs of trauma, asymmetry, and an abnormal breathing pattern.

Auscultate for tachycardia, arrhythmia, murmur, rub, rales, and wheezing.

Palpate for tenderness and subcutaneous emphysema.

Assess for breast tenderness, which could indicate physiologic changes of adolescence or pregnancy. Finally, in children who complain of pain with walking or moving the arms, palpate the lower ribs and perform a hooking maneuver (grasp the rib margins and pull them anteriorly) to see if this reproduces the pain. This finding suggests slipping rib syndrome, a rare disorder of the eighth, ninth, and tenth ribs that causes chest pain and a clicking sound with movement.[33]

Laboratory Studies

For most children with chest pain, diagnostic tests are not of great value. When history and physical examination do not lead to a specific diagnosis for the chest pain, laboratory tests are usually not helpful either. Laboratory studies generally confirm previously known disorders or abnormal findings that are suspected clinically. Chest radiographs and electrocardiograms (ECG) should not be routinely ordered unless indicated by worrisome findings in the history or physical examination (**Table 1**).[1,12,22,34]

Consider a chest radiograph or electrocardiogram when the history reveals acute onset of chest pain (began in the past 2 or 3 days) or if there are specific concerns for pulmonary problems or cardiac disease. In particular, obtain an ECG and chest radiograph if the chest pain occurs with exertion or syncope.[1,5,22,34]

Consider a chest radiograph or ECG when children have a history of heart disease. Chest pain in these children is usually not serious; however, there is often great anxiety

---

Table 1
Worrisome signs and symptoms to prompt further workup in pediatric patients with chest pain (partial list)

Workup	History/Symptom	Sign
Chest radiograph	Fever	Fever
	Cough	Tachypnea, rales, distress
	Shortness of breath	Ill-appearing/sick
	History of trauma	Significant trauma
	Pain wakes from sleep	Extreme tachycardia
	History of drug use (eg, cocaine)	Pathologic auscultation of heart
	Associated with exercise	Absent/decreased breath sounds
	Acute onset of pain	Palpation of subcutaneous air
	Serious medical problems (Marfan, Kawasaki, lupus)	Tall, thin
	Foreign body ingestion (coin, button battery)	Drooling, gagging
ECG	Associated with exercise	Pathologic auscultation of heart
	Associated with syncope	Tachycardia (>180 bpm)
	History of drug use (eg, cocaine)	Ill-appearing/sick
	Consider with fever	Consider with fever

Abbreviations: bpm, beats per minute; ECG, electrocardiogram.
Data from Gokale J, Selbst SM. Chest pain and chest wall deformity. Pediatr Clin North Am 2009;56:49–65.

about the underlying condition. Noninvasive diagnostic studies are reassuring. This group represents only a small percentage of children with chest pain.

Order laboratory studies when children with chest pain have abnormal physical examination findings. A chest radiograph is justified when patients have fever, respiratory distress, and decreased or abnormal breath sounds. Look for an infiltrate, because fever with chest pain is highly correlated with pneumonia. Also, look for cardiomegaly indicating possible pericarditis or myocarditis. Moreover, order an electrocardiogram when children have an abnormal cardiac examination, including unexplained tachycardia, arrhythmia, murmur, rub, or click.

Laboratory studies are probably not necessary in children with chronic pain, a normal physical examination, and no history to indicate cardiac or pulmonary disease. If the family cannot be reassured, consider noninvasive studies to alleviate their anxiety. It is not necessary to obtain an echocardiogram on all children with ill-defined chest pain to look for mitral valve prolapse.[1,12] The significance of this diagnosis and its relationship to the symptom of chest pain is unclear.

It is not usually necessary to obtain radiographic or endoscopic studies to confirm gastroesophageal reflux. When this diagnosis is suspected clinically, begin management empirically. Furthermore, blood counts and sedimentation rates are of limited value unless sickle cell disease, a collagen vascular disease, infection, or malignancy is suspected. Obtain a drug screen for cocaine in an older child with acute pain that is associated with anxiety, tachycardia, hypertension, or shortness of breath. Cardiac enzymes are rarely of value unless there are specific concerns from the history or examination. Refer patients for a 24-hour Holter monitor if an arrhythmia is strongly suspected. Consider an echocardiogram to diagnose structural heart disease (see the article by Masato Takahashi and by Anderson and Vetter elsewhere in this issue for further exploration of this topic). **Box 6** summarizes an approach to children with chest pain.

MANAGEMENT OF CHILDREN WITH CHEST PAIN

Begin specific treatment when a particular etiology for the pain is found, such as pneumonia or asthma. Reassurance, acetaminophen or nonsteroidal antiinflammatory analgesics, and rest are appropriate for most cases of musculoskeletal, psychogenic, or idiopathic pain. Consider use of heat and relaxation techniques to manage pain. When esophagitis is suspected, begin a therapeutic trial of antacids. For pill-induced

---

Box 6
Approach to the child with chest pain

- Assess vital signs and the general appearance of patients to determine if immediate treatment is needed.
- Do not immediately assume pediatric chest pain is cardiac in nature.
- Do not immediately rule out serious pathology in children with chest pain.
- Assess the degree of pain and the impact of pain on the patients' life.
- Determine if the chest pain is part of a chronic underlying condition.
- Consider laboratory studies if the history is concerning or the physical examination is abnormal.
- Avoid expensive, invasive laboratory studies with chronic pain and normal physical examination and benign history.

Box 7
When to refer children with chest pain

- Acute distress
- Significant trauma
- History of heart disease or related serious medical problem
- Pain with exercise, syncope, palpitations, dizziness
- Serious emotional disturbance
- Esophageal foreign body, caustic ingestion
- Pneumothorax, pleural effusion

---

esophagitis, consider endoscopic evaluation to document midesophageal ulcers. Some investigators suggest endoscopy is not always necessary. Instead, discontinue the tetracycline medication and treat with sucralfate.[24] Provide appropriate counseling to patients with chest pain related to minor stress and anxiety.[5,12]

Disposition and Referral

Admit children in severe distress or with abnormal vital signs to the hospital for monitoring, further diagnostic studies, and extended treatment. Refer all patients who have pain with exertion, syncope, dizziness, or palpitations for further evaluation. They may require a Holter monitor, an echocardiogram, exercise stress tests, or pulmonary function tests to look for an arrhythmia, structural heart disease, or exercise-induced asthma. Refer those with a suspected esophageal foreign body to a specialist for rapid removal of the foreign object. Refer patients with serious emotional problems that cannot be easily managed to a psychiatrist. Refer children with chest pain who have known or suspected heart disease to a cardiologist, even though the pain may prove to be unrelated.[12] **Box 7** summarizes the indications for referring children with chest pain.

In all cases, arrange appropriate follow-up, because many children with ill-defined chest pain will have persistent symptoms for many months. Serious organic pathology is unlikely to be found in the future in such patients.[35,36] However, some of these children are kept from participating in their usual activities because of the pain, and some manifest significant psycho-emotional problems or exercise-induced asthma that was not recognized initially.[35]

SUMMARY

Chest pain is a common complaint among children of all ages. It is rarely caused by cardiac disease, but it is important to evaluate for this with a thoughtful history and careful physical examination.[5,12,30] Perform laboratory tests in limited cases. Obtain studies (at least a chest radiograph and electrocardiogram) if the pain is acute in onset; interferes with sleep; is precipitated by exercise; or associated with dizziness, palpitations, syncope, or shortness of breath. Study pain further if children have a history of coin ingestion, trauma, previous cardiac disease, or conditions that put them at risk for developing cardiac pathology. Use caution for those with a history of conditions, such as asthma, Marfan syndrome, or sickle cell disease. Finally, obtain radiographs and an electrocardiogram for those with an abnormal physical examination (fever, respiratory distress, abnormal breath sounds, cardiac murmur, abnormal rhythm or heart sounds, palpable subcutaneous air, or obvious trauma). Reassure and carefully follow (rather than ordering extensive studies) children with chronic chest pain who lack a worrisome

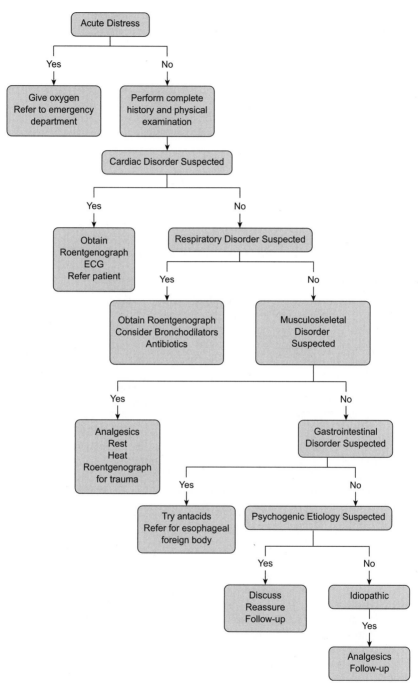

Fig. 1. Approach to the child with chest pain. (*From* Selbst SM. Evaluation of chest pain in children. Pediatr Rev 1986;8(2):56–62; with permission.)

history, appear well, and have a normal physical examination. **Fig. 1** shows an algorithmic approach to children with chest pain.[37]

REFERENCES

1. Selbst SM, Ruddy RM, Clark BJ, et al. Pediatric chest pain: a prospective study. Pediatrics 1988;82:319–23.
2. Massin MM, Bourguignont A, Coremans C, et al. Chest pain in pediatric patents presenting to an emergency department or to a cardiac clinic. Clin Pediatr 2004; 43(3):231–8.
3. Rowe BH, Dulberg CS, Peterson RQ, et al. Characteristics of children presenting with chest pain to a pediatric emergency department. CMAJ 1990;143(5): 388–94.
4. Driscoll DJ, Glicklich LB, Gallen WJ. Chest pain in children: a prospective study. Pediatrics 1976;57:648–51.
5. Cava JR, Sayger PL. Chest pain in children and adolescents. Pediatr Clin North Am 2004;51:1553–68.
6. Selbst SM. Chest pain in children. Pediatrics 1985;75:1068–70.
7. Madhok AB, Boxer R, Green S. An adolescent with chest pain- sequela of Kawasaki disease. Pediatr Emerg Care 2004;20:765–8.
8. Declue TJ, Malone JI, Root AW. Coronary artery disease in diabetic adolescents. Clin Pediatr 1988;27:587–90.
9. Woodward GA, Selbst SM. Chest pain secondary to cocaine use. Pediatr Emerg Care 1987;3:153–4.
10. Washington RL. Sudden deaths in adolescent athletes caused by cardiac conditions. Pediatr Ann 2003;32:751–6.
11. Galioto FM. Child chest pain; a course of action. Contemp Pediatr 2007;24(5): 47–57.
12. Selbst SM. Chest pain in children. Pediatr Rev 1997;18:169–73.
13. Graneto JW, Turnbull TL, Marciniak SA. An unusual cause of chest pain in an adolescent presenting to the emergency department. Pediatr Emerg Care 1997;13:33–6.
14. Roodpeyma S, Sadeghian N. Acute pericarditis in childhood: a 10 year experience. Pediatr Cardiol 2000;21(4):363–7.
15. Leonard EG. Viral myocarditis. Pediatr Infect Dis J 2004;23:665–6.
16. Durani Y, Egan M, Baffa J, et al. Pediatric myocarditis: presenting clinical characteristics. Am J Emerg Med 2009;27:942–7.
17. Freedman SB, Haladyn JK, Floh A, et al. Pediatric myocarditis: emergency department clinical findings and diagnostic evaluation. Pediatrics 2007;6:1278–85.
18. Bullaro FM, Bartoletti SC. Spontaneous pneumomediastinum in children- a literature review. Pediatr Emerg Care 2007;23:28–30.
19. Kahn DA, Kanegaye JT. An adolescent football player with chest pain. Clin Pediatr 2003;42:471–4.
20. Uva JL. Spontaneous pneumothoraces, pneumomediastinum, and pneumoperitoneum: consequences of smoking crack cocaine. Pediatr Emerg Care 1997; 13:24–6.
21. Rajpurkar M, Warrier I, Chitiur M, et al. Pulmonary embolism- experience at a single children's hospital. Thromb Res 2007;119:699–703.
22. Gokale J, Selbst SM. Chest pain and chest wall deformity. Pediatr Clin North Am 2009;56:49–65.

23. Johnson AS, Bolte RG. Pulmonary embolism in the pediatric patient. Pediatr Emerg Care 2004;20:555–60.
24. Palmer KM, Selbst SM, Shaffer S, et al. Pediatric chest pain induced by tetracycline ingestion. Pediatr Emerg Care 1999;15:200–1.
25. Taylor C, Carter F, Poulose J, et al. Clinical presentation of acute chest syndrome in sickle cell disease. Postgrad Med J 2004;80:346–9.
26. Van Karnebeek CD, Naeff MS, Mulder BJ, et al. Natural history of cardiovascular manifestations in Marfan syndrome. Arch Dis Child 2001;84:129–37.
27. Miller A, Texidor TA. "Precordial catch" a neglected syndrome of precordial pain. JAMA 1955;159:1364–5.
28. Gumbiner CH. Precordial catch syndrome. South Med J 2003;96(1):38–41.
29. Wiens L, Sabath R, Ewing L, et al. Chest pain in otherwise healthy children and adolescents is frequently caused by exercise induced asthma. Pediatrics 1992; 90:350–3.
30. Danduran MJ. Chest pain: characteristics of children and adolescents. Pediatr Cardiol 2008;29:775–81.
31. Lipsitz JD, Warner CM, Apfel H, et al. Anxiety and depressive symptoms and anxiety sensitivity in youngsters with noncardiac chest pain and benign heart murmurs. J Pediatr Psychol 2004;29:607–12.
32. Layton K. Fever and "worst pain ever" in the chest: in one ED, out the other. Contemp Pediatr 2006;23(2):18–26.
33. Mooney DP, Shorter NA. Slipping rib syndrome in childhood. J Pediatr Surg 2002; 132:1081–2.
34. Swenson JM, Fischer DR, Miller SA. Are chest radiographs and electrocardiograms still valuable in evaluating new pediatric patients with heart murmurs and or chest pain? Pediatrics 1997;991:1–3.
35. Selbst SM, Ruddy R, Clark BJ. Chest pain in children: follow-up of patients previously reported. Clin Pediatr 1990;29:374–7.
36. Lam JC, Tobias JD. Follow-up survey of children and adolescents with chest pain. South Med J 2001;94:921–4.
37. Selbst SM. Evaluation of chest pain in children. Pediatr Rev 1986;8(2):56–62.

Assessment and Treatment of Psychological Factors in Pediatric Chest Pain

Cassandra J. McDonnell, MA[a], Kamila S. White, PhD[b],*

KEYWORDS

- Chest pain • Pediatric • Recurrent pain • Anxiety
- Psychopathology

ASSESSMENT AND TREATMENT OF PSYCHOLOGICAL FACTORS IN PEDIATRIC CHEST PAIN

Chest pain is a common complaint among the pediatric population. Community surveys indicate that 4% to 10% of students report experiencing chest pain within the past 2 weeks,[1,2] and chest pain or discomfort is the primary complaint of 0.14% to 0.6% of patients in pediatric emergency departments.[2–6] Although most cases are not found to be associated with organic causes, chest pain may be associated with many organic diagnoses that vary widely in morbidity and mortality.[7] As such, a complaint of chest pain or discomfort by a pediatric patient raises the possibility of serious illness and often precipitates a comprehensive medical evaluation.[8] Whatever the diagnostic outcome of this evaluation, psychological assessment and treatment may be relevant for many patients with chest pain.

For patients with causes of organic chest pain that require medical treatment, psychological interventions may facilitate lifestyle changes and adherence to treatment regimens. Psychologists may also assist patients and their families in coping with the stress of a troubling or uncertain prognosis. Treatment of psychological disorders such as depression or anxiety can make pain less burdensome and improve overall quality of life.

This work was partially supported by the University of Missouri-Saint Louis by a Dissertation Fellowship (awarded to C.J.M.) and University Research Funds (awarded to K.S.W.).
The authors have nothing to disclose.
[a] Department of Psychology, University of Missouri-Saint Louis, One University Boulevard, 231 Stadler Hall, St Louis, MO 63121, USA
[b] Department of Psychology, University of Missouri-Saint Louis, One University Boulevard, 212 Stadler Hall, St Louis, MO 63121, USA
* Corresponding author.
E-mail address: whiteks@umsl.edu

Pediatr Clin N Am 57 (2010) 1235–1260
doi:10.1016/j.pcl.2010.09.010
0031-3955/10/$ – see front matter © 2010 Elsevier Inc. All rights reserved.

pediatric.theclinics.com

This article begins by briefly reviewing the medical evaluation of chest pain. The psychological stress that may accompany this process for some patients and families is then discussed, and suggestions are offered about clinical practices that may alleviate some of this stress. General guidelines for diagnosing and alleviating psychological problems and the broad diagnostic categories for most causes of organic chest pain are discussed. Within these categories, specific conditions that may be particularly likely to benefit from psychological consultation are highlighted, and issues to consider during psychological assessment and intervention efforts with these patients are suggested. The phenomenon of medically unexplained chest pain is discussed from a psychological perspective. This discussion illustrates the elusive and complex nature of this condition, critically reviews existing literature on the prevalence of psychopathology within this population, and draws implications for clinical assessment and management.

Medical Evaluation

The most crucial component of chest pain evaluation is a thorough physical examination and comprehensive medical history.[7,9] Patients and parents are likely to be queried about events leading up to, during, and following the episode or episodes of chest pain, as well as details regarding time of onset, frequency, duration, setting, exacerbating and relieving factors, and any other physical symptoms that accompany the chest pain.[7,8] Any relationship between the pain and body positions, activity, meals, trauma, potential foreign body ingestion, menses, and psychological stress may be noted and explored.[7,8] It is recommended that adolescents be asked privately about substance use, including illicit substance use.[7] A typical physical examination of a child or adolescent with a chest pain complaint includes auscultation of the heart and lungs, vital signs, general appearance and state, examination of skin and extremities, range of motion and resistance testing of the upper extremities, and palpation of chest wall, musculature, breasts, sternum, and xiphoid.[7,8] In many cases, a thorough history and physical examination are sufficient to determine the cause.[7] However, some patients are referred for 1 or more specific cardiac, gastrointestinal, or respiratory tests (**Box 1**) based on the presence of accompanying signs and symptoms (**Box 2**).[7,8]

The most serious potential causes of chest pain are cardiovascular and are often a primary concern of children and families seeking medical attention. Diseases of the heart represent a serious public health concern and are the fifth leading cause of death for children aged 1 to 19 years,[21] although most chest pain complaints are not attributable to cardiac problems. Studies report that 1% to 5% of children seen at emergency departments for a primary complaint of chest pain are identified as having a causal heart problem.[3,4] However, the association of chest pain in adults with cardiac disease and myocardial infarction is well known and patients' caregivers are likely to perceive chest pain as heart pain.[22–24] Between 50% and 56% of pediatric patients with chest pain attribute their pain to a heart problem [25,26] and most report a specific fear of heart attack or heart disease.[4] This fear may persist despite education regarding prevalence. Adolescents who report knowing that heart attacks are unlikely in their age group and that chest pain is generally benign nonetheless tend to attribute their own pain to a heart problem.[25]

The fear and concern reported by patients with chest pain and their families reflects perception of chest pain as potentially dangerous. Public health education regarding hypertension and cardiovascular disease in adults may increase younger individuals' awareness of cardiac risk factors and the most dangerous potential implications of chest pain.[5,23] In addition, rare but tragic sudden deaths of local or high-profile young

---

Box 1
Selected psychological factors for chest pain analysis

Pain

    Pain characteristics (ie, frequency, intensity, duration, quality)

    Pain antecedents (eg, exertion, parental separation, interpersonal conflict)

    Interoceptive hypersensitivity (ie, strong emotion, cardiovascular vigilance/attention, pulse checking)

    Pain consequences (eg, pain relief, absenteeism, sick role, attention, secondary gain)

    Factors that alleviate pain

Cognitive understanding

    Fears (eg, fear of pain, intolerance of discomfort, serious illness, heart attack)

    Beliefs about illness (ie, cause of the pain, likelihood of death, losing control)

Behavioral responses

    Interoceptive avoidance (ie, restricted physical engagement, including kinesiophobia)

    Situational avoidance

    Safety behaviors (eg, pulse checking, lucky charms, experiential states)

    Medication use

Social effects

    Quality of life (eg, caregiver role, sibling relationships, family dynamics)

    Academic and peer relations

---

athletes from cardiac ailments are often well publicized. This may increase public estimation of catastrophic cardiac events during childhood and adolescence far beyond actual prevalence rates.[5,27] It is therefore unsurprising that clinicians overwhelmingly report that both patients and their parents may be frightened by chest pain.[8,22,23,28]

Box 2
Selected child self-report measures

Anxiety

    Multidimensional Anxiety Scale for Children (MASC)[10,11]

    Revised Children's Manifest Anxiety Scale (RCMAS)[12,13]

Depression

    Children's Depression Inventory[14,15]

    Reynolds Adolescent Depression Scale[16]

Somatization

    Children's Somatization Inventory[17]

Stress

    Perceived Stress Scale[18]

    Pediatric Quality of Life Inventory[19,20]

When pain persists following a negative medical evaluation, any psychological distress experienced by children and their families also has the potential to persist. According to follow-up questionnaires sent to patients with chest pain of mixed causes and their parents 1 to 2 years after an initial emergency department evaluation, 34 of the 35 cases who reported continuing chest pain also indicated ongoing worry and concern about that pain.[5] Clinicians report that, in some cases, a parent's anxiety regarding a child's chest pain may be such that the child is restricted from participating in sports or strenuous physical activities even after undergoing a medical evaluation with negative results.[27,28] In addition, medical care providers express concern that parental anxiety may drive a certain amount of health care use by pediatric patients with chest pain, and observe that such anxiety may potentially result in more testing than is diagnostically necessary.[4]

Bidirectional Relationship Between Chest Pain and Emotional Distress

The emotional stress observed in patients with chest pain and their caregivers is particularly relevant given that there is the potential for a bidirectional relationship between chest pain and emotional experiences. In addition to experiencing pain related to organic disease, children may experience the bodily sensation of chest pain, tightness, or pressure as part of the physiological arousal that accompanies strong emotional experiences. As such, any emotional distress that a child might feel regarding their pain has the potential to increase the frequency and severity of that pain. Increased pain may in turn be accompanied by increased distress, and so on (**Fig. 1**). For patients who experience intermittent episodes of chest pain that reoccur over an extended period of time, the pain has the potential to become

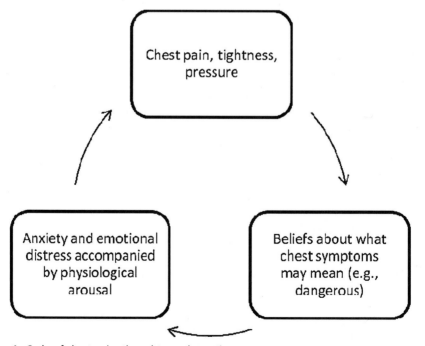

Fig. 1. Cycle of chest pain, thoughts, and emotions.

preoccupying and may provoke increasingly high levels of persistent worry in patients and caregivers.

Working with Emotionally Distressed Patients

Clinicians may be able to address this distress by acknowledging that chest pain can be a frightening physical symptom. Normalizing the distress about chest pain may encourage patients and their caregivers to be receptive to education about actual childhood prevalence rates of feared cardiac events, such as heart attacks or heart disease. Following the medical examination, diagnosis, and treatment recommendations, we suggest that clinicians check with the patient regarding their anxiety and their current attribution for their pain. If uncertainty is apparent, it may be helpful to suggest to the caregiver that some children need continued reassurance and review of the cause of their pain. Referral for psychological consultation is warranted if the child's pain exceeds the level that would be expected based on organic causes.

Consultation and Liaison with Medical Treatment Team

It is wise for the referring clinician/and or treatment team to discuss the concerns about the patient with the consulting psychologist. This consultation facilitates ongoing protections of the child's safety, health, and progress in assessment and treatment planning. Topics of such discussion may include any medical risks, psychological risks (such as suicidality and self-harm), predictors of treatment nonadherence, and any changes in physical symptoms. In addition, the psychologist may be able to discuss the need for other behavioral health–related interventions for problems that the referring physician may not have suggested during the original referral. Some physicians may be less familiar with the benefits of direct referrals to psychologists for the management of psychosocial and behavioral interventions for exercise, risk factor counseling, and risk reduction.

PSYCHOLOGICAL ASSESSMENT AND INTERVENTION OF PATIENTS WITH CHEST PAIN
Assessment

The major goal of psychological assessment of a child with chest pain is to integrate medical symptoms and disease with affective, cognitive, behavioral, and familial functioning within the context of overall well-being. Assessment includes interviews with the child and caregiver and the administration of standardized measures of behavioral and psychological functioning. An initial joint conversation allows for rapport building, observation of child/caregiver interactions, and review of informed consent/assent. Because the child will likely have undergone multiple medical appointments, tests, and procedures related to chest pain, the psychologist should quickly orient the child to the purpose and procedures of the meeting. Younger children may need to be reassured that the psychologist is a doctor who will not be administering shots or other painful physical procedures. If the child has been brought to an outpatient setting, it is helpful to determine his or her understanding of the visit and provide orientation to assessment procedures.

For children with conditions that require adherence to effortful treatment regimens, the joint discussion is an appropriate time to determine the distribution of disease-related tasks (eg, what the child does to take care of the disease, what the caregiver does, what other family members do). It may be helpful to playfully ask the child and caregiver to each identify the hardest and easiest disease-related task. This process can offer insight into family dynamics as well as past or current barriers to treatment adherence. Separate interviews following the combined introduction may facilitate both gathering information and establishing relationships with the child and parent. With adolescents, an individual interview is often beneficial even during a brief consultation.

During interviews with the parent, it can be helpful to begin by assessing the child's typical daily activities, likes, dislikes, and general personality traits. A review of the child's medical history may then ease into discussion of its effect on the family's lifestyle and coping methods. Reviewing caregivers' knowledge about the child's medical health and their perception of the treatment regimen may reveal additional adherence barriers. In some cases, identifying barriers to adherence may be a primary goal of the assessment. Given the myriad individual, familial, and environmental influences on children's lives it is often helpful to conceptualize barriers systemically, while remaining mindful of the transactional relationships that may occur both within and across systems (**Fig. 2**). Expressing empathic, genuine, and nonjudgmental concern for the family may facilitate open and sincere communication from the caregiver.

The form of the child interview will vary depending on the child's chronologic age and developmental level. When the assessment occurs during multiple appointments, it is often beneficial to balance assessment across structured child and parent diagnostic assessment (ie, using structure or semi-structured diagnostic interview schedules for *Diagnostic and statistical manual of mental disorders* [DSM-IV]), behavioral assessment (ie, structured observations, parent-child interactions), and parent evaluation (ie, parent report instruments). It is also

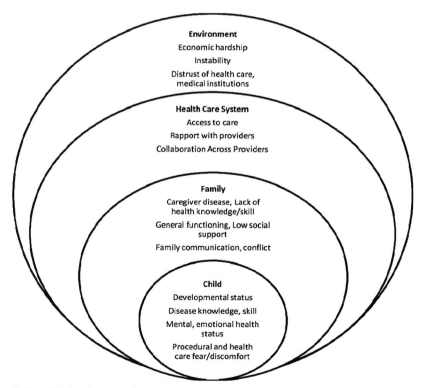

Fig. 2. Possible barriers to adherence.

important to include age-appropriate activities that ensure the child has ample modes to express their pain, coping, and adjustment (eg, verbally, behaviorally, indirectly). For example, it may be helpful to ask children to describe their disease and treatment to assess knowledge and skill level. Asking children to identify a negative aspect of the disease (eg, what they dislike the most about it) may provide insight into both distress levels and adherence barriers. For children whose condition is of recent onset, a discussion of what has changed since their pain began can provide insight into coping and adjustment. Children who have lived with their condition for longer can be asked about what advice or information they would give to a child with a similar condition, and the child's family. Asking a child whether any peers have been told about the child's condition, and if so what their reaction has been, can also suggest information about adjustment. In general, the overall goals of assessment are to determine clinical diagnosis identify the target problem area(s) and conceptualize a treatment plan or recommendation.

Chest Pain Analysis

The child's experience of chest pain is a central focus of assessment. A thorough and detailed understanding of the pain may be best accomplished by beginning with open-ended inquiries (ie, "Tell me a bit about how your chest pain affects your daily life?"), moving on to specific inquiries (ie, "What activities does your pain keep you from doing?"), and eventually progressing to closed-ended inquiries depending on response quality (ie, "Can you run when you have chest pain?"). Beginning with open-ended questions shows caregivers that they are being listened to and can allow children to use creatively descriptive idioms for pain. The form and specificity of subsequent questions are guided by the quality of previous responses. Younger children may need to move quickly into closed-ended questioning. Areas of inquiry can be broadly categorized as pain characteristics, antecedents, alleviating factors, response behaviors, and consequences (see **Box 1**).

Psychiatric Diagnosis

Psychiatric diagnosis is another possible reason for referral. Systematic evaluation of psychopathology can identify difficulties that are causal, exacerbating, or comorbid with chest pain. To this end, the caregiver's concerns about the child should be elicited and the child should be queried about emotional and behavioral functioning. This questioning may be effectively and thoroughly accomplished by administering structured diagnostic interviews. Because some symptoms may be common to both medical and psychiatric diagnoses, queries should be used to differentiate disease symptoms and natural reactions to a medical diagnosis from clinically significant psychopathology. **Box 2** summarizes a few possible child and parent report instruments that may be helpful in screening for and diagnosing psychological difficulties in patients with chest pain.

Intervention

With the exception of a few related medical conditions (eg, asthma), there is a paucity of research evaluating psychological interventions with pediatric patients with chest pain. It is therefore often necessary to adapt protocols developed with physically well children or children with other health conditions to meet the needs of the patient. It is crucial to maintain continuous assessment of patient health and safety as well as symptom improvements and declines. The diverse causes potentially associated with chest pain make it difficult to form generalizations about intervention guidelines. This article provides a few brief general suggestions for promoting positive health behaviors, followed by specific considerations for selected conditions. Clinicians are encouraged to use the references herein as a starting point from which to explore issues that are especially relevant to their own patients.

Promoting Positive Health Behaviors and Reducing Risk Factors

Patients with chest pain but with apparently significant coronary artery disease risk factors or other health compromising behaviors (eg, obesity, physical inactivity, nicotine use) should be referred to appropriate specialists for counseling and/or treatment. The urgency of lifestyle change may vary depending on current health and disease status. Health behaviors particularly relevant to patients with chest pain may include diet and physical activity level. Strategies for eliciting behavior change may include self-monitoring, stimulus control strategies, contingency planning, and breaking long-term treatment goals into discrete components. Older children and adolescents who are ambivalent or negative toward possible behavior change may benefit from motivational interviewing strategies to promote change readiness. In particular, interventions targeting changes in diet and physical activity level often include a familial component because these behaviors often reflect the lifestyle of the family as a whole. Patients with chest pain who are overweight may benefit from lifestyle interventions delivered in a group setting.[29] Children and families who successfully complete health behavior interventions are likely to require some sort of follow-up service to maintain lifestyle changes and changes in health status.[30]

PSYCHOLOGICAL ASSESSMENT AND INTERVENTION CONSIDERATIONS BY DIAGNOSES
Cardiac Chest Pain

Because of the need to rule out cardiac causes in many cases, chest pain is the second most common reason, following heart murmur, for referral to a pediatric cardiologist.[31] On the rare occasions when pediatric chest pain is associated with serious cardiac illness, prompt recognition, evaluation, and intervention are essential to protect against an adverse outcome; conversely, diagnostic error may lead to morbidity or morality.[8] Undergoing an extensive medical evaluation for chest pain may be anxiety provoking for pediatric patients and their families. Patients referred for cardiac testing may experience significant chest pain–related concern during the interim between referral and testing, even if they are reassured that their pain is unlikely to be causally linked to a heart problem. Only 20% of adolescents who are referred from primary care for cardiac evaluation report feeling reassured by a primary care provider, with 30% reporting increased anxiety after their appointment.[25] Therefore, short time intervals between referral and further tests are desirable not only medically[8] but also from a psychological viewpoint.

Research indicates that 6% to 12% of patients with chest pain referred to a pediatric cardiologist for testing will receive a cardiac diagnosis.[3,25,32] Some patients with cardiac diagnoses may benefit from psychological consultation. Cardiac disorders that are not associated with psychopathology per se may nonetheless have significant lifestyle implications that place patients at risk for adjustment difficulties. Patients may be required to refrain from activities such as organized sports or adhere to medication regimens. Patients and families may also need assistance in coping with the emotional ramifications of a heart condition that increases a child's risk of morbidity. Even conditions that are objectively low risk nonetheless have the potential to provoke strong emotional reactions from parents and children.

Congenital Heart Disease

At times, chest pain may occur in patients with a history of congenital heart disease (CHD).[33] CHD may function as an ongoing stressor for both the patient and their family. A meta-analysis of research regarding behavioral functioning in children with CHD suggests that children 10 years or older are rated by parents as having more internalizing and externalizing problem behaviors than healthy controls.[34] The children themselves indicate increased depression.[35] Overall, children with CHD seem especially at risk for internalizing problems during late childhood and early adolescence, such as mood and anxiety disorders, relative to externalizing behavior problems.[34]

Children with more severe CHD may also be at greater risk for cognitive difficulties [34] as well as mild motor deficits and language difficulties.[36,37] Children with surgically corrected CHD may be particularly at risk for academic difficulties.[35] However, little research has been conducted on psychological or academic interventions with this population specifically.[38] These patients may nonetheless benefit from psychological and academic interventions. Overall, CHD is associated with an increased risk for emotional and cognitive difficulties. Emotional difficulties such as anxiety and depression may be especially relevant for older children and adolescents.

Clinical Considerations for Work with Patients with CHD

Psychotherapeutic intervention

Because of an increased risk for general internalizing problems, patients with CHD may benefit from transdiagnostic interventions that focus on emotional regulation.[39] In cases with high anxiety, negative responses to heart sensations may be an important treatment focus. Patients with CHD who report high anxiety are apt to attend to harmless heart-related bodily cues, which may lead to overperception of heart symptoms in the absence of actual heart dysfunction,[40] particularly under stress.[41] In children with congenital heart disease, those who have high anxiety also tend to negatively interpret heart-related physical sensations, and this interpretation bias is partially responsible for the negative effect of anxiety on quality of life.[42] These children may benefit from cognitive interventions to reduce overly negative interpretations of heart sensations[42] in addition to treatment of fear and anxiety-related conditions.

Academic intervention

Children with CHD-related chest pain may experience cognitive and neurologic symptoms that may affect academic, behavioral, and emotional functioning. Patients who report or show difficulty at school may benefit from comprehensive psychoeducational evaluations that include cognitive, language, and motor skills testing to identify the specific domains in which the child needs intervention or accommodation. Some difficulties may be subtle and will become more apparent as children age and academic material becomes more challenging. As such, psychoeducational evaluations should be considered for older patients even without a long standing history of learning difficulties. Children who meet legal criteria for learning or occupational (motor skills) disabilities may receive special education services through individual educational plans. Patients with CHD with other neurodevelopmental impairments may be eligible for individual educational plans based on the presence of other health impairment. Students may also access services via laws, statutes, or policies created to provide services for students with medical problems.

Because knowledge of the cognitive and neurologic correlates of CHD may be specialized, students may benefit from a referral to a pediatric psychologist or neuropsychologist for testing. In such cases, the examiner may need to communicate with staff to explicate the child's difficulties to school officials who may be unfamiliar with

CHD. In circumstances in which specialized services are not available, caregivers should be encouraged to advocate for their children and educate school officials about CHD. Caregivers may also wish to use school nursing staff as a resource during this process, even if the child is not actively receiving medical treatment. Clinicians may assist parents in this process by being available for consultation with school officials.

Mitral Valve Prolapse

Children with mitral valve prolapse (MVP) are often referred for psychological assessment and treatment, partly because of the similarity between the cardiovascular symptoms of the MVP and the manifestations of panic attacks, including palpitations, chest pain, fatigue, dizziness, and a sensation of fainting. Although medical treatment is not indicated for most patients with MVP, it is generally beneficial to collaborate with the cardiologist to help the child and the family to identify what physical symptoms merit calling the physician. This process includes identifying urgent and nonurgent symptoms of concern. Second, the autonomic symptoms associated with MVP can frighten children and their caregivers. In some cases, the symptoms are linked with the presence of anxiety disorders.[43] Both children and their caregivers may benefit from education about MVP, psychoeducation about the physiology of emotions, especially anxiety and panic, and cognitive and behavioral skills in emotion regulation, particularly skills in managing the autonomic symptoms of hyperarousal. For the child with MVP, the intense physical symptoms and the fear and confusion can result in a panic attack. In some cases, children develop an enduring fear of having additional symptoms, and become hypervigilant to the slightest bodily sensation (eg, sensations of warmth, sweaty palms, slight heart rate changes). This fear may trigger the release of stress hormones (those that induce panic attacks), thus initiating and/or escalating a new panic attack. For children with chest pain who also meet diagnostic criteria for an anxiety disorder, the child and caregiver may benefit from a full course of evidence-based treatment of that disorder.[44]

RESPIRATORY-RELATED CHEST PAIN

Studies suggest that 13% to 21% of cases of chest pain in the emergency department are attributable to pulmonary causes,[3,4,45] with asthma alone accounting for 7% of cases.[45]

Asthma

Meta-analysis has indicated that children with asthma have more behavioral difficulties, particularly internalizing behaviors, than healthy controls.[46] Psychosocial factors such as acute and chronic stressors, strong emotions, and family relationships have been identified as relevant to asthma symptoms.[47–50] The psychophysiologic mechanisms responsible for this, although not completely understood, are believed to involve multiple pathways including autonomic airway control, neuroendocrine function, and immune regulations.[51–53]

Clinical Considerations

Consistent with the multifactorial causes of asthma, research supports the usefulness of interdisciplinary treatment teams that integrate various health care domains, including psychology, in managing this condition.[52,54,55] Within the treatment team context, psychologists may help improve symptom control by providing psychoeducation focused on increasing knowledge of asthma and treatment.[56,57] There are many published psychosocial individual, group, and family interventions that have been shown to effectively improve asthma management, maximize treatment adherence, and facilitate cooperation between families and physicians in various inpatient and outpatient settings.[52,58] Evidence-based interventions evaluated in a variety of patient populations include modalities such as motivational interviewing, organizational strategies, problem-solving techniques, and family empowerment.[58–61] There is also a growing literature on implementing such interventions effectively among traditionally underserved populations.[62]

Perhaps because of its high prevalence and effect on public health, there is a substantial evidence base regarding asthma and psychosocial factors on which clinicians may draw when developing individual treatment plans. Because a comprehensive review is beyond the scope of this paper, clinicians are urged to examine this evidence in depth to determine how best to meet the unique assessment and intervention needs of their individual patients with chest pain and asthma comorbidity. Recent reviews such as those by McQuaid and Abramson,[52] Drotar and Bonner,[63] and Tibosch and colleagues[50] may be useful sources of information.

GASTROINTESTINAL EVALUATION AND DIAGNOSES

Gastrointestinal (GI) conditions account for approximately 3% to 4% of cases of chest pain in the emergency department.[3,5] Although there are certain signs and symptoms that call for immediate GI evaluation, research suggests that patients who report chest pain without these markers may nonetheless have test results that indicate a GI cause.[64]

Clinical Considerations

As a group, the GI disorders that may be associated with chest pain in children are heterogeneous in clinical presentation and may be multifactorial in cause. They are often conceptualized from a biopsychosocial perspective,[65] and treatment is regularly interdisciplinary with a focus on maintaining psychosocial quality of life as well as physical health.[66] In general, psychological stress may exacerbate GI symptoms.[67,68] As such, psychosocial treatment with stress management components may be particularly helpful for these patients.[65] Such interventions may also include elements of psychoeducation, relaxation training and biofeedback, and parent training.[65]

MUSCULOSKELETAL CHEST PAIN

It is difficult to estimate the proportion of chest pain cases that are caused by musculoskeletal causes because this is defined variably across studies and may be used as a diagnosis of exclusion or reported in the same category as idiopathic cases.[7] Research suggests that costochondritis is diagnosed in approximately 9% of patients with chest pain in emergency departments,[45] and other musculoskeletal causes are diagnosed in approximately 15% of cases.[45] A traumatic cause is reported in 5% to 15% of cases of chest pain in the emergency department.[3,4,45]

CHEST WALL DEFORMITIES

Congenital chest wall deformities such as pectus excavatum (chest depression) and pectus carinatum (chest protrusion) are at times accompanied by chest pain.[9] Such deformities are estimated to occur in approximately 1 in 400 live births.[69] Children with chest wall deformities may have chest pain secondary to muscle, cardiac, and respiratory difficulties, but there are also certain issues that are unique to this patient group.[9]

Clinical Considerations

Chest wall deformities may result in noticeable cosmetic differences that are potentially distressing for patients and families. Physicians report that chest wall deformities may have significant psychological consequences for patients.[9,70] Preliminary research indicates that 70% to 80% of patients older than 11 years of age report problems such as increased risk for anxiety, shyness, feelings of stigmatization, self-consciousness, and poor body image.[71] These problems are markedly higher in this age group than in younger children.[71] This may reflect increased evidence of appearance differences correlating with physical growth as well as the increased body-focus and self-consciousness that often accompanies early adolescence. Gender may also be relevant to appearance-related distress among these patients. In one study, significantly more girls (68%) than boys (40%) reported being bothered by their chests often or very often.[72] Some patients may require evaluation and treatment of co-occurring clinically significant emotional distress (eg, body image disturbances, social anxiety and avoidance).

Patients and families may also, and perhaps primarily, benefit from supportive treatment as they make decisions regarding treatment. Liaison may be especially important in these cases, because some care providers may underestimate the depth of a patient's and family's concerns regarding the cosmetic aspects and corresponding psychosocial burden of this condition.[73,74] Significantly improved psychosocial functioning has been reported by patients, both girls and boys, and parents following corrective surgery.[72] Because there are few resources associated with this disorder, clinicians may need to be proactive and creative in facilitating patient support and psychoeducation. Patients who lack access to peers with similar conditions may benefit from Internet forums hosted by the Web sites of advocacy groups.

CHEST PAIN IN THE ABSENCE OF ORGANIC DISEASE OR DIAGNOSIS
Terminology

Differences in terminology are a frequent challenge when attempting to integrate research produced by health care providers across different fields and specialties. This challenge is especially pertinent to chest pain. Psychological studies of chest pain tend to use noncardiac chest pain (NCCP) as a descriptor for recurrent chest pain in the absence of cardiac or other organic causes. However, within current medical literature the term NCCP may also be used as a broad category that contains any non–heart-related classifications, including musculoskeletal, pulmonary, and gastrointestinal causes, in addition to nonorganic pain. Chest pain that is nonorganic may be categorized in some studies as idiopathic pain. This term may also be used to reference localized chest wall pain or musculoskeletal pain. In some cases, idiopathic chest pain may also include pain that seems related to psychiatric concerns such as panic attacks or anxiety. Alternatively, pain relating to psychiatric difficulties may be classified as psychogenic, psychological, nonorganic, or functional chest pain. Nomenclature is complicated by the possibility that, in some chest pain cases, there may be more than 1 diagnosis.[75] For an in-depth review of chest pain classification issues, see Ref.[76]

The issue of terminology illustrates the broader point that chest pain in the absence of an acute organic disorder is a nebulously defined and under-researched complaint.[76] Although some cases of nonorganic chest pain may be symptoms of a psychiatric disorder, which have specific diagnostic criteria, other cases may occur in patients without such disorders. Any diagnostic label assigned to these cases, be it idiopathic chest pain, NCCP, or miscellaneous chest pain, may therefore be considered a diagnosis of exclusion that lacks definitive diagnostic criteria. Psychological factors may nonetheless be relevant to these cases. This article simply uses the term chest pain to refer to cases with chest pain that (1) occurs in the absence of a diagnosed or documented organic disorder, (2) may or may not be accompanied by psychopathology, and (3) may or may not be considered a symptom of psychiatric disorder.

Chest Pain and Psychopathology

Etiologic studies suggest that clinically significant psychopathology is present in 5% to 17% of cases of chest pain in the emergency department,[3–6] 4% to 19% of cardiology clinic cases,[22,23,25,77,78] and 30% of general pediatric clinic cases.[79] However, because of methodological issues, these prevalence rates should be applied cautiously. These studies of chest pain include data generated from retrospective chart reviews,[3,5,6,77] or prospectively obtained from emergency department[4] or cardiology clinic examinations.[22,23] Although patients underwent thorough medical testing, researchers seem to have relied on medical records, patient self-identification, parent report, or physician histories for psychiatric diagnosis rather than specific psychological assessment measures. This may have artificially lowered prevalence ratings, particularly in emergency departments, because medical chart reviews indicate that standard chest pain emergency examinations are unlikely to include mental health screening.[80] In addition, identifying potentially complex or indirect relationships between pain and psychological symptoms in emergency or specialty care settings may be challenging, particularly for medical providers who do not specialize in psychological assessment.

In the single study in which psychiatric evaluation is reported, patients were evaluated only if medical records showed a previous history of psychological difficulties,[78] suggesting that patients with new-onset psychopathology may have been excluded. In addition, the nature of the assessment was not clearly explicated. This example illustrates another methodological concern, in that nonstandardized assessment methods (eg, the questions asked by physicians during histories, or the unspecified and potentially variable assessments noted in medical records) may produce variable results. Thus, some of the variance in prevalence of psychiatric symptoms across studies may be attributable to differences in assessment.

Overall, much of the published literature on chest pain and psychiatric comorbidity is not based on valid psychological assessment. It has been speculated that psychopathology was significant, but unnoticed, in a sizable proportion of cases categorized as idiopathic or miscellaneous.[81] Psychiatric symptoms are often relevant to medically unexplained pain complaints such as headache and recurrent abdominal pain,[82–85] and, in one study, adolescent outpatients with chest pain reported as many psychiatric symptoms as patients presenting with headache and abdominal pain.[86] This study is limited by the inclusion chest pain of both organic and non-organic origin and the exclusion of patients with significant psychiatric histories, but nonetheless provides preliminary evidence for the relevance of psychiatric symptoms to chest pain.

Research using psychological assessment suggests an increased rate of psychopathology among patients with chest pain. In 1995, Tunaoglu and colleagues[87] reported that 74% of patients with idiopathic chest pain who were referred to a child psychiatric outpatient clinic for evaluation met DSM-III-R criteria for psychiatric disorder, as only 80% followed through on that referral.[87] The requirement that patients visit a psychiatric clinic to receive psychological evaluation may have resulted in a selection bias. Parents of children with psychiatric symptoms may have been more likely to follow through on this referral than parents of psychiatrically asymptomatic children. However, a conservative estimate that all nonpresenting patients were psychiatrically asymptomatic nonetheless results in a 60% prevalence rate of DSM-III-TR psychiatric disorders.

Because the assessments examined in 1995 by Tunaoglu and colleagues[87] were based on interviews conducted by a single child psychiatrist, diagnostic reliability across subjects is assumed to be high. Nonetheless, the nature of these interviews represents a limitation on these findings. Unstructured psychological assessment may have considerable variability based on factors such as question wording, the order of questioning, and the specific symptoms inquired about. However, this limitation was not applicable to a study conducted by Lipsitz and colleagues[88] in which cardiac patients diagnosed with NCCP were assessed using a structured diagnostic interview, the Anxiety Disorder Interview Schedule for DSM-IV: Child and Parent Versions (ADIS-IV:C-P), which reliably assesses a broad range of anxiety, mood, somatoform, and behavioral disorders and also screens for the presence of developmental and psychotic disorders. These assessments, which were administered in patients' homes, indicated that 59% of patients (N = 27) met criteria for a current DSM-IV axis I psychiatric disorder.[88] In summary, these studies suggest that psychopathology may be more prevalent among cardiac patients with chest pain than was reflected in previous studies.

Clinical Implication

Although further research is needed, clinically significant psychopathology may be more prevalent among patients with chest pain than was previously believed. Clinicians should routinely consider referring patients with recurrent, impairing chest pain for psychological evaluation. Prevalence data suggest that psychological assessment is useful to rule out the presence of psychopathology in patients with chest pain.

Anxiety

Lipsitz and colleagues[88] reported that anxiety disorders were the most common psychiatric diagnoses, with a prevalence rate of 56% for singular anxiety disorders and 30% for 2 or more concurrent disorders. Among this group of patients with anxiety disorders (N = 15), panic disorder (60%) and generalized anxiety disorder (47%) were the most common diagnoses.[88] This finding suggests that some children experience chest pain during panic attacks. However, a significant proportion of patients did not meet criteria for panic disorder, which indicates that some cases of medically unexplained chest pain represent a singular ailment distinct from undiagnosed panic disorder. Anxiety was also the most commonly diagnosed disorder indicated by the interviews conducted by Tunaoglu and colleagues,[87] and was present in 20% of patients. Because this study did not distinguish between psychiatric diagnoses within broad classifications, rates of specific anxiety disorders in this patient sample are unknown. The disparate prevalence rates between these 2 studies may reflect several methodological differences, including sample size, assessment method, and the setting in which the assessment occurred. However, taken together, these studies suggest that anxiety may be particularly relevant to chest pain. This interpretation is somewhat consistent with a previous retrospective review of medical records that attributed 37% of medically unexplained chest pain cases to anxiety based on emergency room exams.[5,6] This interpretation is also is congruent with the frequent association of anxiety with unexplained medical symptoms such as headache, musculoskeletal pain, and abdominal pain in children.[83–85,89]

As discussed previously, cardiac evaluation and testing might be expected to induce a degree of situational anxiety in many children. Interviewing children at home[88] or in an outpatient psychiatric clinic[87] rather than in a medical setting may minimize situational anxiety. However, because patients report chest pain–related worry continuing past medical evaluation,[5] some of the anxiety symptoms reported by pediatric patients with chest pain may be a normative response to evaluation for cardiac symptoms, suggesting the need for controlled studies that examine differences in the prevalence of anxiety between pediatric patients with chest pain and other patients who undergo cardiac evaluations. One such study does indicate that patients who received cardiac evaluation for chest pain report higher levels of general anxiety and more physical anxiety symptoms then patients with benign heart murmurs.[90] The increased general anxiety symptoms reported by patients with chest pain suggest that the anxiety reported by these patients reflects more than specific worry about chest pain and that their anxiety extends to areas unrelated to physical health.[90]

Along with overall levels of anxiety symptoms, certain anxiety-related psychological traits and tendencies may influence a child's experience of chest pain. The finding that more than half of pediatric patients with chest pain perceive their pain as threatening suggests that perception of bodily sensations may be potentially relevant to these patients' experience. The trait tendency to fear anxiety-related physiologic sensations is commonly referred to as anxiety sensitivity. Child and adolescent patients with NCCP report higher anxiety sensitivity than pediatric patients with benign heart murmurs and also report more concern specifically regarding potential physical distress.[90] These patients report levels of anxiety sensitivity that are comparable with levels shown by pediatric patients receiving treatment of an anxiety disorder.[90] Furthermore, fear of physiologic arousal is associated with greater chest pain severity in pediatric patients with NCCP.[81]

Age variance of beliefs regarding chest pain was not reported in this research, and it may be that cognitions regarding chest pain vary across different levels of cognitive development. Although the perception of benign physiologic symptoms as dangerous has been shown in children as young as 6 years,[91] cognitive interpretation of these sensations may change in time. As their fund of physiologic knowledge increases, children are increasingly likely to form thoughts and beliefs about the meaning and dangerousness of their own physical symptoms.[92] In general, children start thinking of health as an interactive, long-term condition sometime between the ages of 11 and 14 years.[93] Older children and adolescents may therefore be more likely than younger children to associate individual symptoms, such as chest pain, with dysfunction of organs or broader physiologic systems, such as the heart or cardiovascular system.

Clinical Implications

Fear and anxiety should routinely be assessed in patients with chest pain referred for psychological evaluation. Many clinicians associate chest pain with panic attacks, and some patients with chest pain may meet diagnostic criteria for panic disorder. Such patients may benefit from evidence-based treatments specifically for panic disorder.[44,94] Cognitive interpretation of bodily sensations, particularly chest pain, may be an important target for intervention. Patients' fear and anxiety may extend to areas unrelated to health, because generalized anxiety disorder also seems prevalent among this group.

Depression

Psychological factors other than anxiety, such as depression, are also regularly associated with medically unexplained pain complaints in children.[84,85,89] Thus far, research regarding pediatric chest pain and depressive symptoms has provided mixed results. In one study, 52% (N = 56) of patients who received psychiatric evaluation met DSM-IV-TR criteria for depression, which was the most common psychiatric diagnosis in this group.[78] However, patients in this study only received psychiatric evaluation they had a significant psychiatric history. It is possible that other psychiatric symptoms would have been more prevalent if all patients with chest pain (N = 300) had received psychiatric evaluation. In one study, adolescent patients with NCCP showed a clinically significant group mean on a standard self-report measure of depressive symptoms.[86] Unstructured psychiatric interviews indicated that 100% of a small (N = 4) sample of cardiac patients with no organic cardiac disorder met criteria for major depressive disorder, although this finding may also reflect that depression was the only type of psychopathology investigated in this study.[95]

In contrast, Tunaoglu and colleagues[90] and Lipsitz and colleagues[81] respectively reported that 15% and 11% of patients met criteria for a depressive disorder. An experimenter-designed questionnaire assessing depressive symptoms in patients in emergency departments failed to show differences across patients whose chest pain was categorized as miscellaneous, psychogenic, idiopathic, traumatic, pulmonary, and chest wall pain.[4] This suggests that depression may be less relevant to pediatric chest pain than other types of psychopathology. Accordingly, on standardized self-report measures, 11% of pediatric patients with NCCP indicate increased levels of depressive symptoms, comparable with the prevalence of depressive symptoms reported by patients with benign heart murmurs.[90,95] However, it may be that there exists a subgroup of pediatric patients with chest pain for whom depression is a notable factor and who would benefit from further study of depressive symptoms within this population. Among pediatric patients diagnosed with NCCP, depression is associated with the frequency and intensity of overall physical symptoms, suggesting that patients with co-occurring NCCP and depressive symptoms may be at risk for greater symptom severity.[81]

Clinical Implication

Although the likelihood that patients with chest pain will meet diagnostic criteria for depression is uncertain based on current research, this is nonetheless an important area for assessment, because patients who do have co-occurring depression may be at increased risk for more severe chest pain.

Somatization

Although most pediatric patients with medically unexplained chest pain do not report additional physiologic symptoms, complaints such as headaches, abdominal pain, fatigue, and dizziness are reported in approximately 30% of cases.[96] Thus, in a minority of cases, chest pain may be 1 symptom of broader somatization difficulties. However, psychological research on the prevalence of broader somatization difficulties among pediatric patients with chest pain is unclear. Tunaoglu and colleagues[87] and Yildirim and colleagues[78] respectively reported that 8% and 25% of patients met criteria for a somatoform disorder, although this disparity may reflect changes in diagnostic criteria, and the larger sample size examined by Tunaoglu and colleagues[87] may have contributed to more within-sample variation in psychiatric symptoms. However, the prevalence of somatoform disorders may also reflect the failure to report variance within diagnostic classes. It is therefore possible that these patients could have received a diagnosis of undifferentiated somatoform disorder based solely on the presence of medically unexplained chest pain for 6 months or more.[97,98] These patients may or may not have reported additional physiologic symptoms. In contrast, Lipsitz and colleagues[88] did not report any somatoform diagnoses based on DSM-IV criteria. Number and severity of other physical symptoms are positively associated with chest pain severity and account for 17% of variance in reported pain severity,[81] so these patients may be at risk for severe chest pain symptoms.

Clinical Implication

In a minority of patients, chest pain may indicate broader somatization tendencies. Because other physical symptoms are associated with increased pain severity, these patients may be especially likely to report functional impairments and may benefit from evidence-based psychological interventions targeting chronic and/or recurrent pain complaints.

Stress

Guidelines for the medical evaluation of pediatric chest pain suggest that physicians inquire about recent individual and family stressors.[7] Asnes and colleagues[79] reported that stressful situations were associated with pain onset in nearly all patients in a group diagnosed with psychogenic chest pain. However, this finding may be largely attributable to the broad definition of stressful situation, which included imagining being separated from a parent, sleeping alone, going to school, and the experience of psychiatric symptoms. Between 25% and 30% of patients report stressful life events such as a death in the family, major illness, accident, family separation, or school change.[77] Because these life events are common within a pediatric population, it is difficult to establish a specific relationship between stress and chest pain based on these findings. Adolescents with idiopathic chest pain do not report a higher frequency of life stressors than patients whose pain is attributable to specific organic causes.[26] Because different individuals may experience variable stress reactions in response to identical events, further research is needed to determine whether there is a relationship between perceived stress and NCCP.

Clinical Implication

In many cases, chest pain may be associated with stress partly because of emotion regulation difficulties. Clinicians may find that physiologic arousal reduction techniques (eg, deep breathing, relaxation) and the cognitive and behavioral skills delivered to target emotion regulation are more productive to reduce chest pain and improve functioning compared with general stress management programs for children with chest pain and stress difficulties.

PSYCHOLOGICAL INTERVENTION WITH PATIENTS WITH CHEST PAIN

Recurrent medically unexplained chest pain is a condition that is perhaps best considered as distinct from pediatric anxiety and other pain disorders because it does not meet the diagnostic criteria for either of these disorders classes. The experience and clinical presentation of recurrent medically unexplained chest pain may share characteristics with both of these broader disorder classes, and it is possible that a child with a pain or anxiety disorder may suffer from chest pain as well. Psychotherapeutic interventions may be useful for children and adolescents suffering recurrent and impairing chest pain.[77,88] It is recommended that psychological assessment and treatment be provided only in the context of the child receiving regular scheduled medical care by a pediatrician.

Effective psychological assessment allows the clinician to conceptualize likely mechanisms underlying the clinical problems and enables the clinician and patient to arrive at shared treatment goals. In some cases, it may be useful to work in partnership with the patients and their families about shared conceptualizations and treatment goals. For instance, caregivers who may be less psychologically minded may not be as open to exploring less-familiar causes, including stress, emotional distress, and psychological disorders including anxiety disorders. If the family is reluctant to consider psychological explanations for their pain, clinicians may find it useful to emphasize the physiologic components of emotion and the bidirectional relationship between emotional distress and physical pain. The cycle of physical pain symptoms precipitating emotions are just as common as the converse. The clinician might introduce the psychological diagnosis not as a new entity or experience but rather as an explanation for, or perhaps even a renaming of, the pain and other symptoms that the child already has. Some families are pleased to learn that the chest pain does not signify a serious medical condition and that it is attributable to a psychological disorder.

At present, we are not aware of any published, empirically supported psychological treatments specifically designed for pediatric patients with chest pain. As a result, psychological interventions with this patient group targeting chest pain are not yet well studied. Because there are currently no psychological treatments specifically designed for, and evaluated with, patients with chest pain, most interventions with this group will be somewhat experimental in nature. Children with ongoing chest pain who meet diagnostic criteria for anxiety or mood-disorders (ie, DSM-IV axis I psychiatric disorders) may be best treated with evidence-based treatments for these conditions first. This systematic approach has a high likelihood of easing their emotional distress and reducing their overall physiologic arousal. Sessions targeting arousal reduction techniques can be tailored to reduce chest pain and distress via deep breathing, progressive relaxation training, and imagery, as appropriate to the child. Older children and adolescents may be especially likely to benefit from a cognitive component of treatment that targets beliefs they may have about their pain. In particular, cognitive and behavioral therapy techniques that are intended to reduce their sensitivity and responsiveness to cardiac-related physical sensations (ie, interoceptive sensitivity to palpitations, dyspnea, dizziness, or exertion) via traditional exposure techniques may be beneficial. Lessening the misinterpretation of possible fears associated with physical sensations may also be a treatment goal. For example, one child who presented for treatment believed that her chest sensations were dangerous and meant that she would have a heart attack. As a result, she avoided all exertion (including exercise, warm showers) and she would often pace herself during her daily activities to avoid rushing or feeling flushed (eg, slowing her gait, opting to walk home by herself after school). Assisting patients to reduce and remove all avoidance behaviors, and any other maladaptive safety devices (sometimes referred to as safety signals), may help patients to regain their sense of safety. Moreover, working with children (and caregivers, as needed) to increase their acceptance and tolerance for anxiety and discomfort will likely benefit them. Exposure techniques are likely advantageous in this patient group, and have found acceptance among other similar samples.[99,100] In nearly all cases, some extent of caregiver involvement facilitates treatment.[101,102]

Patients with clinically significant anxiety disorders may benefit from a recently developed treatment protocol that adapts an empirically supported cognitive behavioral protocol for anxiety specifically for children with medically unexplained pain conditions.[103] This protocol has been piloted with patients with medically unexplained gastrointestinal conditions comorbid with anxiety disorders.[104] Patients with mood difficulties may benefit from empirically supported depression treatments such as interpersonal psychotherapy for depressed adolescents (IPT-A)[105] and cognitive behavioral therapy (CBT).[106] Patients with especially severe chest pain who also experience other somatic complaints may benefit from interventions targeted

Table 1
Prevalence of psychiatric symptoms in patients with chest pain

Authors	Sample	N	Age (y), Range (mean)	Assessment	Outcome
Asnes et al[79]	General	123	4–14[b]	Medical examination	30% categorized as psychogenic chest pain
Diehl[22]	Cardiology	48	[b]	Medical record review, medical examination	12% categorized as psychological chest pain
Evangelista et al[23]	Cardiology	50	5–21[24]	Medical examination	2% categorized as psychogenic
Kashani et al[95]	Cardiology[a]	4	[b]	Psychiatric interview	100% met DSM-III criteria for depression
Lam and Tobias[77]	Cardiology	55	6–20 (14.2)	Reviewed records, asked parents about presumed cause of chest pain during follow-up call	0% initial psychiatric diagnosis; 4% received secondary diagnosis of anxiety or panic
Lipsitz et al[88]	Cardiology[a]	27	8–17 (12.7)	Structured interview	59% met criteria for a DSM-IV axis 1 disorder
Massin et al[3]	Emergency	168	3–15 (10.1)	Medical examination	9% psychogenic chest pain
Rowe et al[4]	Emergency	325	2–18 (11.6)	Medical examination	5% categorized as psychogenic chest pain
Selbst[5]	Emergency	267	1–19[b]	Medical records review	17% categorized as functional (anxiety-related) chest pain
Tunaoglu et al[87]	Cardiology[a]	74	3–16 (11.3 girls, 9.9 boys)	Psychiatric interview	74% report psychiatric symptoms
Yildirim et al[78]	Cardiology	300	3–17 (9.6 girls, 10.4 boys)	Psychiatric if significant psychological history	19% categorized as psychiatric chest pain

[a] Includes only patients with negative medical evaluations.
[b] Specific age range or mean not reported.

specifically for physical pain. Preliminary research suggests that biofeedback may help reduce pain in some patients by reducing overall sympathetic nervous system arousal.[107,108] Progressive muscle relaxation training, deep breathing, imagery, and cognitive restructuring have been incorporated into several programs that specifically target a child's subjective experience of pain.[109,110]

FUTURE DIRECTIONS

Currently, there are several important and largely unexplored questions about the relationship between pediatric chest pain and psychological factors. Further study is needed to explore the direct and indirect influences of psychological factors on outcome variables such as the severity and duration of chest pain. The role that psychological factors may play in chest pain–related impairment is a key area for future research. The extent to which psychological factors are causally related to chest pain in children is not yet established. Further examination of psychopathology within this population is necessary both to clarify the distress experienced by pediatric patients with chest pain and to explore whether psychiatric symptoms might function as risk factors and maintaining variables for medically unexplained chest pain. Thus far, no published research has explored the influence of psychiatric symptoms on the cause and maintenance of pediatric chest pain over time. Longitudinal studies are needed to examine fluctuations of psychopathology in pediatric patients with chest pain and to explore the directionality of the relationship between pain and psychopathology. It is particularly important to determine whether psychiatric symptoms predict future recurrence and severity of chest pain.

Although research indicates that psychological factors are relevant in many pediatric chest pain cases, children with pain complaints are most likely to present to medical settings and may not spontaneously seek out psychological assessment or treatment. The discrepant prevalence of psychiatric symptoms across studies that did and did not use psychological assessment (**Table 1**) suggests that such symptoms may be present but unapparent during examinations in medical settings. This finding highlights the need for specific and reliable guidelines for assessing psychiatric symptoms in pediatric patients with chest pain. There may also be a need for greater integration of behavioral health care providers within emergency and cardiology settings. This integration could significantly contribute to effective assessment and treatment of children with this condition and help to alleviate the emotional distress associated with the experience of chest pain for many children and families.

REFERENCES

1. Rhee H, Miles MS, Halpern CT, et al. Prevalence of recurrent physical symptoms in U.S. adolescents. Pediatr Nurs 2005;31:314–9, 350.
2. Garber J, Walker LS, Zeman J. Somatization symptoms in a community sample of children and adolescents: Further validation of the children's somatization inventory. Psychol Assess 1991;3:588–95.
3. Massin MM, Bourguignont A, Coremans C, et al. Chest pain in pediatric patients presenting to an emergency department or to a cardiac clinic. Clin Pediatr (Phila) 2004;43:231–8.
4. Rowe BH, Dulberg CS, Peterson RG, et al. Characteristics of children presenting with chest pain to a pediatric emergency department. CMAJ 1990;143: 388–94.

5. Selbst SM. Chest pain in children. Pediatrics 1985;75:1068–70.
6. Zavaras-Angelidou KA, Weinhouse E, Nelson DB. Review of 180 episodes of chest pain in 134 children. Pediatr Emerg Care 1992;8:189–93.
7. Thull-Freedman J. Evaluation of chest pain in the pediatric patient. Med Clin North Am 2010;94:327–47.
8. Kocis KC. Chest pain in pediatrics. Pediatr Clin North Am 1999;46:189–203.
9. Gokhale J, Selbst SM. Chest pain and chest wall deformity. Pediatr Clin North Am 2009;56:49–65.
10. Martin AL, McGrath PA, Brown SC, et al. Anxiety sensitivity, fear of pain and pain-related disability in children and adolescents with chronic pain. Pain Res Manag 2007;12:267–72.
11. March JS, Parker JD, Sullivan K, et al. The Multidimensional Anxiety Scale for Children (MASC): factor structure, reliability, and validity. J Am Acad Child Adolesc Psychiatry 1997;36:554–65.
12. Reynolds CR, Paget KD. Factor analysis of the revised children's manifest anxiety scale for blacks, whites, males, and females with a national normative sample. J Consult Clin Psychol 1981;49:352–9.
13. White KS, Farrell AD. Structure of anxiety symptoms in urban children: a test of competing factor analytic models of the revised children's manifest anxiety scale. J Consult Clin Psychol 2001;69:333–7.
14. Kovacs M. The Children's Depression Inventory (CDI). Psychopharmacol Bull 1985;21:995–8.
15. Smucker MR, Craighead WE, Craighead LW, et al. Normative and reliability data for the Children's Depression Inventory. J Abnorm Child Psychol 1986; 14:25–39.
16. Weber S. Factor structure of the Reynolds Adolescent Depression Scale in a sample of school-based adolescents. J Nurs Meas 2000;8:23–40.
17. Walker LS, Beck JE, Garber J, et al. Children's somatization inventory: psychometric properties of the revised form (CSI-24). J Pediatr Psychol 2009;34: 430–40.
18. Cohen S, Kamarck T, Mermelstein R. A global measure of perceived stress. J Health Soc Behav 1983;24:385–96.
19. Varni JW, Limbers CA. The Pediatric Quality of Life Inventory: measuring pediatric health-related quality of life from the perspective of children and their parents. Pediatr Clin North Am 2009;56:843–63.
20. Varni JW, Seid M, Kurtin PS. PedsQL 4.0: reliability and validity of the Pediatric Quality of Life Inventory version 4.0 generic core scales in healthy and patient populations. Med Care 2001;39:800–12.
21. Heron M, Sutton PD, Xu J, et al. Annual summary of vital statistics: 2007. Pediatrics 2010;125:4–15.
22. Diehl AM. Chest pain in children. Tip-offs to cause. Postgrad Med 1983;73: 335–7, 340–332.
23. Evangelista JA, Parsons M, Renneburg AK. Chest pain in children: diagnosis through history and physical examination. J Pediatr Health Care 2000;14:3–8.
24. Gutgesell HP, Barst RJ, Humes RA, et al. Common cardiovascular problems in the young: part I. Murmurs, chest pain, syncope and irregular rhythms. Am Fam Physician 1997;56:1825–30.
25. Kaden GG, Shenker IR, Gootman N. Chest pain in adolescents. J Adolesc Health 1991;12:251–5.
26. Pantell RH, Goodman BW Jr. Adolescent chest pain: a prospective study. Pediatrics 1983;71:881–7.

27. Cava JR, Sayger PL. Chest pain in children and adolescents. Pediatr Clin North Am 2004;51:1553–68.

28. Selbst SM, Ruddy RM, Clark BJ. Chest pain in children: follow-up of patients previously reported. Clin Pediatr (Phila) 1990;29:374–7.

29. Wilfley DE, Tibbs TL, Van Buren DJ, et al. Lifestyle interventions in the treatment of childhood overweight: a meta-analytic review of randomized controlled trials. Health Psychol 2007;26:521–32.

30. Wilfley DE, Stein RI, Saelens BE, et al. Efficacy of maintenance treatment approaches for childhood overweight: a randomized controlled trial. JAMA 2007;298:1661–73.

31. Brenner JI, Ringel RE, Berman MA. Cardiologic perspectives of chest pain in childhood: a referral problem? To whom? Pediatr Clin North Am 1984;31:1241–58.

32. Fyfe DA, Moodie DS. Chest pain in pediatric patients presenting to a cardiac clinic. Clin Pediatr (Phila) 1984;23:321–4.

33. Reddy SR, Singh HR. Chest pain in children and adolescents. Pediatr Rev 2010; 31:1–9.

34. Karsdorp PA, Everaerd W, Kindt M, et al. Psychological and cognitive functioning in children and adolescents with congenital heart disease: a meta-analysis. J Pediatr Psychol 2007;32:527–41.

35. Miatton M, De Wolf D, Francois K, et al. Behavior and self-perception in children with a surgically corrected congenital heart disease. J Dev Behav Pediatr 2007; 28:294–301.

36. Miatton M, De Wolf D, Francois K, et al. Do parental ratings on cognition reflect neuropsychological outcome in congenital heart disease? Acta Paediatr 2008; 97:41–5.

37. Miatton M, De Wolf D, Francois K, et al. Neuropsychological performance in school-aged children with surgically corrected congenital heart disease. J Pediatr 2007;151:73–8.

38. Delamater A, Jent JF. Cardiovascular disease. In: Roberts MC, Steele RG, editors. Handbook of pediatric psychology. New York: Guilford Press; 2009. p. 381–91.

39. Trosper SE, Buzzella BA, Bennett SM, et al. Emotion regulation in youth with emotional disorders: implications for a unified treatment approach. Clin Child Fam Psychol Rev 2009;12:234–54.

40. Karsdorp PA, Kindt M, Everaerd W, et al. Preattentive processing of heart cues and the perception of heart symptoms in congenital heart disease. Behav Res Ther 2007;45:1893–902.

41. Karsdorp PA, Kindt M, Rietveld S, et al. Stress-induced heart symptoms and perceptual biases in patients with congenital heart disease. Int J Cardiol 2007;114:352–7.

42. Karsdorp PA, Kindt M, Rietveld S, et al. Interpretation bias for heart sensations in congenital heart disease and its relation to quality of life. Int J Behav Med 2008; 15:232–40.

43. Filho AS, Maciel BC, Martin-Santos R, et al. Does the association between mitral valve prolapse and panic disorder really exist? Primary Care Companion J Clin Psychiatry 2008;10:38–47.

44. Ollendick TH, King NJ, Chorpita BF. Empirically supported treatments for children and adolescents: cognitive-behavioral procedures. In: Kendall PC, editor. Child and adolescent therapy. New York: Guilford Press; 2006. p. 492–520.

45. Selbst SM, Ruddy RM, Clark BJ, et al. Pediatric chest pain: a prospective study. Pediatrics 1988;82:319–23.

46. McQuaid EL, Kopel SJ, Nassau JH. Behavioral adjustment in children with asthma: a meta-analysis. J Dev Behav Pediatr 2001;22:430–9.
47. Wright RJ, Rodriguez M, Cohen S. Review of psychosocial stress and asthma: an integrated biopsychosocial approach. Thorax 1998;53:1066–74.
48. Wood BL, Klebba KB, Miller BD. Evolving the biobehavioral family model: the fit of attachment. Fam Process 2000;39:319–44.
49. Miller G, Chen E. Unfavorable socioeconomic conditions in early life presage expression of proinflammatory phenotype in adolescence. Psychosom Med 2007;69:402–9.
50. Tibosch MM, Verhaak CM, Merkus PJ. Psychological characteristics associated with the onset and course of asthma in children and adolescents: a systematic review of longitudinal effects. Patient Educ Couns 2010, in press. DOI:10.1016/j.pec.2010.03.011.
51. Wright RJ. Stress and atopic disorders. J Allergy Clin Immunol 2005;116:1301–6.
52. McQuaid EL, Abramson NW. Pediatric asthma. In: Roberts MC, Steele RG, editors. Handbook of pediatric psychology. New York: Guilford Press; 2009. p. 254–70.
53. Expert panel report 3 (epr-3): guidelines for the diagnosis and management of asthma-summary report 2007. J Allergy Clin Immunol 2007;120:S94–138.
54. Bratton DL, Price M, Gavin L, et al. Impact of a multidisciplinary day program on disease and healthcare costs in children and adolescents with severe asthma: a two-year follow-up study. Pediatr Pulmonol 2001;31:177–89.
55. Gupta RS, Weiss KB. The 2007 National Asthma Education and Prevention Program asthma guidelines: accelerating their implementation and facilitating their impact on children with asthma. Pediatrics 2009;123(Suppl 3):S193–8.
56. Clark NM, Brown R, Joseph CL, et al. Effects of a comprehensive school-based asthma program on symptoms, parent management, grades, and absenteeism. Chest 2004;125:1674–9.
57. Bonner S, Zimmerman BJ, Evans D, et al. An individualized intervention to improve asthma management among urban Latino and African-American families. J Asthma 2002;39:167–79.
58. Lemanek KL, Kamps J, Chung NB. Empirically supported treatments in pediatric psychology: regimen adherence. J Pediatr Psychol 2001;26:253–75.
59. Borrelli B, Riekert KA, Weinstein A, et al. Brief motivational interviewing as a clinical strategy to promote asthma medication adherence. J Allergy Clin Immunol 2007;120:1023–30.
60. Canino G, Vila D, Normand SL, et al. Reducing asthma health disparities in poor Puerto Rican children: the effectiveness of a culturally tailored family intervention. J Allergy Clin Immunol 2008;121:665–70.
61. Warman K, Silver EJ, Wood PR. Asthma risk factor assessment: what are the needs of inner-city families? Ann Allergy Asthma Immunol 2006;97:S11–5.
62. Weiss KB. Eliminating asthma disparities: a national workshop to set a working agenda. Chest 2007;132:753S–6S.
63. Drotar D, Bonner MS. Influences on adherence to pediatric asthma treatment: a review of correlates and predictors. J Dev Behav Pediatr 2009;30:574–82.
64. Berezin S, Medow MS, Glassman MS, et al. Chest pain of gastrointestinal origin. Arch Dis Child 1988;63:1457–60.
65. Cunningham CL, Banez GA. Pediatric gastrointestinal disorders: biopsychosocial assessment and treatment. New York: Springer; 2006.

66. Marlais M, Fishman JR, Koglmeier J, et al. Reduced quality of life in children with gastro-oesophageal reflux disease. Acta Paediatr 2010;99:418–21.
67. Banez GA, Cunningham CL. Abdominal pain-related gastrointestinal disorders. In: Roberts MC, Steele RG, editors. Handbook of pediatric psychology. New York: Guilford Press; 2009. p. 403–19.
68. Bennett EJ, Piesse C, Palmer K, et al. Functional gastrointestinal disorders: psychological, social, and somatic features. Gut 1998;42:414–20.
69. Chung CS, Myrianthopoulos NC. Factors affecting risks of congenital malformations. I. Analysis of epidemiologic factors in congenital malformations. Report from the Collaborative Perinatal Project. Birth Defects Orig Artic Ser 1975;11:1–22.
70. Ellis DG. Chest wall deformities in children. Pediatr Ann 1989;18:161–2, 164, 165.
71. Einsiedel E, Clausner A. Funnel chest. Psychological and psychosomatic aspects in children, youngsters, and young adults. J Cardiovasc Surg (Torino) 1999;40:733–6.
72. Kelly RE Jr, Cash TF, Shamberger RC, et al. Surgical repair of pectus excavatum markedly improves body image and perceived ability for physical activity: multicenter study. Pediatrics 2008;122:1218–22.
73. Wheeler R, Foote K. Pectus excavatum: studiously ignored in the United Kingdom? Arch Dis Child 2000;82:187–8.
74. Jaroszewski D, Notrica D, McMahon L, et al. Current management of pectus excavatum: a review and update of therapy and treatment recommendations. J Am Board Fam Med 2010;23:230–9.
75. Coulshed DS, Eslick GD, Talley NJ. Non-cardiac chest pain. Patients need diagnoses. BMJ 2002;324:915.
76. Eslick GD. Classification, natural history, epidemiology, and risk factors of noncardiac chest pain. Dis Mon 2008;54:593–603.
77. Lam JC, Tobias JD. Follow-up survey of children and adolescents with chest pain. South Med J 2001;94:921–4.
78. Yildirim A, Karakurt C, Karademir S, et al. Chest pain in children. Int Pediatr 2004;19:175–9.
79. Asnes RS, Santulli R, Bemporad JR. Psychogenic chest pain in children. Clin Pediatr (Phila) 1981;20:788–91.
80. Porter SC, Fein JA, Ginsburg KR. Depression screening in adolescents with somatic complaints presenting to the emergency department. Ann Emerg Med 1997;29:141–5.
81. Gilleland J, Blount RL, Campbell RM, et al. Brief report: psychosocial factors and pediatric noncardiac chest pain. J Pediatr Psychol 2009;34:1170–4.
82. Campo JV. Functional abdominal pain in childhood: lifetime and familial associations with irritable bowel syndrome and psychiatric disorders. Prim Psychiatry 2007;14:54–68.
83. Campo JV, Bridge J, Ehmann M, et al. Recurrent abdominal pain, anxiety, and depression in primary care. Pediatrics 2004;113:817–24.
84. Campo JV, Fritsch SL. Somatization in children and adolescents. J Am Acad Child Adolesc Psychiatry 1994;33:1223–35.
85. Egger HL, Costello EJ, Erkanli A, et al. Somatic complaints and psychopathology in children and adolescents: stomach aches, musculoskeletal pains, and headaches. J Am Acad Child Adolesc Psychiatry 1999;38:852–60.
86. Kislal FM, Kutluk T, Cetin FC, et al. Psychiatric symptoms of adolescents with physical complaints admitted to an adolescence unit. Clin Pediatr 2005;44: 121–30.

87. Tunaoglu FS, Olgunturk R, Akcabay S, et al. Chest pain in children referred to a cardiology clinic. Pediatr Cardiol 1995;16:69–72.

88. Lipsitz JD, Masia C, Apfel H, et al. Noncardiac chest pain and psychopathology in children and adolescents. J Psychosom Res 2005;59:185–8.

89. Liakopoulou-Kairis M, Alifieraki T, Protagora D, et al. Recurrent abdominal pain and headache–psychopathology, life events and family functioning. Eur Child Adolesc Psychiatry 2002;11:115–22.

90. Lipsitz JD, Masia-Warner C, Apfel H, et al. Anxiety and depressive symptoms and anxiety sensitivity in youngsters with noncardiac chest pain and benign heart murmurs. J Pediatr Psychol 2004;29:607–12.

91. Weems CF, Hammond-Laurence K, Silverman WK, et al. Testing the utility of the anxiety sensitivity construct in children and adolescents referred for anxiety disorders. J Clin Child Psychol 1998;27:69–77.

92. Muris P, Hoeve I, Meesters C, et al. Children's perception and interpretation of anxiety-related physical symptoms. J Behav Ther Exp Psychiatry 2004;35:233–44.

93. Hergenrather JR, Rabinowitz M. Age-related differences in the organization of children's knowledge of illness. Dev Psychol 1991;27:952–9.

94. Ollendick TH. Panic disorder in children and adolescents: new developments, new directions. J Clin Child Psychol 1998;27:234–45.

95. Kashani JH, Lababidi Z, Jones RS. Depression in children and adolescents with cardiovascular symptomatology: the significance of chest pain. J Am Acad Child Psychiatry 1982;21:187–9.

96. Rowland TW, Richards MM. The natural history of idiopathic chest pain in children: a follow-up study. Clin Pediatr (Phila) 1986;25:612–4.

97. American Psychiatric Association. Task Force on DSM-IV. Diagnostic and statistical manual of mental disorders. Washington, DC: American Psychiatric Association; 2000. DSM-IV-TR.

98. American Psychiatric Association. Work group to revise DSM-III. Diagnostic and statistical manual of mental disorders. Washington, DC: American Psychiatric Association; 1987. DSM-III-R.

99. White KS. Assessment and treatment of psychological causes of chest pain. Med Clin North Am 2010;94:291–318.

100. Spinhoven P, Van der Does AJ, Van Dijk E, et al. Heart-focused anxiety as a mediating variable in the treatment of noncardiac chest pain by cognitive-behavioral therapy and paroxetine. J Psychosom Res 2010;69(3):227–35.

101. Barrett PM, Dadds MR, Rapee RM. Family treatment of childhood anxiety: a controlled trial. J Consult Clin Psychol 1996;64:333–42.

102. Chambers CT. The role of family factors in pediatric pain. In: McGrath PJ, Finley GA, editors. Pediatric pain: biological and social context. Seattle (WA): IASP Press; 2001. p. 99–130.

103. Reigada LC, Fisher PH, Cutler C, et al. An innovative treatment approach for children with anxiety disorders and medically unexplained somatic complaints. Cogn Behav Pract 2008;15:140–7.

104. Masia-Warner C, Reigada LC, Fisher PH, et al. CBT for anxiety and associated somatic complaints in pediatric medical settings: an open pilot study. J Clin Psychol Med Settings 2009;16:169–77.

105. Mufson LH, Dorta KP, Olfson M, et al. Effectiveness research: transporting interpersonal psychotherapy for depressed adolescents (IPT-A) from the lab to school-based health clinics. Clin Child Fam Psychol Rev 2004;7:251–61.

106. Asarnow JR, Jaycox LH, Tompson MC. Depression in youth: psychosocial interventions. J Clin Child Psychol 2001;30:33–47.

107. Humphreys PA, Gevirtz RN. Treatment of recurrent abdominal pain: components analysis of four treatment protocols. J Pediatr Gastroenterol Nutr 2000;31:47–51.

108. Sowder E, Gevirtz R, Shapiro W, et al. Restoration of vagal tone: a possible mechanism for functional abdominal pain. Appl Psychophysiol Biofeedback 2010;35(3):199–206.

109. Walco GA, Ilowite NT. Cognitive-behavioral intervention for juvenile primary fibromyalgia\ syndrome. J Rheumatol 1992;19:1617–9.

110. Dahlquist LM, Nagel MS. Chronic and recurrent pain. In: Roberts MC, Steele RG, editors. Handbook of pediatric psychology. New York: Guilford Press; 2009. p. 153–70.

Cardiac Ischemia in Pediatric Patients

Masato Takahashi, MD

KEYWORDS

- Congenital heart disease • Kawasaki disease
- Coronary artery anomaly • Coronary artery ostial stenosis

Children and teenagers are frequently brought to primary care physicians with complaints of chest pain. In the minds of the patients, their parents, and their physicians, thoughts of a cardiac event with an unpleasant outcome are often conjured up in such situations. If a child experiences chest pain while he or she is on the school grounds, the teachers and school officials may become alarmed, demanding an immediate medical consultation. There is prevailing fear of sudden death or cardiac disability among lay people as well as medical professionals. This fear of chest pain in a child is triggered by our vivid experience with an adult who suffered acute coronary syndrome or news reports of a high-profile case of sudden cardiac death in a young athlete. Atherosclerotic heart disease as a basis for myocardial ischemia in children is very rare. The great majority of chest pain experienced by children and teenagers are noncardiac in origin. Cardiac ischemia in children is usually not an isolated disease in an otherwise normally formed coronary artery, but is part of more complex congenital or acquired diseases. Myocardial infarction in a child is seldom manifested as classic pressure-like angina pectoris, but may take nonspecific symptoms such as unusual irritability, nausea and vomiting, abdominal pain, shocked state, syncope, seizure, or sudden unexpected cardiac arrest. Some patients may develop silent nonfatal infarction.[1] Although cardiac ischemia is not a frequent occurrence, it must be recognized as a serious, life-threatening event. Pediatricians must be aware of these conditions, and stand ready to take prompt and appropriate actions to avoid irreversible consequences. This article lists and characterizes major causes of cardiac ischemia in children, describes signs and symptoms of each, and provides therapeutic considerations.

DEFINITION AND BACKGROUND

The word ischemia is derived from two Greek roots: *ischō*, to keep back, plus *haima*, blood. Myocardial ischemia implies inadequate perfusion of the myocardium usually as a result of coronary artery obstruction anywhere along the course of the epicardial

Childrens Hospital Los Angeles, University of Southern California Keck School of Medicine, 4650 Sunset Boulevard, Los Angeles, CA 90027, USA
E-mail address: mtakahashi@chla.usc.edu

Pediatr Clin N Am 57 (2010) 1261–1280
doi:10.1016/j.pcl.2010.09.007
0031-3955/10/$ – see front matter © 2010 Elsevier Inc. All rights reserved.

pediatric.theclinics.com

artery from the ostium in the aorta to the minute intramyocardial branches. Obstruction may be due to intrinsic narrowing of the vessel lumen due to thickening of the wall, presence of thrombus within its lumen, extrinsic compression of the vessel from a nearby structure, kinking or stretching of the artery itself, or abnormal vasoreactivity or spasm.

Typically, in a normal subject, there are two coronary arteries arising from the right- and left-facing sinuses of Valsalva. The right coronary artery (RCA) typically courses along the right atrioventricular groove adjacent to the tricuspid valve ring and reaches the posterior crux of the heart. It gives off branches sequentially to the sinus node, right atrium, right ventricle (RV), atrioventricular node, and posteroinferior wall of the left ventricle (LV) in a majority of patients (so-called right dominant pattern). The main trunk of left coronary artery (LCA) tunnels under the main pulmonary artery and, as it resurfaces, bifurcates into the left anterior descending artery (LAD) and the left circumflex artery (LCX). The LAD courses on the anterior surface of the LV along the attachment of the ventricular septum to the free wall, supplying blood to the LV anterior wall and about two-thirds of the ventricular septum. The LCX courses along the left atrioventricular groove just outside the mitral valve ring, and gives off a large branch to the lateral wall of the LV. In a minority of patients the LCX crosses the posterior crux of the heart and extends into the posterior descending artery (so-called left dominant coronary pattern).

Embryologically, primordial coronary vessels are formed by endothelial precursor cells migrating from the liver and form networks of channels along the differentiating epicardium of the heart tube. These primitive vessels penetrate into the myocardium. These ingrowing vessels merge, acquire smooth muscle coats, and transform themselves into arteries.[2] The main right and left arterial channels eventually connect to the aorta. In normal subjects, there are no well-developed connections (collateral arteries) linking the RCAs and LCAs. Intercoronary collaterals may develop rapidly, especially in young children, when one of the major arteries is blocked by disease process.

Coronary arteries provide oxygen and fuel (in the form of glucose and free fatty acid) to actively contracting myocardial cells. Because increased tension within the ventricular walls during systole impedes blood flow, most of the coronary blood flow occurs during diastole. Thus, the aortic diastolic pressure is an important determinant of coronary perfusion. Any pathologic condition that lowers the diastolic pressure, such as aortic insufficiency or presence of an abnormal run-off from the aorta (eg, patent ductus arteriosus or arterovenous fistula) tends to have a negative impact on coronary perfusion.

CLASSIFICATION

Coronary artery diseases which form the basis of myocardial ischemia in children may be classified in terms of cause. Major classes include (1) congenital anomalies of the coronary arteries, (2) coronary artery complications associated with congenital heart disease, (3) coronary artery sequelae of Kawasaki disease, and (4) myocardial ischemia associated with hypertrophic cardiomyopathy (**Box 1**).

CONGENITAL ANOMALIES OF THE CORONARY ARTERIES
Anomalous Origin of the Left Coronary Artery from the Pulmonary Artery (ALCAPA) or Bland-White-Garland Syndrome

This particular anomaly is most likely come to the attention of a primary care physician in an infant between a few weeks to 12 months of age (**Fig. 1**). There are a few patients with this anomaly who remain symptom-free and survive until adulthood. The

---

Box 1
Classification of cardiac ischemia in children

Congenital coronary artery anomalies

    Anomalous origin of LCA from the pulmonary artery (ALCAPA; Bland-White-Garland syndrome)

    Origin of a coronary artery from the wrong aortic sinus with its course between the aorta and the pulmonary artery

Coronary artery complications associated with congenital heart disease

    Coronary artery obstruction after arterial switch operation for D-transposition of the great arteries

    Coronary artery complication after repair of tetralogy of Fallot

    Coronary artery ostial stenosis associated with supravalvar aortic stenosis (Williams syndrome)

    Coronary artery obstruction associated with pulmonary atresia with intact ventricular septum

Coronary artery sequelae of Kawasaki disease

    Thrombotic occlusion of large coronary artery aneurysm

    Coronary artery stenosis at ends of large aneurysm

    Obliterative coronary arteritis without large aneurysm (rare)

Myocardial ischemia associated with hypertrophic cardiomyopathy

Myocardial ischemia associated with cocaine use

---

prevalence of this anomaly is 1 in 300,000 live births. The predominant symptoms in infancy include pallor, sweatiness, rapid breathing, and episodes of extreme fussiness during feedings. Given early detection and prompt referral to a tertiary care facility, this rare congenital anomaly can be surgically corrected and the patient may survive with a good quality of life. Failure to diagnose this problem on a timely manner may result in early death due to congestive heart failure. Although this condition was known to pathologists as far back as the 19th century, its first rather graphic clinical description was published by Bland and colleagues[3] in 1933. The LCA originates from the main pulmonary artery, and follows the usual distribution and branching pattern. During the fetal life and immediate neonatal period, blood flows into the LCA in a normal forward direction owing to relatively high pulmonary artery diastolic pressure. However, after the postnatal drop in pulmonary vascular resistance, the RV can no longer generate high enough pressure to drive blood forward into the myocardium. Thus, myocardial ischemia ensues over the LCA territory. Myocardial ischemia, in turn, stimulates development of collateral arteries bridging between the RCA and the LCA. In a few exceptional patients, intercoronary collaterals develop rapidly and adequately, so that the LV myocardium remains viable. However, in a majority of patients, the LV will suffer severe ischemic damage.

Physical examination may show tachypnea, tachycardia, and pale cool and sweaty skin. One may hear distant heart tones and systolic murmur over the cardiac apex due to mitral regurgitation. The chest radiograph may show cardiomegaly with or without signs of passive pulmonary congestion. The ECG may suggest ischemic change or infarction pattern over the left anterior wall. Echocardiogram may show dilated poorly contracting LV with dyskinetic or akinetic anterolateral wall and ventricular septum. Careful color Doppler flow mapping may reveal flow in the LCA directed toward the

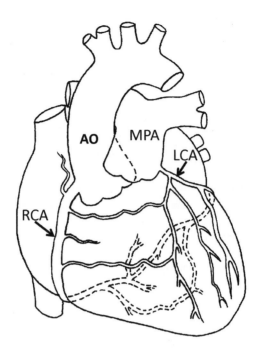

Fig. 1. Schematic diagram representing ALCAPA. ALCAPA, anomalous origin of the left coronary artery from the pulmonary artery; AO, ascending aorta; LCA, left coronary artery; MPA, main pulmonary artery; RCA, right coronary artery.

main pulmonary artery. Cineangiography with dye injection into the ascending aorta will demonstrate opacification of a dilated RCA, which will give off collateral arteries at various points along its route to the LCA (**Fig. 2**). The direction of the flow in the LCA is retrograde and drains into the main pulmonary artery.

Differential diagnosis of ALCAPA includes acute myocarditis, cardiomyopathy, and severe forms of left heart obstruction such as congenital aortic stenosis or coarctation of the aorta.

Management
History of episodic respiratory distress with effort such as feeding, physical findings of pallor, wheezing, tachycardia, and ECG findings of ischemic changes and chest radiograph evidence of cardiomegaly with passive congestion raise an index of suspicion for this diagnosis. Definitive diagnosis relies on imaging studies such as echocardiography or cineangiography. A 2D-echocardiographic image of the LCA alone may be misleading, because there may be false continuity between the aorta and LCA. However, with color Doppler interrogation with Nyquist limit set to a low velocity, flow signal may detect retrograde direction of LCA flow with continuity to the main pulmonary artery, which is characteristic of this lesion. The life-threatening nature of this anomaly demands judicious medical stabilization and rapid transportation to a tertiary pediatric facility, so that surgery is performed. Currently, the preferred surgical approach is removal of the ALCAPA and reimplantation into the aorta. Because of ischemic myocardial injury, the postoperative course may be quite stormy due to hypotension and frequent arrhythmia. In some patients, extracorporeal membrane oxygenator support may be necessary until LV function recovers sufficiently. After a two coronary artery system is established and

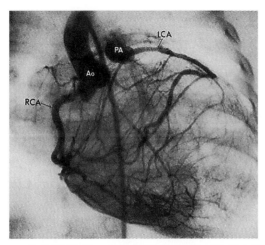

Fig. 2. Cineangiogram of ALCAPA. The catheter tip is in the AO. The RCA is dilated. There are numerous collateral vessels between RCA and LCA. LCA opacifies retrograde and empties into the main pulmonary artery (PA). ALCAPA from the main pulmonary artery is redundant.

the patient survives the postoperative period, his or her myocardial function may improve steadily.[4] However, depending on the size of infarcted fibrotic segment and surrounding peri-infarct ischemic area in the myocardium, the patient must be carefully monitored for recurrent ventricular arrhythmia. A patient with a large devitalized myocardial segment forming an aneurysm is particularly vulnerable to sudden onset of ventricular tachycardia or fibrillation months or years later. These patients may require Holter monitoring and, if indicated, an implantable defibrillator.

Origin of a Coronary Artery from the Wrong Aortic Sinus with its Course Between the Aorta and the Pulmonary Artery

Unfortunately, these cardiac anomalies seldom give warnings before a catastrophic event, frequently on an athletic field. They are often diagnosed postmortem after sudden unexpected cardiac death in athletes, and are the second most frequent cause of such death behind hypertrophic cardiomyopathy.[5] Of the two types of anomalies depicted in **Fig. 3**, the origin of the LCA from the right aortic sinus is more frequently lethal. The prevalence of sudden athletic field deaths due to all causes is estimated to be 0.5 per 100,000 per year among high school age athletes in the United States.

Postmortem examinations have shown an acute angle take-off of the anomalous coronary artery with a slit-like ostium located in the inappropriate aortic sinus. The proximal course of the anomalous artery lies between the aorta and pulmonary artery. It may be intramural (within the muscular layer of the aortic wall itself) or free in the space between the great arteries. Typically no atheromatous plaques have been found. Such an anomalous coronary artery may be able to provide adequate myocardial perfusion at rest such that the patients are asymptomatic. However, during strenuous activities, because of the narrow slit-like orifice, the intramural or interarterial course of the vessel, the aberrant coronary artery may be incapable of providing coronary blood flow commensurate with the subject's demand for increased myocardial perfusion, thus producing sudden ischemia, which in turn may lead to onset of ventricular fibrillation or cardiac standstill. Systolic engorgement of the aorta and the pulmonary artery due to increased stroke volume may further compromise the coronary artery caliber.

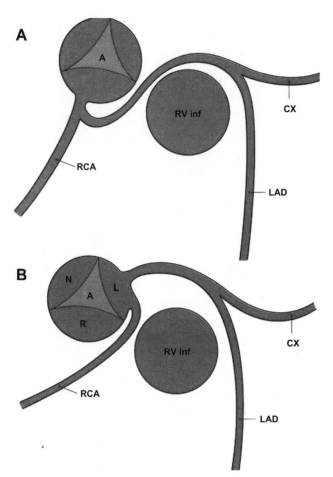

Fig. 3. Two types of aberrant coronary artery from "wrong sinuses." Each shows the aortic valve with its 3 sinuses, right ventricular infundibulum, and two coronary arteries. Top of the diagram is posterior, bottom is anterior, left of the diagram is right side, right of the diagram left side. (*A*) Origin of the LCA from the right sinus of Valsalva, coursing between the aorta and the pulmonary artery. Although in this diagram, the two coronary arteries share a common ostium, actual cases vary in anatomy. Sometimes the LCA ostium is slit-like. The initial segment of LCA may be intramural (embedded within the aortic wall). (*B*) Origin of the RCA from the left sinus, coursing between the two great arteries. L, left coronary sinus; N, noncoronary sinus; R, right coronary sinus; RV inf, right ventricular infundibulum. (*From* Lieberthson R. Congenital anomalies of the coronary arteries. In: Gatzoulis MA, Webb GD, Daubeney PEF, editors. Diagnosis and management of adult congenital heart disease. Philadelphia: Churchill Livingstone; 2003. p. 425–31; with permission.)

Management

These anomalies are rarely suspected or diagnosed in life. ECG or stress tests may not yield abnormal results. Some of the athletes have noted syncope or chest pain in the preceding 24 months of the final catastrophic event. If healthy young patients complain of such symptoms, they should be explored carefully, including imaging studies for coronary arteries first with transthoracic echocardiography specifically focused on coronary artery origins. If the patient's body habitus does not allow clear visualization of his or her coronary arteries, multidetector CT scan will demonstrate clear images albeit at the cost of added expense and radiation exposure. Also, it is highly recommended that when an echocardiogram is ordered for a young patient for any other clinical indications, the interpreting cardiologist and the sonographer verify origins and distributions of the RCAs and LCAs. This is not yet a uniformly established standard for sonographers, but every now and then an aberrant coronary artery is incidentally discovered.

Surgical "unroofing" of the intramural coronary artery segment to move coronary orifice to a more normal position and at the same time widen the orifice area has been done successfully.[6]

CORONARY ARTERY COMPLICATIONS ASSOCIATED WITH CONGENITAL HEART DISEASE
Coronary Artery Obstruction After Arterial Switch Operation for D-Transposition of the Great Arteries

Complete transposition (or D-transposition) of the great arteries (DTGA) is one of the more common cyanotic heart disease with prevalence of 20 to 30 per 100,000 live births. Without prompt treatment, about 90% of these babies will die within the first year of life. This anomaly may exist alone or in association with a ventricular septal defect, coarctation of the aorta, or other cardiac anomalies. Because of low oxygen saturation noted by bedside pulse oximetry, the patient should receive echocardiography or be referred to a cardiologist within a few days after birth. Once diagnosed, a baby with DTGA can be stabilized using prostaglandin infusion and transported to a tertiary facility. There, the patient undergoes either balloon atrial septostomy (Rashkind procedure) or is brought directly to the operating room for an arterial switch procedure.

As part of this operation the surgeons truncate both great arteries near their origins from the ventricles, and move the RCAs and LCAs from the original aorta to the new aorta (native main pulmonary artery root). There are at least nine anatomic variations in the way the two coronary arteries arise from the native aorta.[7] Since the inception of arterial switch operations in the mid-1980s, congenital heart surgeons have improved the technique of transposing coronary arteries. In cases of "usual" coronary artery pattern (RCA from the posterior right-facing aortic cusp and LCA from the posterior left-facing cusp) the surgeon will remove the RCAs and LCAs from the old aortic root together with a small piece of surrounding aortic wall (so-called button), and move them to the new aortic root. In patients with more complex or unusual coronary pattern the surgeon must use innovative techniques of switching the coronary arteries. In those patients with unusual coronary artery distribution, there appears to be a higher risk of postoperative ischemia due to kinking or stretching of the arteries. Most of the survivors of the arterial switch operation are asymptomatic. Nevertheless, some patients, especially those with originally unusual coronary artery distribution, have had less-than-normal coronary flow reserve.[8,9] The clinical significance of these findings is not fully understood.

Management
It is important to encourage survivors of the arterial switch operation to seek periodic cardiac evaluation on a life-long basis. Also, the primary care physician should emphasize heart healthy life-style and dietary habits in these children so as to minimize accumulation of coronary risk factors as they grow into adolescence and adulthood. Those who have demonstrated coronary obstruction require more frequent and intensive follow-up evaluations.

Coronary Artery Damage Associated with Repair of Tetralogy of Fallot

Tetralogy of Fallot (TOF) is the most frequently encountered cyanotic heart disease. Its prevalence is estimated to be 26 to 48 per 100,000 live births. Timing of corrective surgery is dictated by several anatomic features. In the presence of pulmonary atresia, marked hypoplasia of the pulmonary arteries or presence of large collateral arteries from the aorta to the pulmonary arteries, the patient may have to undergo one or more palliative operations before corrective surgery is done.

Corrective surgery for TOF includes patch-closure of the ventricular septal defect and widening of the right ventricular outflow tract by infundibular muscle resection combined with either a patch placement across the pulmonary valve annulus (so-called transannular patch) or use of a prosthetic conduit from the RV to the pulmonary artery. There are known aberrant coronary artery patterns associated with TOF. Origin of the anterior descending branch from RCA has been reported to occur in 5% of TOF patients.[10] A large conus branch, or an accessory LAD present in about 15% of TOF patients, runs across the face of the right ventricular outflow tract (infundibulum) and may be inadvertently damaged during the surgery. If such an arterial branch subtends a large myocardial territory, the patient may suffer from clinically significant myocardial infarction and myocardial conduction delay, both of which may reduce the overall cardiac function in the future. In general, postoperative TOF patients are more likely to develop global RV or LV dysfunction, right heart enlargement, right bundle branch block, and sustained or intermittent arrhythmia than to develop localized myocardial ischemia or myocardial infarction.[11]

Management

Patients with postoperative tetralogy must be followed, by a cardiologist experienced in congenital heart disease, at regular intervals on a life-long basis for surveillance of the right ventricular size and function, volume overloading due to pulmonary regurgitation, and propensity for cardiac arrhythmia. In addition they should be given the same advice as the aforementioned DTGA patients; that is, the need for heart healthy life-style.

Coronary Artery Ostial Stenosis Associated with Supravalvar Aortic Stenosis (Isolated or in Association with Williams Syndrome)

Supravalvar aortic stenosis (SVAS) is caused by localized or diffuse narrowing of the ascending aorta starting at the junction between the sinuses of Valsalva and the tubular portion of the ascending aorta (**Fig. 4**). It may occur alone or in association with pulmonary artery stenosis. It is often a cardiac phenotype of Williams syndrome. The genotype of Williams syndrome is deletion of 7q11.23, the segment that includes elastin gene.[12] Prevalence of Williams syndrome is estimated to be 1 in 20,000 live births, and is characterized by SVAS, peripheral pulmonary artery stenosis, developmental delay, and social and friendly personality traits. There are at least four factors in this condition which contribute to myocardial ischemia. First, deficiency of elastin in the aortic wall causes loss of Windkessel effect, whereby part of the energy carried by the ejecting blood is stored during systole and released back during diastole. Without it there is wider pulse pressure and low diastolic pressure, impairing coronary perfusion. Second, deficiency of elastin also causes proliferation of smooth muscle cells in the arterial walls, causing medial thickening of the aorta and its branches, including coronary arteries. This has an effect of increasing impedance to forward aortic flow. Third, development of obstructive supravalvar ridge further increases LV afterload and stimulates LV myocardial hypertrophy. Pulmonary artery obstruction, likewise, causes RV hypertrophy. Biventricular hypertrophy tends to increase oxygen demand. Fourth, abnormally shallow sinuses of Valsalva with prominent ridge restrict

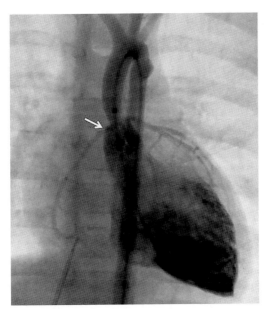

Fig. 4. Cineangiogram of supravalvar aortic stenosis. Contrast injection was made with the catheter tip in the LV. Note abrupt narrowing of the junction between and sinuses of Valsalva and the tubular portion of the ascending aorta. The two coronary arteries arise at the junction. Commissures between the aortic valve leaflets are located near or at the sinotubular junction. Valve motion may interfere with coronary inflow. In some cases, anatomic stenosis of one or both coronary ostia occurs. The white arrow indicates right coronary ostium.

excursion of the aortic leaflets. The valve leaflets are thus unable to fully open into positions paralleling the blood flow axis, and may obstruct the coronary ostia. Duration of diastole may be shortened owing to prolonged systolic ejection time, reducing myocardial perfusion. Exposure of the coronary arteries to high pressure proximal to the aortic stenosis may contribute to progressive coronary artery pathology. Ostia of the coronary arteries, especially the left coronary ostium frequently becomes stenotic. There have been reports of sudden death of patients, presumably due to sudden myocardial ischemia. Risk of sudden death in this condition is estimated to be 1/1000 patient years as compared with 0.01–0.04/1000 patient years in general population. This risk does not appear to correlate with the severity of aortic obstruction but appears to be related to bilateral ventricular hypertrophy and coronary artery stenosis.[13] Furthermore, sudden death in Williams syndrome and, to a lesser extent, in isolated SVAS have occurred during cardiac catheterization or noncardiac operation under sedation or general anesthesia.[13] Based on analysis of 19 cases of sudden cardiac deaths in Williams syndrome, Bird and colleagues[14] concluded that presence of biventricular outflow tract obstruction combined with coronary artery abnormalities carried the highest risk of sudden death.

Management
In this condition, potential for myocardial ischemia exists without overt hemodynamic abnormalities. Thus, the patient may not show any alarming symptoms. ECG or echocardiographic findings may be insensitive for prediction of sudden ischemic event. Thus, completely elective surgery needs to be weighed against this possibility.

Traditionally, surgical correction in the form of patch aortoplasty, more recently symmetric patch technique of Brom, is considered, when the pressure gradient from the LV to the ascending aorta exceeds 40 to 50 mmHg. Whereas adequate imaging of the coronary arteries is desirable either by cardiac catheterization and or less invasive multidetector CT scan or MRI, these tests in themselves carry greater than usual risks. Repair of coronary oxtail stenosis is challenging but it has been done successfully.[15]

Coronary Artery Obstruction Associated with Pulmonary Atresia with Intact Ventricular Septum

Hypoplastic right heart syndrome is characterized by an abnormally small RV, which is unable to support normal pulmonary blood flow on its own accord (**Fig. 5**). Tricuspid atresia and pulmonary atresia are two major variants of this syndrome. A subset of pulmonary atresia with intact ventricular septum with a patent but small tricuspid valve may produce a network of vascular channels (called sinusoids) communicating the right ventricular lumen to one or both of the pericardial coronary arteries. With systemic or suprasystemic systolic pressure within the right ventricular cavity, blood flow in these fistulous connections may compete with the normal coronary blood flow originating in the ascending aorta. Sometimes, these competing blood coronary streams may cause tortuosity, severe intimal proliferation with obstruction, such that portions of the myocardium may be dependent on the RV-originated coronary flow (so-called RV-dependent coronary circulation).[16]

Patients with pulmonary atresia and intact ventricular septum usually undergo an initial surgical palliation in the form of modified Blalock-Taussig shunt with or without pulmonary valvotomy. This latter procedure is to allow resumption of some RV pumping function. In some centers, pulmonary valvotomy may be done as a transcatheter intervention.

Those patients who do not have any functioning RV, in effect, have single ventricle physiology, and are consigned to eventual Fontan procedure, whereby both superior and inferior vena cava (SVC, IVC) are anastomosed to the pulmonary artery. On the other hand, those with a relatively mild degree of RV hypoplasia and amenable to

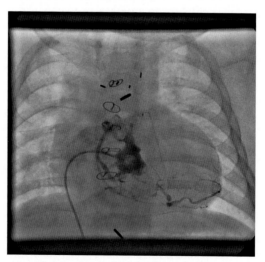

Fig. 5. Cineangiogram with injection inside the hypoplastic RV with pulmonary atresia. Sinusoids connecting RV to both coronary arteries are clearly seen.

pulmonary valvotomy may receive only Glenn anastomosis between the SVC and right pulmonary artery, so that only the blood return from IVC is pumped by the small RV into the pulmonary artery (so-called one-and-a-half ventricle repair). Pulmonary valvotomy may produce sudden decompression of the RV pressure. If such a patient has an unsuspected RV-dependent coronary circulation with no adequate aorta-originated blood supply to a portion of the myocardium, that patient may suffer from myocardial ischemia and heart failure as a result. In some cases, thrombosis within the abnormal coronary artery has caused myocardial infarction. Coronary artery stenosis associated with pulmonary atresia may be progressive over time, so that the patients with demonstrated sinusoidal connection between RV and epicardial coronary arteries should have follow-up imaging studies. In some cases, heart transplantation may be the only viable therapy.

Management

The subset of patients with hypoplastic right heart syndrome with known coronary artery stenosis or complete occlusion need to be followed closely for any progressive myocardial ischemia, and the patients and families must be made aware of the increased risk of cardiac events in the future. However, most patients with pulmonary atresia with intact septum, who undergo a Fontan operation have good short- and intermediate-term survival.

Coronary Artery Sequelae of Kawasaki Disease

Kawasaki disease (KD) is an immune-mediated vasculitis affecting medium-sized arteries, most prominently coronary arteries. Epidemiologic findings suggest that KD is triggered by one or more widely distributed infectious agents in a genetically predisposed child.[17] It attacks mostly children under 5 years of age, more in males than females with a ratio of 1.5 to 1. The highest prevalence is found among children of East Asian backgrounds (Japanese, Korean, and Chinese), the lowest among white children, and intermediate among African American children. The disease occurs most frequently in the winter and spring in temperate zone countries.[18,19]

Despite extensive searches for a specific causal agent by many investigators in the 33 years since the original description of the disease,[20] no cause has been established. Currently prevailing theory is that there is genetic propensity in a segment of population to develop vasculitic cascade through expression of proinflammatory proteins and promoters, triggered by one or more ubiquitous infectious agents either viral or bacterial in nature. A consortium of researchers are involved in genome-wide search for a set of mutations coding for these host factors.[17,21]

Diagnosis is made by fulfillment of principal clinical criteria. Diagnosis of KD requires the presence of fever lasting 5 or more days, and at least four of the five following physical findings, without another explanation:

Conjunctival injection, usually without discharge
Oral mucous membrane changes, such as red, cracked, dry lips or strawberry tongue
Peripheral extremity changes, including erythema of palms or soles, edema of hands or feet
Rash (nonvesicular)
Cervical lymphadenopathy (at least one lymph node >1.5 cm in diameter).

About 15% of the patients do not fulfill four of the five requisite criteria, and are classified as atypical or incomplete Kawasaki disease. Recent management guidelines copublished by the American Heart Association and the American Academy of Pediatrics,[22] show a diagnostic algorithm using acute phase reactants (elevated C-reactive protein and erythrocyte sedimentation rate) and supplementary laboratory tests serum albumin less than 3 g/dL, anemia for age, elevated alanine aminotransferase, and platelet count after 7 days greater than 450,000/mm³ to assist clinicians to arrive at a working diagnosis of KD within 7 to 10 days of fever onset. This should allow that intravenous immunoglobulin and aspirin therapies may be instituted in time to prevent coronary artery sequelae. This diagnostic strategy appeared to be useful in identifying 97% of the patients within the time window for intravenous immunoglobulin (IVIG) treatment according to a retrospective chart review of nearly 200 patients with typical and incomplete KD patients from four centers.[23]

Before the widespread use of IVIG therapy, about 20% of the KD patients developed coronary artery aneurysms. With timely (within 10 days of fever onset) IVIG treatment, the prevalence of aneurysms has been reduced to about 5% and, most importantly, giant aneurysms (>8 mm in diameter) prevalence has been reduced to less than 1%. Approximately 50% of the aneurysms, particularly small-to-medium sized aneurysms (3–6 mm in diameter) undergo a process of regression such that the coronary artery lumen becomes normal.[24] However, this regression seems to be the result of migration of smooth muscle cells from outer layers into the intimae and subsequent proliferation forming a thick neointima. Thus, these regressed arteries possess abnormal wall thickness and reduced response to various vasodilators.

Myocardial ischemia occurs in patients with KD owing to occlusion or critical narrowing of one or more coronary arteries through three different mechanisms.

Thrombotic Occlusion of Coronary Artery Aneurysm

The earliest stage of KD is characterized by microangiitis of many organs, including the skin and mucous membranes. Ten to 12 days into the illness, panvasculitis of major coronary arteries begins. In some patients, the coronary arterial walls, weakened by inflammation, yields to expansile force of the arterial pressure, and becomes an aneurysm. A combination of resultant flow stagnation, activated procoagulant endothelium, and increased number and activity of platelets collaborate to produce thrombotic occlusion, leading to myocardial infarction (**Fig. 6**). Patients with aneurysm diameter greater than 8 mm (giant aneurysm) are more likely to develop thrombotic occlusion starting in the acute of illness.[25] Myocardial infarction is most likely to occur within the first year after onset of KD.[1,25]

Management

Patients with large coronary artery aneurysms can be protected from thrombosis with anticoagulant therapy using warfarin (with a target international normalized ratio of 2.0–2.5) and aspirin 3 to 5 mg/kg per day.

Some patients develop thrombosis within the coronary artery lumen despite anticoagulation. Recognized in time, such a patient may be rescued with thrombolytic therapy using tissue plasminogen activator or another agent, followed by heparin infusion. With early detection of coronary artery aneurysms and timely treatment with IVIG, there has been a dramatic decrease in the number of giant aneurysms and acute myocardial infarction during the acute illness. Once the occluding thrombus becomes organized, and there are no adequate collateral vessels to ameliorate ischemia, coronary artery bypass graft may be the only solution. Attempts to surgically remove or trim down the giant aneurysm have met with mixed results thus far.

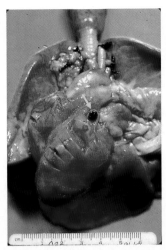

Fig. 6. Autopsied heart of a 3-month-old girl who died of myocardial infarction 3 weeks after the onset of Kawasaki disease. Both coronary arteries had formed giant aneurysms (*arrow* shows aneurysmal left coronary artery filled with clot). The LCA aneurysm was completely occluded with old and fresh clots.

Coronary Artery Stenosis Due to Neointimal Proliferation

During the subacute phase of the disease, there is neointimal thickening as a result of migration of smooth muscle cells and fibroblasts from media to intima of the vessel wall. Fifty percent or more of the original coronary artery aneurysms undergo complete regression or normalization of the lumen size, although both the wall structure and vasoreactivity of the coronary artery segment remains abnormal. Similar process may occur locally at the entrance or exit point of the aneurysm, causing localized stenosis. When the stenosis becomes severe, this may cause myocardial ischemia. Again, depending on whether there are enough collateral channels to compensate for the ischemia, some type of revascularization procedure should be considered.

Management

Bypass graft surgery using arterial grafts have been successful. Kitamura and colleagues[26] reported a graft patency rate of 95% over 20 years in a cohort of 114 children and adolescents. However, the cardiac event-free rate has declined over time. Percutaneous balloon angioplasty alone is unlikely to succeed in the presence of dense scar tissue and calcification. Rotational ablation with or without stent placement has been used with short-term success in Japan.[27] However, there were cases of restenosis or formation of new aneurysms at the site of intervention, often requiring repeat intervention or surgical revascularization (**Fig. 7**).

Obliterative Coronary Arteritis Without Large Aneurysm

This is a rare complication of KD with only a few reported cases.[28–30] Typically, the patient is known to develop diffuse mild-to-moderate coronary artery dilation. In time, the coronary arteries appear to undergo regression, then acute chest pain, respiratory distress or abdominal pain occurs, and the patient dies unexpectedly. Postmortem examination would show almost complete obliteration of the coronary artery lumen due to excessive proliferation of neointimal cells surrounded by copious intracellular matrix (**Fig. 8**).

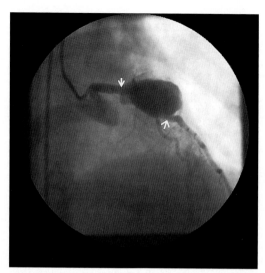

Fig. 7. Cineangiogram showing a giant aneurysm of the LAD of 2-year-6-month-old boy 5 months after the onset of Kawasaki disease. The two arrows indicate entrance and exit points of the saccular aneurysm, where localized stenosis may occur due to intimal proliferation.

Management

Because this process occurs diffusely over long segments of arteries, currently there is no effective therapy. In cases, where the obliterative process is confined to a short segment, surgical treatment may be improvised on a case-by-case basis.

Myocardial Ischemia Associated with Hypertrophic Cardiomyopathy

Hypertrophic cardiomyopathy (HCM) is a genetically determined myocardial hypertrophy far exceeding the degree of LV hypertrophy necessary to sustain the usual amount of work load (**Fig. 9**). Its incidence is estimated to be as high as 0.2% of population in all ages.[31] However, it is relatively rare in the pediatric population. Typically the onset is gradual and full clinical manifestation may not occur until the teenage years and young adulthood. There is global hypertrophy of ventricular walls, but hypertrophy is often quite remarkable in the ventricular septum.

In a subset of patients, there is dynamic obstruction of the left ventricular outflow tract due to the combination of asymmetric septal hypertrophy (ASH) and abnormal systolic anterior motion (SAM) of the mitral anterior leaflet. These morphologic changes can be easily diagnosed by routine echocardiography. ECG almost always shows abnormal left ventricular hypertrophy accompanied by ST segment and T wave changes, indicative of global ischemia. Microscopically, there is extensive disarray of myocardial muscle fibers. As the disease advances, there will be increasing fibrosis within the myocardium probably related to a relative paucity of intramyocardial nutrient arteries. Occasionally, there is an associated myocardial bridge, in which a segment of an epicardial major coronary artery, most typically the LAD, tunnels through the myocardium for a short distance. During systole, myocardial contraction may "pinch off" that section of the coronary artery lumen, and may cause decreased flow. The role of myocardial bridge in causation of myocardial ischemia is being debated.[32,33] Intramyocardial fibrosis may be delineated by MRI using late gadolinium enhancement imaging technique relatively early in the course of HCM.[34] This

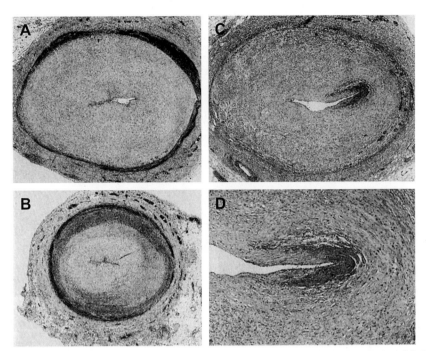

Fig. 8. Photomicrograms of epicardial coronary arteries of a 4-year-old boy with a febrile illness with conjunctivitis, pharyngitis, rash, and lymphadenopathy 7 months before death, followed by multiple episodes of abdominal pain requiring repeated hospital admissions. There is diffuse severe fibrointimal proliferation with marked luminal narrowing of (A) the left main, (B) LCX, and (C) RCA. (D) The right coronary artery demonstrated a small thrombus (high magnification). Multiple areas of medial destruction as well as infiltrating numerous CD4+ and CD8 + T lymphocytes and rare B cells. (From Burke AP, Virmani R, Perry LW, et al. Fatal Kawasaki disease with coronary arteritis and no coronary aneurysms. Pediatrics 1998;101:109; with permission.)

technique makes use of the phenomenon in which intravenously injected gadolinium chelate lingers in fibrous tissue long after its level in the surrounding metabolically active tissue has declined. Its application began in patients with myocardial infarction due to coronary artery disease.

Patients with severe HCM may be asymptomatic or may show a variety of symptoms, including easy fatigue, chest pain (ranging from sharp transient atypical pain to typical angina pectoris), palpitations, and syncope. This diagnosis should always be considered when a young athlete or teenager complains of chest pain with exertion. Sudden cardiac death due to HCM is estimated to be 2% to 4% per year. It is the leading cause of sudden cardiac death in young athletes. The cause of death is attributed to onset of ventricular fibrillation due to localized myocardial ischemia.

In a subset of patients, there is dynamic obstruction of the left ventricular outflow tract due to a combination of ASH and abnormal SAM. These morphologic changes can be easily diagnosed by routine echocardiography.

Management
A β-adrenergic blocking agent is the mainstay of therapy for HCM. Its effects include reducing myocardial oxygen consumption and ameliorating hyperdynamic myocardial contraction, thus reducing the outflow tract pressure gradient. Those patients with

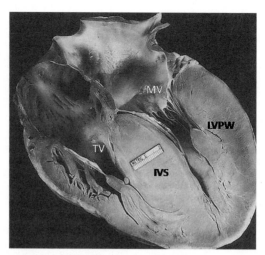

Fig. 9. Autopsy photo of an adult with hypertrophic cardiomyopathy. The heart has been sectioned to show atrial and ventricular septa, mitral (MV) and tricuspid valves (TV). Note marked hypertrophy of the interventricular septum (IVS) and the LV posterior wall (LVPW), and moderate hypertrophy of the RV. (*From* Sorajja P, Nishimura RA. Hypertrophic cardiomyopathy. In: Gatzoulis MA, Webb GD, Webb, et al, editors. Diagnosis and management of adult congenital heart disease. Philadelphia: Churchill Livingstone; 2003. p. 425–31; with permission.)

dynamic LV outflow obstruction may benefit from surgical myotomy and myectomy. Those patients considered to be at high risk of sudden death may received implantable cardiac defibrillators.

Acute Coronary Syndrome Associated with Cocaine Use

Abuse of illicit drugs has become a major problem that pediatricians cannot avoid in their teenage patients. Although many street drugs and prescription drugs taken by patients without medical supervision may cause cardiovascular-related problems, cocaine stands out as the drug most likely to cause direct myocardial ischemia and death. An estimated 8 million individuals use it on a regular basis in the United States. As many as 25% of patients that present to urban hospitals with nontraumatic chest pain have detectable cocaine or its metabolites in their urine. Cardiovascular effects of cocaine may be due to inhibition of presynaptic uptake of adrenergic neurotransmitters, resulting in tachycardia, hypertension, and coronary artery spasm. Chronic use of cocaine is associated with accelerated atherosclerosis, endothelial dysfunction, and increased inflammatory markers, which may lead to acute coronary syndrome.[35,36] Cocaine toxicity may precipitate seizures, and respiratory and circulatory depression. Cocaine is also highly pyrogenic because of increased muscular activity. Heat loss is inhibited by the intense vasoconstriction. Cocaine-induced hyperthermia may cause muscle cell destruction and myoglobinuria resulting in renal failure.

Acute coronary syndrome is associated with chest pain (typical or atypical), ST-segment elevation of ischemic type on presentation, and elevation of troponin or creatinine kinase MB fraction within 24 hours of presentation.

Management
Patients presenting with chest pain should receive careful history-taking (including crucial social history) and physical examination. Patients with chest pain related to

cocaine often present with agitation, anxiety, tachycardia, and hypertension. Toxicologic screening must be done if drug abuse is suspected. The patient should be observed in the ICU or cardiac care unit. Treatment should include benzodiazepine, aspirin, supplementary oxygen, and an ACE-inhibitor. In addition, a calcium channel blocker such as diltiazem is useful to counteract or prevent coronary vasospasm. There is controversy regarding the use of a β-adrenergic blocker in this setting, because of fear that possible overactive α-adrenergic effect of cocaine may cause hypertension and coronary vasospasm. Hoskins and colleagues[37] have reported that labetalol, a balanced α and β blocker has shown favorable outcomes in terms of improvements in hemodynamics as well as inflammatory markers.

GENERAL STRATEGY FOR MANAGEMENT OF CARDIAC CRISIS WITH POSSIBLE MYOCARDIAL ISCHEMIA

Although myocardial ischemia is not an everyday pediatric problem, it may presents itself unexpectedly and, therefore, it causes an inordinate amount of confusion and anxiety for those called upon to manage it. First, early recognition of the problem is important.

Infants with severe myocardial ischemia such as those with ALCAPA may, in its early stage, show episodic pain and distress but gradually change into persistent symptoms of heart failure with progressive respiratory distress, tachycardia, and failure to thrive. A heart murmur is either absent or only faintly audible. Heart tones are often distant, reflecting weakened myocardial contractility. Grunting and retractions may be present. When a cardiac problem is suspected, the primary care physician must obtain basic studies, including chest radiograph and ECG. If these tests show abnormal findings, the patient must be referred promptly to a pediatric cardiologist. Initial echocardiogram should focus on evaluation of cardiac chamber size and function as well as presence or absence of pericardial effusion. More detailed echocardiographic examination can be undertaken by the cardiologist, looking for specific diagnosis.

Upon witnessing a patient with cardiorespiratory distress, the physician must first establish adequate airway and support ventilation. Then, proceed to evaluate the presence and quality of peripheral pulses, to determine whether full-scale cardiopulmonary resuscitation is needed. After having ruled out more common problems such as heat exhaustion, asthmatic attacks or panic attacks, the physician must entertain the possibility of a cardiac event. Inappropriate tachycardia, hypotension, and anxiety may be a tip-off. Chest pain may or may not be present. In young children, myocardial ischemia may cause nausea, vomiting, and abdominal pain.

If an older child is brought in with a cardiorespiratory crisis, airway, breathing, and cardiac function must be immediately assessed, and supportive or resuscitative measures must be taken. After a team of care-givers has been organized, the clinician must obtain a careful history exploring suspected heart disease, past cardiac surgery, or possible prolonged febrile illness accompanied by skin rash, conjunctivitis, and oral mucous membrane lesions (possible missed Kawasaki disease).

The physician must explore possible recent syncope or seizure (especially any without warning). After establishing some rapport with the patient, the physician must also ask, as delicately as possible, about substance use, for the purpose of eliciting specific drugs involved.

The physician must also explore the possible family history of syncope, seizures, or sudden cardiac deaths especially among the first-degree relatives. In examining the patient, begin by looking for obvious dimorphisms, such as Williams syndrome.

The patient's distress must be alleviated with supplemental oxygen and analgesics, as needed. Basic 12-lead ECG, chest radiograph, and echocardiogram may further elucidate the problem. Venipuncture to start a peripheral intravenous line should be combined with obtaining creatinine phosphokinase subfractions and troponin levels, as well as other routine laboratory tests. These biomarker levels and ECG must be repeated periodically to establish a time course of myocardial damage.

If cocaine or other recreational drug use is suspected, toxicologic screening tests should be obtained.

Judicious incremental fluid management is important to remedy hypovolemia and, at the same time, prevent overloading the weakened heart.

When cardiac ischemia is strongly suspected, a pediatric cardiologist must be consulted. A speedy transfer to a tertiary care center must be arranged. The primary task of the pediatric cardiologist is to arrive at an accurate anatomic and physiologic diagnosis as to the cause of ischemia and plan a definitive therapeutic course to remove its source. In many cases surgical therapy is clearly indicated. In other situations, medical management can be adopted while surgical options are being weighed.

REFERENCES

1. Kato H, Ichinose E, Kawasaki T. Myocardial infarction in Kawasaki disease: clinical analysis in 195 cases. J Pediatr 1986;107:59–63.
2. Mikawa T, Fischman DA. Retroviral analysis of cardiac morphogenesis: discontinuous formation of coronary vessels. Proc Natl Acad Sci U S A 1992;89:9504–8.
3. Bland EF, White PD, Garland J. Congenital anomalies of the coronary arteries: report of an unusual case associated with cardiac hypertrophy. Am Heart J 1933;8:787–801.
4. Ojala T, Salminen J, Happonen JM, et al. Excellent functional result in children after correction of anomalous origin of left coronary artery from the pulmonary artery—a population-based complete follow-up study. Interact Cardiovasc Thorac Surg 2010;10(1):70–5.
5. Maron BJ, Gohman TE, Aeppli D. Prevalence of sudden cardiac death during competitive sports activity in Minnesota high school athletes. J Am Coll Cardiol 1998;32:1881–4.
6. Romp RL, Herlong JR, Landolfo CK, et al. Outcome of unroofing procedure for repair of anomalous aortic origin of left or right coronary artery. Ann Thorac Surg 2003;76:589–95.
7. Wernovsky G, Sanders SP. Coronary artery anatomy and transposition of the great arteries. Coron Artery Dis 1993;4:148–57.
8. Turner DR, Muzik O, Forbes TJ, et al. Coronary diameter and vasodilator function in children following arterial switch operation for complete transposition of the great arteries. Am J Cardiol 2010;106(3):421–5.
9. Angeli E, Formigari R, Napoleone CP, et al. Long-term coronary artery outcome after arterial switch operation for transposition of the great arteries. Eur J Cardiothorac Surg 2010. [Epub ahead of print].
10. Need LR, Powell AJ, del Nido P, et al. Coronary echocardiography in tetralogy of Fallot: diagnostic accuracy, resource utilization and surgical implications over 13 years. J Am Coll Cardiol 2000;36:1371–7.
11. Khairy P, Aboulhosn J, Gurvitz MZ, et al. Alliance for Adult Research in Congenital Cardiology (AARCC). Arrhythmia burden in adults with surgically repaired tetralogy of Fallot. A multi-institutional study. Circulation 2010;122(9):868–75.
12. Rodriguez-Revenga L, Badenas C, Carrio A, et al. Elastin mutation screening in a group of patients affected by vascular abnormalities. Pediatr Cardiol 2005;26: 827–31.

13. Burch TM, McGowan FX, Kussman BD, et al. Congenital supravalvar aortic sten-osi and sudden death associated with anesthesia: what's the mystery? Anesth Analg 2008;107:1848–54.
14. Bird LM, Billman GF, Lacro RV, et al. Sudden death in Williams syndrome: report of ten cases. J Pediatr 1996;129:926–31.
15. Inan BK, Ucak A, Gullu AU, et al. Left main coronary artery and supravalvar aortic stenosis in adult: treatment with ostial patchplasty and modified Brom procedure. J Card Surg 2009;24:299–300.
16. Dauberry PE, Delaney DJ, Anderson BH, et al. Pulmonary atresia with intact ventricular septum: range of morphology in a population-based study. J Am Coll Cardiol 2002;39:1670–9.
17. Burgner D, Davila S, Breunis WB, et al. A genome-wide association study iden-tifies novel and functionally related susceptibility Loci for Kawasaki disease. PLoS Genet 2009;5(1):e1000319.
18. Taubert KA. Epidemiology of Kawasaki disease in the United States and world-wide. Prog Pediatr Cardiol 1997;6:181–5.
19. Nakamura Y, Yashiro M, Uehara R, et al. Epidemiologic features of Kawasaki disease in Japan: results from the nationwide survey in 2005–2006. J Epidemiol 2008;18:167–72.
20. Kawasaki T, Kosaki F, Okawa S, et al. A new infantile acute febrile mucocutaneous lymph node syndrome (MLNS) prevailing in Japan. Pediatrics 1974;54:271–6.
21. Onouchi Y, Tamari M, Takahashi A, et al. A genomewide linkage analysis of Kawasaki disease: evidence for linkage to chromosome 12. J Hum Genet 2007;52(2):179–90.
22. Newburger JW, Takahashi M, Gerber MA, et al. Diagnosis, treatment, and long-term management of Kawasaki disease: a statement for health professionals from the committee on Rheumatic fever, Endocarditis, and Kawasaki disease, Council on Cardiovascular Disease in the Young, American Heart Association. Pediatrics 2004;114:1708–33.
23. Yellen ES, Gauvreau K, Takahashi M, et al. Performance of 2004 American Heart Association recommendations for treatment of Kawasaki disease. Pediatrics 2010;125(2):e234–41.
24. Takahashi M, Mason W, Lewis A. Regression of coronary artery aneurysms in patients with Kawasaki syndrome. Circulation 1987;75:387–94.
25. Kato H, Ichinose E, Yoshioka F, et al. Fate of coronary artery aneurysms in Kawa-saki disease: serial coronary angiographic and long-term follow-up study. Am J Cardiol 1982;49:21758–66.
26. Kitamura S, Tsuda E, Kobayashi J, et al. Twenty-five-year outcome of pediatric coronary artery bypass surgery for Kawasaki disease. Circulation 2009;120: 60–8.
27. Akagi T. Interventions in Kawasaki disease. Pediatr Cardiol 2005;26:206–12.
28. McConnell ME, Hannon DW, Steed RD, et al. Fatal obliterative coronary vasculitis in Kawasaki disease. J Pediatr 1998;133:259–61.
29. Kuijpers TW, Bioezeveld M, Achterhuis A, et al. Longstanding obliterative panar-teritis in Kawasaki disease: lack of cyclosporine A effect. Pediatrics 2003;112: 986–92.
30. Burke AP, Perry LW, Li L. Fatal Kawasaki disease with coronary arteritis and no coronary aneurysms. Pediatrics 1998;101:102–12.
31. Maron BJ, Gardin JM, Flack JM, et al. Assessment if the prevalence of hypertro-phic cardiomyopathy in a general population of young adults: echocardiographic analysis of 4111 subjects in the CARDIA Study. Circulation 1995;92:785–9.

32. Algeria JR, Herrmann J, Holms DR Jr, et al. Myocardial bridging. Eur Heart J 2005;26:1159–68.

33. Calabrò P, Bianchi R, Caprile M, et al. Contemporary evidence of coronary atherosclerotic disease and myocardial bridge on left anterior descending artery in a patient with a non obstructive hypertrophic cardiomyopathy. J Cardiovasc Med (Hagerstown) 2009. [Epub ahead of print].

34. Aquaro GD, Masci P, Formisano F, et al. Usefulness of delayed enhancement by magnetic resonance imaging in hypertrophic cardiomyopathy as a marker of disease and its severity. Am J Cardiol 2010;105:392–7.

35. Kloner RA, Hale S, Alker K, et al. The effects of acute and chronic cocaine use on the heart. Circulation 1992;85:407–19.

36. Dominguez-Rodriguez A, Abreu-Gonzáles P, Ejuanes-Grau C, et al. Oxidative stress and inflammatory markers in cocaine users with acute coronary syndrome. Med Clin (Barc) 2010;134:152–5.

37. Hoskins MH, Leleiko RM, Ramos JJ, et al. Effects of labetalol on hemodynamic parameters and soluble biomarkers of inflammation in acute coronary syndrome in patients with cocaine use. J Cardiovasc Pharmacol Ther 2010;15:47–52.

Myocarditis and Pericarditis in Children

Yamini Durani, MD[a,b],*, Katie Giordano, DO[b],
Brett W. Goudie, MD[c]

KEYWORDS

• Myocarditis • Pericarditis • Pediatric

Myocarditis and pericarditis must be considered in a select group of pediatric patients with chest pain. The typical characteristics of chest pain in myocarditis and pericarditis are described in **Box 1**. Chest pain can be present or absent in both disease entities. The diagnosis of myocarditis and pericarditis can often be elusive, thus the clinician must maintain a high index of suspicion and understand these disease entities have variable clinical presentations. The presentation of myocarditis may range from mild chest pain and tachypnea to fulminant disease with severe cardiovascular instability, or even sudden death. When myocarditis presents as more subtle disease, the diagnosis may be missed if it is not considered in the initial differential diagnosis. Such patients are often diagnosed after the disease has progressed or even postmortem on autopsy after unexpected death. Myocarditis is an important diagnosis to consider, as it is one of the most common causes of new onset heart failure in previously healthy pediatric patients.[1] Pericarditis can present in an acute or chronic manner and ranges clinically from positional chest pain to cardiac tamponade. Vague symptoms including cough, dyspnea, abdominal pain, vomiting, and fever may be associated with pericarditis depending on the cause.[2] Many patients with pericarditis have a benign course; however, a subset may develop complications including recurrent or constrictive pericarditis.[3,4]

The authors have nothing to disclose.
[a] Department of Pediatrics, Thomas Jefferson University, 1025 Walnut Street, Jefferson Medical College, Philadelphia, PA 19107, USA
[b] Division of Emergency Medicine, Alfred I. duPont Hospital for Children, 1600 Rockland Road, Wilmington, DE 19899, USA
[c] Division of Cardiology, Department of Pediatrics, The Nemours Cardiac Center, Alfred I. duPont Hospital for Children, 1600 Rockland Road, Wilmington, DE 19899, USA
* Corresponding author. Division of Emergency Medicine, Alfred I. duPont Hospital for Children, 1600 Rockland Road, Wilmington, DE 19899.
E-mail address: ydurani@nemours.org

Pediatr Clin N Am 57 (2010) 1281–1303
doi:10.1016/j.pcl.2010.09.012   pediatric.theclinics.com
0031-3955/10/$ – see front matter © 2010 Elsevier Inc. All rights reserved.

> **Box 1**
> **Characteristics of chest pain**
>
> *Myocarditis*
>
>   Pain is variable, ranging from severe to mild or even absent
>
>   Caused by ischemia and myocardial damage
>
>   Crushing substernal chest pain with radiation
>
>   Worse with exertion
>
> *Pericarditis*
>
>   Sharp stabbing pain caused by rubbing of irritated pericardium
>
>   Pain relieved by sitting up and leaning forward
>
>   Worse in supine position
>
>   Worse with respirations

This article reviews the clinical aspects of myocarditis and pericarditis, and is intended to help the clinician evaluate and manage such cases, as a possible cause of chest pain in the pediatric population.

MYOCARDITIS

Definition

Myocarditis is the inflammation of the myocardium, which is the muscular wall of the heart. Myocarditis may also extend to the pericardium and endocardium. It can be caused by a variety of mechanisms from viral infection to cardiotoxic drugs. The end result of all causes of myocarditis is some degree of cardiac dysfunction ranging from mild subclinical effects, arrhythmias, heart failure, cardiogenic shock, to sudden death. Based on the severity of illness, myocarditis can be classified into 3 clinical categories: acute, fulminant, and chronic.[5] The milder subclinical cases of myocarditis may have spontaneous resolution and go unrecognized by clinicians. In fulminant disease the patients present in extremis with overt cardiogenic shock. The chronic cases may progress to dilated cardiomyopathy.

The gold standard of diagnosis is endomyocardial biopsy. Despite many advances, this procedure presents an inherent risk to the patient and is not often sensitive, so the initial diagnosis of acute myocarditis is dependent on clinical evidence and suspicion as well as a variety of noninvasive tests, which are discussed in this article.

Epidemiology

The precise incidence of myocarditis is not known. Many cases may be subclinical or even difficult to diagnose given the nonspecific clinical symptoms early in the disease process and the lack of sensitivity of endomyocardial biopsy, which ranges from 10% to 63%.[6] In a recent retrospective study from a Canadian pediatric tertiary care center, the estimated prevalence of pediatric myocarditis was 0.5 cases per 10,000 emergency department visits.[7] Myocarditis was diagnosed in 0.3% of patients seen in the cardiology service of a pediatric tertiary care center in the United States in a 23-year period. During this same period a higher incidence of 1.15% was found on autopsy.[8]

Because many cases are unrecognized, epidemiologic data are often found from autopsy studies. The higher incidence of myocarditis found on autopsies is shown by studies of patients who died of suspected sudden infant death syndrome (SIDS). Evidence of myocarditis on autopsy was found in 16% to 20% of infants with suspected SIDS.[9–11] Myocarditis is also an important cause of sudden death in adolescents and young adults.[12] A review of sudden cardiac death in adolescents found myocarditis to be the cause in up to 17% of cases.[13] Thus, although myocarditis is generally believed to be a rare disease, it is still an important cause of morbidity and mortality in pediatric patients.

It is widely accepted that myocarditis may progress to dilated cardiomyopathy. This occurs via direct myocyte injury from pathogens such as viruses and by the ongoing inflammatory response of the host.[14,15] In an epidemiologic study of pediatric cardiomyopathies in the United States, the investigators found that 27% of cases of dilated cardiomyopathy were secondary to viral myocarditis.[16]

Myocarditis is usually a sporadic disease caused by viruses. The most commonly reported epidemics of myocarditis have been caused by coxsackie viruses.[8] During outbreaks of this virus in Europe in 1965, 5% to 12% of patients infected with coxsackie virus B had cardiac manifestations of their disease.[8,17–19]

Causes

Although a wide range of causes are possible, most cases of myocarditis in the United States and Western Europe are caused by viral infections.[20] Often the inciting agent causing myocarditis is not identified. Advances in molecular techniques have enabled the increased detection of viruses in endomyocardial biopsy samples.

Enteroviruses, particularly coxsackie viruses, have been the most commonly identified pathogens. Other common viruses include parvovirus B19, human herpesvirus 6 (HHV6), influenza, parainfluenza, and adenovirus (**Box 2**) provides a list of many but not all the causes of myocarditis. Myocarditis is also prevalent in patients with human immunodeficiency virus (HIV); 1 study reported that HIV was present in 52% of patients and was a common cause of left ventricular systolic dysfunction in these patients.[21–23] During the recent pandemic of novel H1N1 influenza A virus, there were also reports of fulminant myocarditis caused by this virus in children. It is suggested that this strain of influenza may be more prone to causing myocarditis.[24]

Other infectious agents such as bacteria, parasites, and fungi have been known to cause myocarditis less frequently.[25] *Borrelia burgdorferi* is the causative agent in Lyme disease and is also known to cause manifestations of myocarditis, particularly atrioventricular conduction abnormalities. *Trypanosoma cruzi* infection is more common in areas of Central and South America.[25] Drugs are also known to cause myocarditis via hypersensitivity reactions or direct cardiotoxic effects (eg, chemotherapeutic agents).

Pathogenesis

Research on murine models has largely contributed to what is known about the pathogenesis of myocarditis in humans. It is well established that primary injury occurs to the myocardium directly by the inciting agent, such as a virus entering the myocyte and replicating, leading to focal necrosis and inflammation of the myocardium (**Fig 1**).[14,26] Next, host inflammatory mediators such as macrophages, natural killer (NK) cells, interleukins, tumor necrosis factor (TNF)-α are produced and function to limit viral replication. Experimental mice models with less of an acute immune response have more severe myocarditis.[14,15,27] T cells also mediate ongoing injury to the myocardium by further stimulating cytokine release; this marks the most severe phase of myocardial damage, which is usually 7 to 14 days after the initial injury by the pathogen.[28,29] Cytokines can circulate and persist in the host for weeks, leading to the

Box 2
Causes of myocarditis

Viral

   Enteroviruses (coxsackie A and B, echovirus, polio)

   Adenovirus

   Influenza A and B

   Cytomegalovirus

   Respiratory syncytial virus

   Herpes simplex virus

   Human herpesvirus 6

   Varicella virus

   Human immunodeficiency virus

   Mumps

   Rubella

   Hepatitis viruses

   Epstein-Barr virus

Bacterial

   Meningococcus

   Streptococcus

   Klebsiella

   Diphtheria

   Tuberculosis

Spirochetal

   Borrelia burgdorferi

   Leptospira

Rickettsial

   Rickettsia ricketsii

   Rickettsia tsutsugamushi

Protozoal

   Trypanosoma cruzii

   Toxoplasmosis

Parasitic

   Ascaris

   Echinococcus

   Visceral larva migrans

Fungal

   Actinomycosis

   Coccidioidomycosis

   Histoplasmosis

   Candida

Toxic

   Scorpion

   Radiation

   Bee sting

Drugs

   Sulfonamides

   Chemotherapeutic agents

   Phenytoin

   Isoniazid

Autoimmune

   Rheumatic fever

   Inflammatory bowel disease

   Systemic lupus erythematosus

Data from Refs.[8,25,27]

ongoing inflammatory response and contributing to ongoing myocyte injury and inflammation. Cytokines limit cardiotoxic effects of the pathogen and can have a negative inotropic effect on the heart. The degree of myocyte injury and inflammatory response determines the severity of symptoms and degree of cardiac dysfunction. Thus, there is a wide clinical range of presentations in patients with myocarditis.

In murine models a variety of host factors (nutrition, exercise, genetics, immune state) also contribute to the susceptibility of the host to the inciting agent.[14] Specific receptors for coxsackie virus and adenovirus have been identified on human myocytes, which possibly accounts for the higher incidence of myocarditis in infections

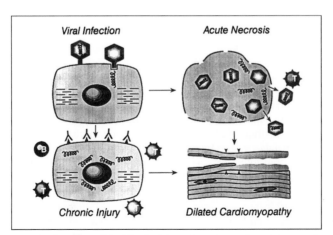

Fig. 1. Pathogenesis of myocarditis. The inciting virus enters the myocyte after interaction with a cellular receptor. Subsequently, cardiomyocyte necrosis and damage occurs leading to acute myocarditis. Progression to dilated cardiomyopathy may occur depending on the host inflammatory response. (*Reprinted from* Liu PP. New concepts in myocarditis: crossroads in the 1990s. Prog Pediatr Cardiol 1992;1:37–47; with permission.)

with these pathogens, which are the most common causative agents in myocarditis.[15,30]

As mentioned earlier, myocarditis can also progress to dilated cardiomyopathy (DCM), as shown by murine models and epidemiologic studies.[14,31] In DCM systolic function is compromised from dilated ventricles, leading to heart failure. In a study of 1426 children with DCM, the most common known cause of DCM was myocarditis in 16% of patients.[32] It is hypothesized that persistent myocyte injury occurs as a result of incomplete clearance of the pathogen, and the persistence of infection leads to an ongoing host inflammatory response causing progression of myocarditis to DCM.[33,34]

Clinical Presentation

Children with myocarditis present with a variable spectrum of clinical disease. Suspicion for the initial diagnosis of myocarditis is highly dependent on the history and physical examination. Many cases may present with mild nonspecific prodromal symptoms typical of a viral illness and the cardiac manifestations of their illness may be subtle. In cases of fulminant myocarditis, children present with overt cardiovascular collapse and shock. Acute myocarditis may also cause sudden unexpected death in children, with preceding symptoms that are minimal or seemingly benign. In 2 retrospective studies of patients less than 20 years old who died suddenly and unexpectedly, 35% to 53% actually had prodromal symptoms that were not believed to be related to cardiac disease.[13,35] A study of pediatric patients with myocarditis also found that 83% were not diagnosed at the first presentation to a clinician and required 2 or more visits to a medical provider before suspicion of myocarditis.[36]

By history, the patient may have complaints that are associated with other common pediatric illnesses such as respiratory tract infections and gastroenteritis. Prodromal symptoms that children often present with include vomiting, diarrhea, fever, shortness of breath, respiratory symptoms, poor feeding, myalgias, fatigue, chest pain, and syncope. In a retrospective review of the presenting clinical characteristics of pediatric patients with myocarditis, the most common presenting symptoms were shortness of breath (69%), vomiting (48%), poor feeding (40%), upper respiratory symptoms (39%), fever (36%), and lethargy (36%).[36] In a second study of clinical presentations, all children who presented with chest pain were more than 10 years of age.[7]

On physical examination clinicians should look for signs of cardiac dysfunction. Respiratory distress may be caused by heart failure causing pulmonary venous congestion. An S3 or S4 gallop may be present, which is caused by decreased ventricular function and dilatation. Murmurs associated with mitral valve and tricuspid valve insufficiency are also associated with ventricular dysfunction. The cardiac chambers dilate in response to dysfunction, with the secondary effect of mitral and tricuspid valve annular dilation, thus leading to incomplete coaptation of the valve leaflets. Tricuspid and mitral valve regurgitation further volume load the heart, creating a positive feedback loop that leads to ever-worsening atrioventricular valve regurgitation. Severe mitral regurgitation and left atrial dilation can cause intermittent compression on the left bronchus, leading to further respiratory compromise. Cardiovascular instability caused by heart failure from myocarditis may also manifest as hypotension, poor pulses, poor perfusion, and a compensatory tachycardia. Other signs of heart failure include hepatomegaly, poor urine output, and altered sensorium. It is commonly believed that patients with myocarditis frequently have tachycardia out of proportion to fever or hydration status; however, 1 study found 66% of children actually had a normal heart rate at initial presentation. The patients in this study most commonly presented with the following physical examination findings: tachypnea (60%), heptomegaly (50%), respiratory distress (47%), fever (36%), and abnormal lung examination (34%).[36]

Chest pain can be present or absent in myocarditis. When present, especially in association with increased troponin levels, the pain can be similar to adult ischemia with anterior chest pressure pain radiating to the neck and arms. As with other causes of ischemic chest pain, the pain of myocarditis worsens with activity or exercise, but does not vary with respiration. Patients with pancarditis (myocarditis and pericarditis) more typically present with precordial chest pain, with pain more prominent in the supine position. Deep breathing or coughing can exacerbate pericardial pain, which is improved in the sitting position.

Diagnostic Evaluation

The diagnosis of myocarditis is initially based on the clinical picture, particularly heart failure or arrhythmia preceded by a prodrome of flulike symptoms and respiratory difficulty. There are several invasive and noninvasive tests that can further support the diagnosis.

The gold standard for diagnosis of myocarditis is endomyocardial biopsy (EB). The Dallas criteria is a standardized classification system used to make the diagnosis of active myocarditis based on the presence of inflammatory cellular infiltrates and myocyte necrosis on pathology specimens from EB. Diagnosis based on biopsy is known to have a variable and low sensitivity because the disease process is patchy and the because of the variability of analysis of biopsy specimens between observers. In pediatric patients, only 20% to 40% have confirmation on EB.[37] EB can help isolate infectious pathogens using molecular techniques, such as amplification of viral genome via polymerase chain reaction (PCR) and in situ hybridization. However, there is more of a focus on noninvasive modalities to diagnose myocarditis because of inherent risks associated with EB, particularly risk of perforation or tricuspid valve injury, which may be higher in younger patients.[38] The diagnosis of myocarditis is thus usually based on the clinical picture with support of noninvasive tests to reach the final diagnosis, rather than biopsy proven disease.

Electrocardiogram (EKG) is a simple noninvasive initial test performed in suspected cases of myocarditis. Retrospective pediatric studies have found abnormal EKGs in 93% to 100% of patients with myocarditis.[7,36] Sinus tachycardia with low-voltage QRS complexes and inverted T waves are the most typical findings on EKG. Other abnormalities that may be present include ventricular hypertrophy, ST segment changes, premature ventricular or atrial beats, arrhythmias (supraventricular tachycardia, ventricular tachycardia), heart block, and infarct patterns (**Figs. 2** and **3**).

Chest radiographs are usually abnormal, showing evidence of cardiomegaly and pulmonary venous congestion caused by heart failure. Abnormal chest radiographs have been found in 60% to 90% of pediatric cases with myocarditis.[7,36]

Typical laboratory tests include complete blood count (CBC), erythrocyte sedimentation rate (ESR), and C-reactive protein (CRP) to look for markers of inflammation. However, there is wide variability in their sensitivity. Other tests to search for pathogens include blood culture, PCR of tracheal aspirates particularly in intubated patients, specific viral titers in blood, nasal culture, and rectal culture particularly for isolation of enteroviruses. Despite extensive testing, often a pathogen is not identified.

Adult studies demonstrate that cardiac specific troponins are more sensitive than conventional cardiac enzymes in providing support for the diagnosis of myocarditis in clinically suspected cases.[39] Cardiac troponin T (TnT), is a cardiac specific protein, and has been found to be increased in pediatric myocarditis, with a sensitivity of 71%

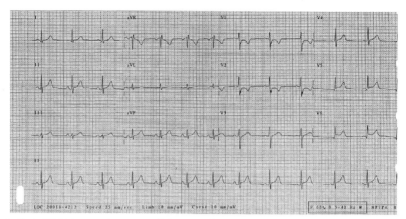

Fig. 2. Early EKG changes in myocarditis. Note the ST segment increase in V4, 5, 6. (*Courtesy of* Nemours Cardiac Center, Wilmington, DE.)

and specificity of 86% at a cut-off level greater than 0.052 ng/mL.[40,41] The data in pediatrics are still limited and this represents an opportunity for future research.

Echocardiography should be performed in suspected cases to assess cardiac function, presence of any wall motion abnormalities, and valvular insufficiency.[41] In most cases of myocarditis the echocardiogram is abnormal. Findings in myocarditis are variable and include left ventricular or biventricular dysfunction, dilation, and wall motion abnormalities. Other findings include mitral and tricuspid valve regurgitation and atrial enlargement (**Fig. 4**).[41,42] Echocardiography may also help to distinguish between fulminant and acute myocarditis. In fulminant myocarditis the left ventricle has normal diastolic dimensions and increased septal thickness and the reverse is true for acute myocarditis. This distinction is important because patients with fulminant myocarditis have a better long-term prognosis.[43] The left ventricle of a patient

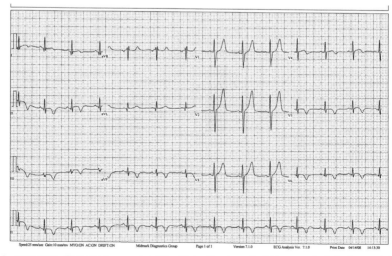

Fig. 3. Late EKG changes in myocarditis. Note the inverted T waves in inferior and lateral leads. (*Courtesy of* Nemours Cardiac Center, Wilmington, DE.)

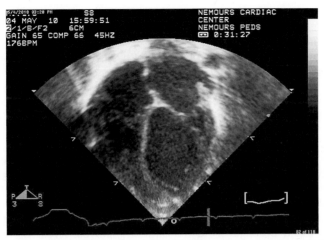

Fig. 4. Echocardiogram of patient with myocarditis. This apical 4-chamber still frame reveals mild LV and LA dilation seen at the time of initial diagnosis of acute myocarditis. Real-time loop shows diminished LV systolic function (not displayed). (*Courtesy of* Nemours Cardiac Center, Wilmington, DE.)

with acute onset myocarditis has typically not yet undergone significant dilation, and usually is characterized by diminished wall motion with decrease shortening or ejection fraction. A patient with chronic burnt-out myocarditis, or dilated cardiomyopathy, will typically have a comparatively more dilated left ventricle with some degree of mitral regurgitation caused by dilation of the valve annulus. These patients with chronic myocarditis may demonstrate surprisingly few symptoms of heart failure despite miserable left ventricular dysfunction, given the accommodative effects of left ventricular dilation.

Cardiac imaging is proving to be an important noninvasive diagnostic tool. Cardiac magnetic resonance imaging (CMRI) with delayed enhancement sequences using gadolinium as the contrast agent identifies areas of myocardial inflammation globally, so it does not have the same limitations as EB, given that myocarditis tends to be a patchy disease histologically.[44] Reported sensitivity of CMRI in visualizing areas of myocarditis is 100% and specificity is 90%.[45,46] The pattern of contrast enhancement is usually on the lateral wall. CMRI can also be used to guide EB by identifying diseased areas of the myocardium for biopsy, which subsequently increases the diagnostic yield of EB.

Treatment

The initial goal of treatment is to manage heart failure and arrhythmias, and achieve cardiovascular stability. Supportive care is the mainstay of therapy. The care should be guided with the expertise of a pediatric cardiologist. Depending on the severity of cardiac dysfunction the patient may only require minimal support and intervention; others with congestive heart failure or fulminant disease may need to be managed in an intensive care unit. Generally, initial medical therapy may include inotropes, diuretics, afterload reducers, antiarrhythmics, digoxin, aldosterone inhibitors, anticoagulation, and beta-blockers after the patient is stabilized. Digoxin should be used with caution, as it may enhance the formation of proinflammatory mediators. Mechanical ventilation may be necessary to reduce metabolic demands and strain on the heart by decreasing afterload. Management of arrhythmias may require some patients to have an implanted defibrillator. Some patients may require the support of extracorporeal membrane oxygenation (ECMO) or ventricular assist devices (VAD), particularly in cases of fulminant myocarditis or persistent arrhythmia leading to severe hemodynamic instability. If a particular infectious pathogen is identified antimicrobial and antiviral therapy should be directed to treat the infection. Bed rest and other strategies to help minimize oxygen demand and consumption are beneficial. Blood products should be reserved for severely anemic patients because exposure to these can cause antibody formation against potential donor hearts.[47]

Because the host's immune response causes much of the myocyte injury in myocarditis, therapies targeting the host immune system have been studied, although this remains a controversial area of treatment. Intravenous immunoglobulin (IVIG) is the most widely accepted immunomodulating therapy and is commonly used in the treatment of myocarditis. Standard dosing with IVIG is typically 2 g/kg per 24 hours. Research studies have demonstrated variable outcomes in children treated with IVIG. Drucker and colleagues[48] demonstrated improved 1-year survival and left ventricular function in 21 children treated with IVIG. Haque and colleagues[49] also demonstrated a higher survival rate but no significant difference in left ventricular function in a sample of 12 pediatric patients treated. However, a randomized control trial of 62 adults did not show a significant improvement in survival or left ventricular function in patients treated with IVIG.[50] A systematic review of all pediatric and adult studies concluded there is currently insufficient evidence in the literature to support the routine use of IVIG for treatment of acute myocarditis.[51]

The use of other immunosuppressive therapies such as corticosteroids, azathioprine, cyclosporine, antilymphocyte antibody (muromonab [OKT3]) and anti-TNF-α antibody is controversial and currently data in pediatrics are limited. Patients with myocarditis caused by autoimmune disease will most likely benefit from immunosuppressive therapy.[47] In a systematic review of the use of immunosuppressive therapy in children with acute myocarditis, the investigators recommended that a large multicenter, randomized, controlled trial be performed to more clearly define the role of such therapies in the treatment regimen.[52]

Mechanical support devices such as VADs are considered in patients who have developed cardiomyopathy or have severely compromised cardiac output despite medical therapies. They can be used long-term either as a bridge to recovery or orthotopic heart transplantation.[47] Although ECMO is not a long-term option, it is a short-term option to support smaller children in whom VADs would otherwise not be available because of size.[37] Survival rates up to 89% have been reported in children with cardiomyopathy who were supported by a VAD or ECMO as they awaited heart transplant.[53]

Prognosis

There is still much to learn about the true prognosis of myocarditis, because many cases are undiagnosed and the incidence of disease is thus not known. The main outcomes are complete recovery, progression to DCM, and death. In a study of 41 children with myocarditis the following outcomes were found: 27 (66%) recovered, 4 (10%) had incomplete recovery, 5 (12%) died, and 5 (12%) received a heart transplant.[54] Another study of 62 children with myocarditis and DCM caused by myocarditis reported that 54 (87%) of patients survived.[36] The proportion of children who develop DCM is not fully known; case reports have documented 12% to 40% progressing to DCM.[27,55,56] Patients with fulminant myocarditis have a better long-term prognosis, even though these patients have more hemodynamic instability at initial presentation. Heart transplant is an option for patients with disease that has progressed to cardiomyopathy. According to a Pediatric Heart Transplant study, 5-year survival is reported to be 70% in children with cardiomyopathy who had an orthotopic heart transplant.[53,57]

PERICARDITIS
Epidemiology

A patient with symptoms of pericarditis can present to a health care provider in many clinical settings; including but not limited to primary care office, emergency department, cardiologist, rheumatologist, or nephrologist. Acute pericarditis is a common and frequent disease and should be considered in the differential diagnosis of chest pain.[58] Although the course is often benign and self-limiting, it can be complicated by a pericardial effusion, pericardial constriction, or recurrent pericarditis.[3]

In 2007, the incidence of acute pericarditis in adult hospitalized patients was 0.1% and was seen in 5% of patients in the emergency department.[59] The incidence of evidence of pericarditis at autopsy is reported to be 1% to 5%.[3,60] Chronic idiopathic pericarditis is a complication in approximately 25% of all cases of acute idiopathic pericarditis.[61]

The Anatomy

The pericardium is a double layer of fibroserous covering of the heart extending to the great vessels. The inner serosal layer of the pericardium adheres to the myocardium forming the epicardium. The 2 layers are 1- to 2-mm thick and normally contain 15 to 35 mL of pericardial fluid. This fluid provides lubrication during contraction of the heart. The blood supply originates from the internal mammary arteries and the innervation stems from the phrenic nerve.[3] The pericardium has several functions: to fix the heart to the mediastinum, act as a barrier to the spread of infection from the lungs to the heart, prevent extreme dilation of the heart during sudden increase of intracardiac volume, equalize the compliance between right and left heart, and reduce friction between the heart and surrounding structures.[3,62,63]

Pathophysiology

The inflammation of the pericardium is caused by infiltration of granulocytes and lymphocytes, with an increase of antibodies found in the pericardial fluid.[60] There is local vasodilatation and increased vascular permeability, thus allowing proteins and free fluid to leak into the pericardial space.[62] The pericardium helps determine the filling of the heart, equalizing pressures between the right and left heart. When the pressure within the pericardium increases, either by effusion or constriction, the ventricular interdependence is exaggerated. Although changes in systemic blood volumes only change the intrapericardial pressures minimally, abrupt or large increases in systemic volume can exceed the pericardial reserve, and exert constraints to cardiac filling during diastole and increase systemic and pulmonary pressures. If untreated, pericarditis can severely impede cardiac output and shock develops.[2,3]

Causes

The cause of pericarditis can be divided into 2 categories: infectious and noninfectious. The noninfectious causes include immunoreactive, metabolic, neoplastic, and traumatic (**Box 3**).[3] Many times a cause is not defined and such cases are considered idiopathic.[59] According to the literature, 40% to 86% of the cases of pericarditis are

| **Box 3** |
| **Causes of pericarditis** |

Viral

   Enteroviruses (coxsackie A and B)

   Adenovirus

   Influenza A and B

   Varicella virus

   Human immunodeficiency virus

   Mumps

   Epstein-Barr virus

Bacterial

   Streptococcus (*Streptococcus pneumoniae, Streptococcus pyogenes, Streptococcus viridans*)

   Meningococcus

   Staphylococcus (*Staphylococcus aureus, Staphylococcus epidermidis*)

   Mycoplasma pneumoniae

   Haemophilus influenzae

   Tularemia

   Salmonella

   Spirochetes

   Coxiella burnitii

   Mycobacterium tuberculosis

   Listeria monocytogenes

Parasitic

   Toxoplasmosis

   Echinococcosis

Fungal

   Actinomycosis

   Histoplasmosis

Metabolic/endocrine

   Uremia

   Hypothyroidism

   Chylopericardium

Hematologoy/oncology

   Bleeding diathesis

   Malignancy (primary and metastatic)

   Radiotherapy

Autoimmune

   Rheumatoid arthritis

   Rheumatic fever

   Systemic lupus erythematosus

Systemic sclerosis

Sarcoidosis

Wegener granulomatosis

Sjögren syndrome

Reiter syndrome

Ankylosing spondylitis

Polymyositis

Giant cell arteritis

Behçet syndrome

Churg-Strauss syndrome

Thrombotic thrombocytopenic purpura

Scleraderma

Other

Idiopathic

Trauma (penetrating or blunt injury)

Iatrogenic (catheter related)

Postoperative (cardiac surgery, thymecotomy)

Familial Mediterranean fever

Smallpox vaccination

Pancreatitis

Loffler syndrome

Stevens-Johnson syndrome

Data from Refs.[3,64,66–69]

idiopathic.[64] Many idiopathic cases are believed to be viral in origin.[3] Despite an extensive workup when the clinical course is complicated, the cause still remains unknown.[65] Confirmation of viral pathogens is difficult because of the invasive nature of diagnosis.[64] Viral cause can be presumed if the patient had a recent upper respiratory infection, exudative effusion, responds to antiinflammatory treatments, and has no recurrence.

Bacterial pericarditis, also known as purulent pericarditis, accounts for about 5% of the cases of pericarditis. Bacteria can infect the pericardium via hematogenous spread or direct extension from adjacent structures, mainly the lungs.[3,70] Infectious pericarditis can cause a thick pericardial effusion, requiring an invasive procedure for drainage. Children have been reported to develop purulent pericarditis spontaneously or with a concurrent infection.[71] The onset of symptoms is often rapid and fatal if left undiagnosed and untreated.[66] Before the widespread use of antibiotics the most commonly identified bacterial pathogen causing pericarditis was *Streptococcal pneumonia*.[72] Pericarditis should still be considered in the hypotensive patient with any pneumococcal infection.[73] Currently *Staphylococcus aureus* is the most common cause of bacterial pericarditis.[70]

Until a vaccine was developed, *Haemophilus influenza* type B was also known to cause purulent pericarditis. Now the once less-virulent nontypable *H influenza* is responsible for more invasive diseases including pericarditis.[72]

Meningococcal disease accounts for 6% to 16% of all cases of purulent pericarditis. Mechanisms of infection include hematogenous seeding, an immune-mediated reaction, or isolated meningococcal pericarditis. Reactive meningococcal pericarditis is believed to be an immunologic phenomenon occurring during the convalescent period; tamponade is common and the pericardial fluid is sterile. Isolated meningococcal pericarditis often occurs in young patients and should be considered in the differential diagnosis of patients with presumed viral or idiopathic pericarditis not responding to conventional treatment.[74]

Mycobacterium tuberculosis accounts for about 4% of the cases of purulent pericarditis and 7% of the cases of cardiac tamponade.[3] The HIV epidemic has contributed to an increase in the cases of tuberculosis and thus an increase in tuberculous pericarditis.[75] Constrictive pericarditis is chronic fibrous thickening or calcification of the pericardium which is usually caused by tuberculosis but may also occur after idiopathic pericarditis.[3] Chronic pericarditis is commonly seen with tuberculosis.[64] An inflammatory response occurs with tuberculous pericarditis, resulting in significant morbidity and mortality caused by effusive and constrictive disease despite antitubercular treatment.[76] Historically, pericardial effusions related to tuberculosis and H influenza are difficult to drain by pericardiocentesis and early pericardiectomy should be considered if initial drainage fails to relieve symptoms.[71]

Neoplasms can cause pericarditis via hematogenous or lymphatic spread, and local tumor invasion. Rarely, pericarditis is caused by a primary cancer.[3] Pericardial effusion is common with neoplastic pericarditis and is often grossly bloody.[65,71] Approximately 50% of malignant effusions present with cardiac tamponade.[71] Failure to respond to treatment with nonsteroidal antiinflammatory drugs (NSAIDs) within 1 week, recurrence of pericarditis, or tamponade on presentation should prompt consideration of neoplastic pericardial effusion.[59]

Radiation treatment of a mediastinal mass causes acute pericarditis but may also progress to constrictive pericarditis.[3] The overall incidence of cancer and radiation therapy has increased, subsequently there has been an increased occurrence of malignant pericarditis. Mortality is high in patients with radiation-induced pericarditis.[77]

Traumatic pericarditis can be caused by any direct blunt or penetrating injury to the pericardium. Percutaneous intervention such as catheterization, pacemaker placement, surgical ablation, and esophageal foreign bodies can also cause penetrating pericardial injury.[3]

Clinical Presentation

Although pericarditis is an uncommon cause of chest pain in the pediatric population, it is one of the first symptoms to occur in cases of true pericarditis.[4] The pain is located over the precordium and can radiate to the left shoulder. It is often described as a stabbing, positional pain, worse when supine and relieved when sitting upright or leaning forward. Common associated symptoms in young children include cough, dyspnea, abdominal pain, vomiting, and fever.[2] No specific clinical feature is useful to differentiate the various causes; diagnosis is based primarily on the history.[59]

Physical examination findings include pericardial friction rub, muffled heart sounds, narrow pulse pressures, tachycardia, neck vein distension, and increased pulsus paradoxus.[2] Pericardial friction rub is pathognomonic for pericarditis. It can be heard best at the left lower sternal border, during expiration, while leaning forward.[3,60] Friction rub is evident with a small pericardial effusion, whereas muffled heart sounds are noted with larger pericardial effusions. Pulsus paradoxus is caused by an exaggerated decrease of systolic arterial pressure during inspiration. A blood pressure drop of greater than 20 mm Hg in a child with pericarditis is suggestive of possible cardiac tamponade.[2] Fluid, which collects slowly, can be accommodated by the pericardium stretching and volumes as high as 2 L have been noted.[3,62] Acute onset of a similar amount of pericardial fluid is poorly tolerated.

Patients with a clinically significant pericardial effusion can be critically ill at presentation. In a 10-year survey of 46 patients, mostly adults, the investigators found that the most common presenting symptoms of a pericardial effusion were breathlessness (90%), chest pain (74%), cough (70%), abdominal pain (61%), and unexplained fever (28%). Pulsus paradoxus was 100% specific for pericardial effusion.[78] Guven and colleagues[79] found similar findings in the pediatric population, noting that large pericardial effusions are uncommon in children and most presented with fever, chest pain, dyspnea, and tachycardia. Beck's triad is pathognomonic for cardiac tamponade and consists of jugular venous distension, hypotension, and muffled heart sounds.[3] Peripheral signs of poor cardiac output associated with cardiac tamponade includes pallor, cold extremities, agitation, decreased consciousness, prolonged capillary refill time, and a compensatory tachycardia.[79]

Constrictive pericarditis presents with symptoms of right heart failure. Physical examination findings may include pulsatile hepatomegaly, decreased apical impulse, early diastolic heart sound referred to as a pericardial knock, and increased jugular venous pressure.[3,80]

Diagnostic Evaluation

Electrocardiogram, chest radiograph, and echocardiogram are useful in the diagnosis of pericarditis. Most patients with acute pericardial disease do not require an extensive workup to determine the exact cause because their clinical course is often benign and self-limited.[65]

EKGs are abnormal in 90% of patients with pericardial disease.[62] EKG changes occur in stages as the disease progresses. The initial changes noted in the first few hours to days include diffuse ST segment increase in leads I, II, III, aVL, aVF, and precordial leads V_2-V_6; ST segment decrease in aVR and V_1; and PR decrease in most leads (**Fig. 5**).[81] Next, the ST and PR intervals normalize but T waves flatten and soon invert. Late in the disease course the EKG may normalize but T wave inversions may become permanent (**Fig. 6**).[60] The evolution of pericardial effusion causes low-voltage QRS segments to develop as a result of the dampening effect of pericardial fluid.[2] In constrictive pericarditis the EKG shows low voltages and nonspecific ST segment changes.[3]

The chest radiograph is often normal in acute pericarditis. A large pericardial effusion must be present to cause cardiomegaly on chest radiograph. Approximately 250 mL of fluid within the pericardium is needed to increase the cardiac size giving a water bottle silhouette (**Fig. 7**).[2,3,82] The presence of pericardial calcifications strongly suggests constrictive pericarditis and is described as an egg shell appearance.[3,82]

Echocardiogram is the diagnostic modality of choice to diagnose pericardial effusion associated with pericarditis (**Fig. 8**), but may be normal if there is minimal fluid accumulation or the fluid is loculated in an area that is not visualized. Therefore, a normal echocardiogram cannot completely exclude pericarditis. In the critically ill patient, in whom cardiac tamponade is suspected, an echocardiogram can provide a lifesaving diagnosis.[60,63] When there is concern for constrictive pericarditis, an echocardiogram is used to evaluate the thickness of the pericardium and provide dynamic information regarding movement variations with respiration to differential constrictive pericarditis from restrictive myocarditis.[3,80]

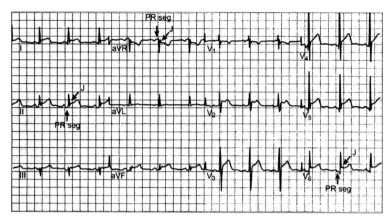

Fig. 5. Early EKG changes in pericarditis. This EKG shows typical EKG findings in early pericarditis, with J point changes and PR depression. Also noted is pronounced ST segment increases in II, avF, V2-6. (*Reprinted from* Spodick DH. Pericardial diseases. In: Braunwald E, Zipes DP, Libby P, editors. Heart disease. 6th edition. Philadelphia: WB Saunders; 2001. p. 1823; with permission.)

Cardiac computed tomography (CT) and cardiac MRI (CMRI) are adjunctive imaging modalities when the echocardiogram findings are inconclusive or nondiagnostic. They are indicated when a pericardial effusion is believed to be loculated, hemorrhagic, or pericardial thickening is suspected. CT attenuation measurements enable further

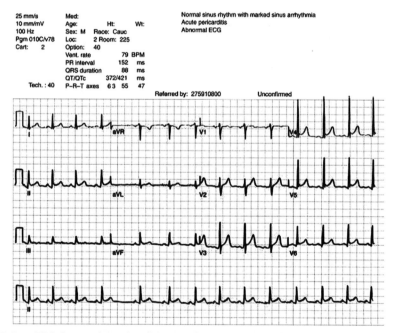

Fig. 6. Late EKG changes in pericarditis. EKG demonstrates late findings in acute pericarditis. (*Courtesy of* Ohio Chapter, American College of Emergency Physicians. *Reprinted from* Jouriles NJ. Pericardial and myocardial disease. In: Marx JA, Hockberger RS, Walls RM, editors. Rosen's emergency medicine. 7th edition. London: Mosby; 2009. p. 1054–68; with permission.)

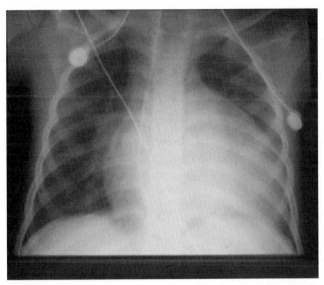

Fig. 7. Water bottle silhouette. This chest radiograph shows marked cardiomegaly, also known as a water bottle silhouette, which is seen in the presence of large pericardial effusions. Also note the associated pulmonary edema from associated high left atrial and left ventricular filling pressures. (*Courtesy of* Dr Steven M. Selbst, Wilmington, DE.)

characterization of the pericardial fluid, which can assist in diagnosis and determination of cause. Fluid attenuation close to that of water is consistent with a simple effusion, if greater than water it is suggestive of either malignancy, hemopericardium, purulent exudate, or effusion associated with hypothyroidism. Cardiac CT and CMRI are also useful in differentiating pericarditis with a small effusion, constrictive pericarditis, and restrictive cardiomyopathy.[63]

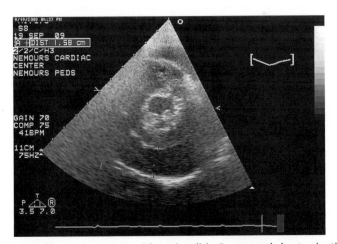

Fig. 8. Pericardial effusion in patient with pericarditis. Parasternal short axis still frame of EKG of patient with a large 1.6-cm pericardial effusion. The left ventricle in systole is seen in cross-section, with papillary muscles at 4 and 8 o'clock. (*Courtesy of* Nemours Cardiac Center, Wilmington, DE.)

In most cases, pericarditis has a benign clinical course and responds well to treatment despite not knowing the cause. Laboratory studies have not played a significant role in diagnosing the cause of pericarditis. Samples from the blood, throat, and rectum can be collected for culture, if clinically warranted, but are of low yield.[64] Further investigation searching for a specific cause is warranted in patients with an abnormal clinical course including cardiac tamponade at presentation, failure to respond to treatment with NSAIDs within 1 week, and recurrence of pericarditis. Cardiac enzymes maybe increased in patients with EKG changes that may be suggestive of myocardial cell damage.[83]

Pericardiocentesis is an invasive procedure that is both therapeutic and diagnostic. Indications include cardiac tamponade, concern for purulent effusion, and concern for malignancy. It is not routinely performed for diagnostic purposes and therefore many cases are labeled idiopathic.[64] The fluid collected can be evaluated for cell count, glucose, protein, lactic dehydrogenase, Gram stain, bacterial and viral cultures, and PCR for infectious pathogens. Purulent hypercellular effusion is associated with bacterial pericarditis; fibrous/serofibrous effusion with lymphocyte predominance is associated with viral pericarditis; fibrous/serofibrous effusion is associated with immunoreactive pericarditis; and hemorrhagic effusion is associated with trauma, tuberculosis, and malignancy.[3]

Treatment

Most patients with acute pericardial disease have a self-limited clinical course and are not difficult to manage and treat even when the cause remains unknown.[65] The goal of treatment is to control inflammation and decrease pain. NSAIDs are the drug of choice, with ibuprofen as first-line treatment.[60] Colchicine has been added to therapy in recurrent cases or in patients not tolerating NSAIDs. Corticosteroids are reserved for severe cases and refractory cases, because there is a risk of reactivating infection and chronic recurrent pericarditis.[3] Bacterial pericarditis is associated with high morbidity and mortality especially if diagnosis and treatment are delayed. If bacterial pericarditis is suspected initial treatment should involve an antistaphylococcal agent until more information is known. In the event of pericardial tamponade, rapid intravenous fluid administration can be lifesaving until the pericardiocentesis is performed.

Although pericardiocentesis is both diagnostic and therapeutic, it is not indicated for routine investigation secondary to its low yield. Indications for pericardiocentesis include purulent pericarditis and evidence of cardiac tamponade.[78] The procedure has been performed since the mid-nineteenth century. A needle is inserted at the left side of the xiphoid process and directed cephlad in a 45° angle to the left, directed toward the left shoulder. EKG monitoring, fluoroscopy, or echocardiographic guidance should be used during the procedure.[71] The complication rate ranges from 4% to 50% despite monitoring, and includes myocardial puncture, atrial and/or ventricular arrhythmia, severe vasovagal episode, and pneumothorax.[78] Pericardiectomy, or surgical removal of the pericardium, is often recommended for purulent pericarditis because of the thick consistency of the effusion and is the treatment of choice for constrictive pericarditis. In cases of constrictive pericarditis a pericardiectomy should be performed early in the clinical course for better prognosis.[4,66] Mortality in children is less than adults likely secondary to a better preoperative physiologic state and physiologic reserve in children.[4]

Prognosis

The clinical course for acute pericarditis is generally benign and self-limited.[3] Approximately 60% recover in 1 week and 80% in 3 weeks.[60] Complications include pericardial effusion, pericardial constriction, and recurrent pericarditis. It is difficult to predict which patients will have complications, but increased risk has been related to female gender, large effusion, cardiac tamponade, or failure to improve with NSAIDs.[59] Up to 30% of patients have recurrent pain and friction rub.[3] Use of cortico-steroids has been linked to recurrent pericarditis and are reserved for use in select cases.[59]

SUMMARY

Myocarditis and pericarditis are rare but important causes of pediatric chest pain. The diagnostic criteria, clinical course, causes, and treatment of acute and chronic myocarditis are reviewed, with particular attention to differentiating the features of acute infection from early dilated cardiomyopathy. Supportive therapy remains the standard of care for pump dysfunction. The identification and treatment of pericarditis with associated large pericardial effusion can be lifesaving. This article reviews the important clinical features that might lead the clinician to diagnose either myocarditis or pericarditis and thus separate the few patients with either of these conditions from the legions of children with noncardiac chest pain.

ACKNOWLEDGMENTS

The authors wish to thank Ms Kristina Flathers for her valuable assistance in the preparation of the manuscript.

REFERENCES

1. Calabrese F, Rigo E, Milanesi O, et al. Molecular diagnosis of myocarditis and dilated cardiomyopathy in children: clinicopathologic features and prognostic implications. Diagn Mol Pathol 2002;11:212–21.
2. Bernstein D. Diseases of the myocardium and pericardium - chapter 440: diseases of the pericardium. In: Kliegman R, Behrman R, Jenson H, et al, editors. Nelson's textbook of pediatrics. 18th edition. Philadelphia: WB Saunders; 2007. p. 1972–5.
3. Troughton RW, Asher CR, Klein AL. Pericarditis. Lancet 2004;363(9410):717–27.
4. Thompson JL, Burkhart HM, Dearani JA, et al. Pericardiectomy for pericarditis in the pediatric population. Ann Thorac Surg 2002;88:1546–50.
5. Knowlton KU, Savoia MC, Oxman MN. Myocarditis and pericarditis. In: Mandell GL, Bennett JE, Douglas RG, editors. Mandell, Douglas and Bennett's principles and practice of infectious diseases. 7th edition. Philadelphia: Churchill Livingstone/Elsevier; 2010. p. 1153–61.
6. Cooper LT, Baughman KL, Feldman AM, et al. The role of endomyocardial biopsy in the management of cardiovascular disease: a scientific statement from the American Heart Association, the American College of Cardiology and the European Society of Cardiology. Circulation 2007;116:2216–33.
7. Freedman SB, Haladyn JK, Floh A, et al. Pediatric myocarditis: emergency department clinical findings and diagnostic evaluation. Pediatrics 2007;120: 1278–85.
8. Friedman RA, Schowengerdt KO, Towbin JA. Myocarditis. In: Garson A, Bricker JT, Fisher DJ, et al, editors. The science and practice of pediatric cardiology. 2nd edition. Baltimore (MD): Williams & Wilkins; 1998. p. 1777–94.
9. Rasten-Almqvist P, Eksborg S, Rajs J. Myocarditis and sudden infant death syndrome. APMIS 2002;110:469.

10. Rajs J, Hammarquist F. Sudden infant death in Stockholm. A forensic pathology study covering ten years. Acta Paediatr Scand 1988;77:812.
11. Shatz A, Hiss J, Arensburg B. Myocarditis misdiagnosed as sudden infant death syndrome (SIDS). Med Sci Law 1997;37(1):16–8.
12. Denfield SW, Garson A. Sudden death in children and young adults. Pediatr Clin North Am 1990;37:215–31.
13. Noren GR, Staley NA, Bandt CM, et al. Occurrence of myocarditis in sudden death in children. J Forensic Sci 1977;22:188–96.
14. Kawai C. From myocarditis to cardiomyopathy: mechanisms of inflammation and cell death. Circulation 1999;99:1091–100.
15. Leonard E. Viral myocarditis. Pediatr Infect Dis J 2004;23:665–6.
16. Lipshultz SE, Sleeper LA, Towbin JA, et al. The incidence of pediatric cardiomyopathy in two regions of the United States. N Engl J Med 2003;348:1647–55.
17. Grist NR. Viruses and myocarditis. Postgrad Med J 1972;48:746–9.
18. Grist NR, Bell EJ. A six-year study of coxsackievirus B infections in heart disease. J Hyg 1974;73:165–72.
19. Helin M, Sarola J, Lapinleimu K. Cardiac manifestations during a Coxsackievirus B5 epidemic. BMJ 1968;3:97.
20. Bowles NE, Bowles KR, Towbin JA. Viral genome detection and outcome in myocarditis. Heart Fail Clin 2005;1:407–17.
21. Anderson DW, Virmani R, Reilly JM, et al. Prevalent myocarditis at necropsy in the acquired immunodeficiency syndrome. J Am Coll Cardiol 1988;11:792–9.
22. Bowles NE, Kearney DL, Ni J, et al. The detection of viral genomes by polymerase chain reaction in the myocardium of pediatric patients with advanced HIV disease. J Am Coll Cardiol 1999;34:857–65.
23. Keesler MJ, Fisher SD, Lipshultz SE. Cardiac manifestations of HIV infection in infants and children. Ann N Y Acad Sci 2001;946:169–78.
24. Bratincsak A, El-Said HG, Bradley JS, et al. Fulminant myocarditis associated with pandemic H1N1 Influenza A virus in children. J Am Coll Cardiol 2010;55:928–9.
25. Cooper LT. Myocarditis. N Engl J Med 2009;360:1526–38.
26. Liu PP. New concepts in myocarditis: crossroads in the 1990s. Prog Pediatr Cardiol 1992;1:37–47.
27. Feldman AM, McNamara D. Myocarditis. N Engl J Med 2000;343:1388–98.
28. Kearney MT, Cotton JM, Richardson PJ, et al. Viral myocarditis and dilated cardiomyopathy: mechanisms, manifestations, and management. Postgrad Med J 2001;77:4–10.
29. Kishomoto C, Kuribayashi K, Masuda T, et al. Immunological behavior of lymphocytes in experimental viral myocarditis: significance of T lymphocytes in the severity of myocarditis and silent myocarditis in BALB/c-nu/nu mice. Circulation 1985;71:1247–54.
30. Demmler GJ, Myocarditis. In: Long SS, Pickering LK, Prober CG, editors. *Principles and Practice of Pediatric Infectious Diseases.* 2nd edition. Philadelphia: Churchill Livingston; 2003. p. 258–61.
31. Dec GW, Palacios IF, Fallon JT, et al. Active myocarditis in the spectrum of acute dilated cardiomyopathies. Clinical features, histologic correlates, and clinical outcome. N Engl J Med 1985;312:885–90.
32. Towbin JA, Lowe AM, Colan SD, et al. Incidence, causes, and outcomes of dilated cardiomyopathy in children. JAMA 2006;296:1867–76.
33. Wee L, Liu P, Penn L, et al. Persistence of viral genome into late stages of murine myocarditis detected by polymerase chain reaction. Circulation 1992;86:1605–14.

34. Kyu B, Matsumori A, Sato Y, et al. Cardiac persistence of cardioviral RNA detected by polymerase chain reaction in a murine model of dilated cardiomyopathy. Circulation 1992;86:522–30.
35. Drory Y, Turetz Y, Hiss Y, et al. Sudden unexpected death in persons less than 40 years of age. Am J Cardiol 1991;68:1388–92.
36. Durani Y, Egan M, Baffa J, et al. Pediatric myocarditis: presenting clinical characteristics. Am J Emerg Med 2009;27:942–7.
37. Levi D, Alejos J. Diagnosis and treatment of pediatric viral myocarditis. Curr Opin Cardiol 2001;16:77–83.
38. Pophal SG, Sigfusson G, Booth KL, et al. Complications of endomyocardial biopsy in children. J Am Coll Cardiol 1999;34:2105–10.
39. Lauer B, Niederau C, Kuhl U, et al. Cardiac troponin T in patients with clinically suspected myocarditis. J Am Coll Cardiol 1997;30:1354–9.
40. Soongswang J, Durongisitkul K, Ratanarapee S, et al. Cardiac troponin T: its role in the diagnosis of clinically suspected acute myocarditis and chronic dilated cardiomyopathy in children. Pediatr Cardiol 2002;23:531–5.
41. Levine MC, Klugman D, Teach SJ. Update on myocarditis in children. Curr Opin Pediatr 2010;22:278–83.
42. Pinamonti B. Echocardiographic findings in myocarditis. Am J Cardiol 1988;62: 285–91.
43. Felker GM, Boehmer JP, Hruban RH, et al. Echocardiographic findings in fulminant and acute myocarditis. J Am Coll Cardiol 2000;36:227–32.
44. Goitein O, Matetzky S, Beinart R, et al. Acute myocarditis: noninvasive evaluation with cardiac MRI and transthoracic echocardiography. AJR Am J Roentgenol 2009;192:254–8.
45. Mahrholdt H, Goedecke C, Wagner A, et al. Cardiovascular magnetic resonance assessment of human myocarditis: a comparison to histology and molecular pathology. Circulation 2004;109:1250–8.
46. Olimulder MA, van Es J, Galjee MA. The importance of cardiac MRI as a diagnostic tool in viral myocarditis-induced cardiomyopathy. Neth Heart J 2009;17:481–6.
47. Levi D, Alejos J. An approach to the treatment of pediatric myocarditis. Paediatr Drugs 2002;4:637–47.
48. Drucker NA, Colan SD, Lewis AB, et al. Gamma-globulin treatment of acute myocarditis in the pediatric population. Circulation 1994;89:252–7.
49. Haque A, Bhatti S, Siddiqui F. Intravenous immune globulin for severe acute myocarditis in children. Indian Pediatr 2009;46:810–1.
50. McNamara DM, Rosenblum WD, Janosko KM, et al. Intravenous immune globulin in the therapy of myocarditis and acute cardiomyopathy. Circulation 1997;95:2476–8.
51. Robinson JL, Hartling L, Crumley E, et al. A systematic review of intravenous gamma globulin for therapy of acute myocarditis. BMC Cardiovasc Disord 2005;5:12.
52. Hia CP, Yip WC, Tai BC, et al. Immunosuppressive therapy in acute myocarditis: an 18 year systematic review. Arch Dis Child 2004;89:580–4.
53. Levi D, Marelli D, Plunkett M, et al. Use of assist devices and ECMO to bridge pediatric patients with cardiomyopathy to transplantation. J Heart Lung Transplant 2002;21:760–70.
54. English RF, Janosky JE, Ettedgui JA, et al. Outcomes for children with acute myocarditis. Cardiol Young 2004;14:488–93.
55. Kuhl U, Schultheiss HP. Viral myocarditis: diagnosis, aetiology and management. Drugs 2009;69:1287–302.

56. D'Ambrosio A, Patti G, Manzoli A, et al. The fate of acute myocarditis between spontaneous improvement and evolution to dilated cardiomyopathy: a review. Heart 2001;85:499–504.

57. Morrow RW. Cardiomyopathy and heart transplantation in children. Curr Opin Cardiol 2000;15:216–23.

58. Imazio M, Demichelis B, Parrini I, et al. Day hospital treatment of acute pericarditis: a management program for outpatient therapy. J Am Coll Cardiol 2004; 43:1042–6.

59. Imazio M, Cecchi E, Demichelis, et al. Indicators of poor prognosis of acute pericarditis. Circulation 2007;115:2739–3744.

60. Jouriles NJ. Pericardial and myocardial disease. In: Marx JA, Hockberger RS, Walls RM, editors. Rosen's emergency medicine. 7th edition. London: Mosby; 2009. p. 1054–68.

61. Peterlana D, Puccetti A, Simeoni S, et al. Efficacy of intravenous immunoglobulin in chronic idiopathic pericarditis: report of 4 cases. Clin Rheumatol 2005;24:18–21.

62. Humphreys M. Pericaridal conditions: signs, symptoms and electrocardiogram changes. Emerg Nurse 2006;4:30–6.

63. Wang ZJ, Reddy GP, Gotway MB, et al. CT and MRI imaging of pericardial disease. Radiographics 2003;23(Spec No):S167–80.

64. Levy PY, Corey R, Berger P, et al. Etiologic diagnosis of 204 pericardial effusions. Medicine 2003;82:385–91.

65. Permanyer-Miralda G, Sagrista-Sauleda MD, Soler-Soler J. Primary acute pericardial disease: a prospective series of 231 consecutive patients. Am J Cardiol 1985;5:623–30.

66. Hayavadana Rao RV, Raveenthiran V. Choice of drainage procedures in paediatric pyopericardium: a 30 year experience. Trop Doct 2005;35:200–4.

67. Dalla Pozza R, Hartl D, Bechtold S, et al. Recurrent pericarditis in children: elevated cardiac autoantibodies. Clin Res Cardiol 2007;96:168–75.

68. Masood SA, Kiel E, Akingbola O, et al. Cardiac tamponade and pleural effusion complicating varicella: a case report and literature review. Pediatr Emerg Care 2008;24:777–81.

69. Esposito S, Faelli M, Tagliabue C, et al. Mycoplasma pneumonia pericarditis and cardiac tamponade in a 7 year old girl with cystic fibrosis infection. Infection 2006;34:355–6.

70. Bhaduri-McIntosh S, Prasad M, Moltedo J, et al. Purulent pericarditis caused by group A streptococcus. Tex Heart Inst J 2006;33:519–22.

71. Moores DW, Dziuban SW Jr. Pericardial drainage procedures. Chest Surg Clin N Am 1995;5:359–73.

72. Elwood RL, DeBaisi RL. Purulent pericarditis caused by non-typeable *Haemophilus influenzae* in a pediatric patient. Diagn Microbiol Infect Dis 2008;62:113–5.

73. Blohm ME, Schroten H, Heusch A, et al. Acute purulent pericarditis in pneumococcal meningitis. Intensive Care Med 2005;3:1142.

74. Nkoski J, Thakrar A, Kumar K, et al. Meningococcal serotype Y myopericarditis. Diagn Microbiol Infect Dis 2009;63:223–7.

75. Hakim JG, Ternouth I, Mushangi E, et al. Double blind randomised placebo controlled trial of adjunctive prednisolone in the treatment of effusive tuberculous pericarditis in HIV seropositive patients. Heart 2000;84:183–8.

76. Wiysonge CS, Ntsekhe M, Gumedze F, et al. Contemporary use of adjunctive corticosteroids in tuberculous pericarditis. Int J Cardiol 2008;124:388–90.

77. Devaleria PA, William MD, Baumgartner WA, et al. Current indications, risks and outcome after pericardiectomy. Ann Thorac Surg 1991;52:219–24.

78. Gibbs CR, Watson RDS, Singh SP. Management of pericardial effusion by drainage: a survey of 10 year's experience in City Centre General Hospital serving a multiracial population. Postgrad Med J 2000;76:809–13.
79. Guven H, Bakiler AR, Ulger Z. Evaluation of children with a large pericardial effusion and cardiac tamponade. Acta Cardiol 2007;62:129–33.
80. Chen C, Lin M, Wu E. Clinical manifestations and outcomes of constrictive pericarditis in children. J Formos Med Assoc 2005;104:402–7.
81. Spodick DH. Pericardial diseases. In: Braunwald E, Zipes DP, Libby P, editors. Heart disease. 6th edition. Philadelphia: WB Saunders; 2001. p. 1823.
82. Lieng LH, Oh JK, Breen JF, et al. Calcific constrictive pericarditis: is it still with us? Ann Intern Med 2000;132:444–50.
83. Karjalamen J, Heikkila J, Helsinki MD. Acute pericarditis; myocardial enzyme release as evidence for myocarditis. Am Heart J 1986;11:546–52.

Arrhythmogenic Causes of Chest Pain in Children

Brett R. Anderson, MD, MBA[a], Victoria L. Vetter, MD, MPH, MSHP[b],*

KEYWORDS

• Chest pain • Arrhythmia • Pediatric

Arrhythmias are common causes of chest pain of cardiac origin in children, both with and without structural heart disease. Children frequently describe feelings of "chest pain" when experiencing not only myocardial ischemia, but also a multitude of other "discomforts," such as those associated with palpitations, irregular heart beats, or even abdominal pain, as young children often have difficulty localizing pain. Thus, a broad differential is necessary when evaluating chest pain in children.

Although chest pain in adults often heralds myocardial infarctions, these are uncommon in children. Chest pain in children, if it is of cardiac origin, however, and especially if it is from an arrhythmia, can signal an impending cardiac arrest. The greatest challenge is to distinguish cardiac chest pain from the multitude of noncardiac causes, including musculoskeletal, pulmonary, and gastrointestinal, and anxiety. This is best accomplished with a thorough and systematic evaluation plan.

EVALUATION OF CHEST PAIN IN CHILDREN

A careful history of the present illness, including associated signs and symptoms; type, location, and duration of pain; and positions or activities that make the pain better or worse should be ascertained (**Box 1**). Past medical, surgical, and family histories should include cardiac conditions and the use of drugs or potential exposure to drugs, either prescription or recreational. Chest pain associated with exercise, palpitations, shortness of breath, diaphoresis, lightheadedness, syncope, or positive medical, surgical, or familial cardiac history is particularly concerning for arrhythmias. Physical examination should include cardiac palpation for the presence of cardiac

The authors have nothing to disclose.

[a] Division of Pediatric Cardiology, Morgan Stanley Children's Hospital of New York-Presbyterian, Columbia University Medical Center, 3959 Broadway, CHN2, New York, NY 10032, USA

[b] Division of Pediatric Cardiology, The Children's Hospital of Philadelphia, University of Pennsylvania School of Medicine, 34th and Civic Center Boulevard, Philadelphia, PA 19104, USA

* Corresponding author.

E-mail address: vetter@email.chop.edu

Pediatr Clin N Am 57 (2010) 1305–1329

doi:10.1016/j.pcl.2010.09.005

Box 1
Questions to ask when evaluating chest pain

1. Is the chest pain acute or chronic?

2. How often does the pain occur?

3. Where is the pain located?

4. What is the quality of the pain? Is it sharp, dull, squeezing, or pressing?

5. Does it radiate? Especially to the jaw or left arm?

6. How long does the pain last?

7. What makes the pain occur?

8. Is it activity related?

9. What makes the pain resolve?

10. What medications do you take to relieve the pain?

11. Do you have palpitations, skipped, or fast heart beats?

12. Are there other associated symptoms?

13. Do you get lightheaded or dizzy?

14. Do you ever faint?

15. Are you more fatigued lately, especially with exercise or when you have chest pain?

16. Are you short of breath when you have the chest pain or at other times?

17. Is the pain precipitated or increased by breathing or movement?

18. Is the pain less when sitting or lying down?

19. Is the pain worse when touching the area of the chest that hurts?

20. What type of exercise have you been doing lately?

21. Have you been lifting weights?

22. What else would you like to tell me about your chest pain?

23. Does anyone else in your family have chest pain?

24. Are you worried about anything or are there recent stresses in your life?

---

enlargement; thrills or heaves; auscultation for murmurs, clicks, rubs, or gallops; and inspection for signs and symptoms of congestive heart failure, such as pulmonary congestion with wheezes and rales, jugular venous distension, edema, and/or liver enlargement. Abnormalities on cardiac examination may indicate structural heart disease or congestive heart failure. Signs of heart failure may be the result of a primary structural defect or secondary to decreased output, as the result of arrhythmia. Of note, arrhythmias and myocardial ischemia in infants and young children may manifest as colic or irritability or other signs or symptoms of congestive heart failure.

LABORATORY AND OTHER TESTS TO EVALUATE CHEST PAIN OF ARRHYTHMIC ORIGIN
Electrocardiogram

The electrocardiogram (ECG) should be used to determine the presence of an abnormal heart rate or rhythm and the type of abnormality. It can also identify the presence of ischemia. An ECG is recommended in any child with chest pain who has an underlying cardiac disorder, in those with any suspicion of an arrhythmia, and in all those who present with syncope or chest pain during exercise.

Echocardiogram

The echocardiogram (ECHO) is used to evaluate the structure and function of the heart. It should be used to clarify any suspected structural or functional cardiac disorder in a child presenting with chest pain.

Exercise Stress Test

The exercise stress test (EST) can document the occurrence of arrhythmia with exercise, as well as determine cardiopulmonary performance. The presence of chest pain during the exercise test, in the absence of arrhythmias or without ST-T wave changes suggestive of ischemia, makes a cardiac cause of the chest pain unlikely.

Event Monitors

A variety of event monitors that can be used to record the ECG during a symptom are available. Some of these monitors transmit or record continuously. Others require activation by the patient. These recordings can be used to correlate symptoms of chest pain with the rhythm and heart rate at the time of the symptom.

Laboratory Tests

All adults with acute chest pain that is suggestive of cardiac origin will have troponin and other cardiac enzymes tested, often with serial tests obtained to look for evidence of damage to myocardial cells. Patients who have been in rapid cardiac arrhythmias for long periods of time may have abnormal values, so care must be taken with interpretation in these instances. It is possible that a child can experience a myocardial infarction and that it can lead to arrhythmias and chest pain. If this is suspected, troponin levels should be obtained.

Magnetic Resonance Imaging, Computed Tomography Angiography, Catheterization, or Electrophysiological Study

Magnetic resonance imaging (MRI), computed tomography (CT) angiography, catheterization, or electrophysiological study tests should be ordered after consultation with a pediatric cardiologist to look for specific cardiac conditions.

ASSOCIATED ARRHYTHMIAS

The most common arrhythmias associated with chest pain in children are supraventricular tachycardias (SVTs); however, other arrhythmias, such as atrial flutter (A Flutter), atrial fibrillation (A Fib), premature ventricular contractions (PVCs), ventricular tachycardia (VT), and bradycardias have been reported to result in chest pain in the pediatric population (**Box 2**). Chest pain associated with arrhythmias generally results from decreased cardiac output and resultant myocardial ischemia. The likelihood of experiencing chest pain in association with arrhythmias is shown in **Table 1**.

This article discusses the most common etiologies of arrhythmogenic chest pain in the young. As children with structural heart disease and/or previous cardiac surgery have particularly high risk of arrhythmias and are more susceptible to the adverse physiologic effects of arrhythmias, special attention is paid to this population throughout the article. Mechanisms, evaluations, and treatments of arrhythmias are discussed briefly.

Box 2
Arrhythmogenic causes of chest pain

Supraventricular tachycardias

    Reentrant tachycardias

        Atrioventricular reentrant tachycardias

        Atrioventricular nodal reentrant tachycardias

    Atrial flutter

    Atrial fibrillation

    Ectopic tachycardias

        Ectopic atrial tachycardia

        Multifocal atrial tachycardia

        Junctional ectopic tachycardia

Premature ventricular contractions

Ventricular tachycardia

Bradycardias

    Sinus node dysfunction

    Atrioventricular nodal block

SUPRAVENTRICULAR TACHYCARDIAS
Atrioventricular Reentrant SVT

General information

SVT are the most common pediatric rhythm disturbances. They are estimated to occur in as many as 1 in 1000 to 1 in 2500 children. Fifty percent of children with SVTs present in infancy. SVTs are arrhythmias that originate above the ventricles and involve the atria, atrioventricular (AV) node, and/or one or more accessory bypass

---

Table 1
Likelihood of experiencing chest pain

AVNRT	+++
AVRT	+++
AF	++
Afib	++
EAT	+
MAT	±
JET	±
Bradycardias	+
Sinus node dysfunction	+
Complete or 3° AV nodal block	++
Arrhythmia with congenital heart disease	++++

Abbreviations: AF, atrial flutter; Afib, atrial fibrillation; AV, atrioventricular; AVNRT, atrioventricular nodal reentrant tachycardia; AVRT, atrioventricular reentrant tachycardia; EAT, ectopic atrial tachycardia; JET, junctional ectopic tachycardia; MAT, multifocal atrial tachycardia; ++++, commonly associated; +++, often associated; ++, sometimes associated; +, occasionally associated; ±, rarely associated.

tracts. More than 90% of clinically significant SVTs involve one or more accessory pathways between the atria and ventricles (AV reentrant tachycardias [AVRT]) or within the AV node (AV nodal reentrant tachycardias [AVNRT]).[1] These pathways result in reentrant circuits, through which electrical impulses repeatedly propagate, resulting in recurrent stimulation of the ventricles. Two-thirds of these AV reentrant arrhythmias involve concealed pathways. One-third involves manifest pathways, such as those seen in Wolff-Parkinson-White syndrome (WPW) or other forms of preexcitation. Fifteen percent of all SVTs are AVNRTs, whereas 30% of SVTs in adolescents are from AVNRTs. The remaining 10% of SVTs are automatic atrial or junctional tachycardias, the result of either enhanced automaticity or triggered automaticity. They are referred to as ectopic rhythms and arise from either the atria or AV junction.[2]

In children, A Fib and A Flutter are collectively responsible for 10% of non-postoperative SVTs and 40% of postoperative SVTs. Junctional ectopic tachycardia (JET), in non-postoperative patients, represents fewer than 1% of SVTs.[3] Multifocal or chaotic atrial tachycardia (MAT), ectopic atrial tachycardia (EAT), A Fib, A Flutter, and JET are SVTs, although in the clinical setting they are often thought of and treated as distinct entities.

Presentation
Of children presenting with chest pain of cardiac origin, 33% to 67% are reported to have SVT.[3,4] The presentation of SVT in children can vary greatly, depending on the child's developmental age, ability to communicate symptoms, duration of the arrhythmia, mechanism of the particular SVT, and underlying cardiac pathology and physiology, especially in the presence of congenital heart disease. Infants more often present with irritability, feeding intolerance, or other signs or symptoms of congestive heart failure.[5] Although most older children have minor symptoms at presentation, 50% of infants with SVT that persists for more than 48 hours develop heart failure.[6]

Older children typically present with palpitations, lightheadedness, and dizziness, or symptoms of fatigue, but chest pain is not uncommon and heart failure, or sudden cardiac death, can occur. In older children, WPW syndrome, in particular, confers a small but real risk of sudden cardiac death: 0.25% per year in patients without structural heart disease and 1% per year in children with structural heart disease.[7]

The more frequent occurrence of chest pain in this paroxysmal tachycardia can be explained by its sudden onset, resulting in a rapid drop in blood pressure. Over time, the blood pressure gradually increases as reflexes attempt to normalize the physiology, even when the child remains in SVT, and symptoms of chest pain may resolve. The severity of the symptoms depends on the rate of the SVT and the underlying cardiac pathophysiology, function, and structure.

SVT occurs with a trimodal age distribution. Half of children present with SVT before 1 year of age. The next peak occurs in adolescence. The third peak occurs between the ages of 6 and 9 years. More than 75% of infantile SVT clinically regresses spontaneously by 1 year of age, yet up to one-third will recur later in life, with a mean age of recurrence of 8 years. Those with WPW are more likely to have persistent SVT. In children who first present after 1 year of age, only 15% regress spontaneously.[8]

Associated factors and etiology
Most SVT occurs spontaneously, but often may present in association with fever, illness, or stimulant medications. To date, no genes have been identified that are associated with SVT. However, 7% of children with SVT, and 20% of children with WPW syndrome, have a first-degree relative with documented SVT.[9] Therefore, evaluation of a child with chest pain and recent illness, stimulant use, or family history of SVT should raise concern for this arrhythmia.

Most children with SVT have structurally normal hearts, but 9% to 32% of children with structural heart disease will experience SVT. There is a strong association between SVT and congenital heart disease (CHD), as seen in children with WPW and Ebstein anomaly, single ventricle disease, congenitally corrected transposition of the great arteries (L-TGA), or heterotaxy syndromes[1,6] with up to 20% of patients with Ebstein anomaly having WPW.[10]

Evaluation

A 12- or 15-lead ECG should be included in the evaluation of any child with suspected SVT to differentiate it from other arrhythmias and to evaluate the specific mechanism of the SVT. The ECG of children in reentrant SVT may resemble sinus tachycardia, but with a fixed rate, and with P waves that are difficult to discriminate or that have an abnormal axis (**Fig. 1**). Reentrant SVTs are distinguished from sinus tachycardia by an abrupt onset and termination. This sudden change is the very factor that makes this arrhythmia likely to be associated with chest pain.

For infants, the rate of reentrant SVT is typically 220 to 320 bpm. In older children, it is typically 160 to 280 bpm. Automatic or ectopic SVT, in contrast, is characterized by more rate variability and by phases of warm-up and cool-down, which make it less likely to cause symptoms of chest pain.

For patients in SVT, an ECG should be recorded while administering abortive therapy, such as adenosine, to assist in diagnosis. ECGs of patients with WPW, while in sinus rhythm, demonstrate the classic "delta wave," a gradual upslope in the QRS complex, formed as the impulse propagates rapidly through the accessory pathway, and then more slowly through the ventricular myocardium.[10] However, the diagnosis of SVT in children who do not have WPW can be difficult when children are in sinus rhythm; children without WPW with SVT typically have normal resting ECGs when not experiencing their tachycardias. Those with EAT or JET may have slower ectopic atrial or junctional rhythms when not in tachycardia, suggesting that the arrhythmia may be an ectopic tachycardia. Twenty-four-hour ambulatory (Holter) monitors or trans-telephonic event monitors are useful methods to capture the arrhythmia events and correlate them with symptoms of chest pain. If a Holter or event monitor repeatedly shows normal sinus rhythm during periods of chest pain, it is unlikely that the

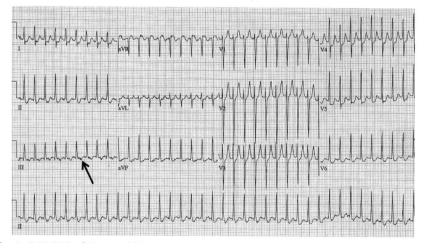

Fig. 1. SVT. ECG of 7-year-old boy with SVT at 230 bpm. Note regular narrow QRS rhythm. Arrow denotes retrograde P wave.

chest pain is secondary to arrhythmia. It should be noted, however, that symptoms of chest pain could correlate with episodes of sinus tachycardia and ST or T-wave abnormalities, which could indicate myocardial ischemia for reasons other than arrhythmia. Exercise testing can be helpful when evaluating children with symptoms of chest pain associated with activity.

Treatment
Treatment of SVT is divided into short-term, acute abortive, and long-term, chronic preventive, therapies. See **Tables 2** and **3** for treatment options. Treatments may include vagal maneuvers (such as ice to the face, carotid massage, Valsalva maneuvers, or headstand), medications, dietary restrictions, or catheter ablations. Synchronized cardioversion should be used for hemodynamically unstable SVT starting with a dose 0.5 J/kg and doubling, up to 4.0 J/kg. Once the arrhythmia resolves, chest pain generally stops immediately. If the arrhythmia is associated with myocardial ischemia or congestive heart failure, however, the chest pain may persist, dissipating more gradually as these conditions improve.

Table 2
Pharmacologic agents for acute treatment of supraventricular tachycardia and ventricular tachycardia

Arrhythmia	Agent	Initial Treatment (IV)
VT (1st line)	Lidocaine	1–2 mg/kg IV bolus every 5–15 min IV infusion: 20–50 μg/kg/min
	Amiodarone	Day 1: 2.5–5.0-mg/IV push over 10 min every 6 h May repeat dose in 10 minutes and as needed up to a total of 15 mg/kg for the first 12–24 hours; maximum dosage: 1050 mg/d Day 2 and subsequent days: 2.5 mg/kg/dose over 10 min every 4–6 hours as needed; not to exceed a total daily dosage of 15 mg/kg/d or 720 mg/d
VT (2nd line)	Magnesium	0.25 mEq/kg over 1 min, followed by 1 mEq/kg over 5 h Especially for torsades de pointes
SVT or 2nd line VT	Amiodarone	As above
	Procainamide	5 mg/kg over 5–10 min or 10–15 mg/kg over 30–45 min Infusion: 20–100 μg/kg/min
	Esmolol	IV load: 200–500 μg/kg/min over 2–4 min Increase in 50–100-μg/kg/min increments (max dose = 1000 μg/kg/min) Maintenance infusion: 50–200 μg/kg/min
	Propranolol	0.05–0.1 mg/kg over 5 min every 6h
SVT	Adenosine	50–100 μg/kg, increase by 50 μg/kg every 2 min to 400 μg/kg or 12 mg
	Digoxin	Dose is age dependent. IV dose is 75% of oral dose. Give in 3 doses (1/2 TDD, 1/4 TDD, 1/4 TDD) Preterm infant: 10–20 μg/kg TDD oral Term newborn-adolescent: 30–40 μg/kg TDD oral to maximal TDD of 1.0–1.5 mg (IV = 3/4 oral dose) Oral maintenance: 10 μg/kg/d every 12 h
	Phenylephrine	100 μg/kg bolus; infusion: 10 μg/kg/min
	Verapamil[a]	0.05 mg/kg–0.30 mg/kg over 3–5 min (Max dose = 10 mg)

Abbreviations: IV, intravenous; VT, ventricular tachycardia; SVT, supraventricular tachycardia; TDD, total digitalizing dose.
[a] Not for use in those younger than 1 year.

Table 3
Chronic pharmacologic agents for supraventricular and ventricular tachycardia

Arrhythmia	Agent	Dose (Oral)
SVT	Digoxin	
	Load in 3 doses	(1/2 TDD, 1/4 TDD, 1/4 TDD)
	Preterm infant:	10–20 µg/kg TDD
	Term newborn-adolescent:	30–40 µg/kg TDD oral to maximal TDD of 1–1.5 mg (IV = 3/4 oral dose)
	Verapamil	Oral maintenance: 10 µg/kg/d q12 h 2–8 mg/kg/d twice a day
VT	Phenytoin	Loading dose: 10–20 mg/kg/d q12 h × 2 d Maintenance: 5–10 mg/kg/d q12 h
	Mexiletine	5–15 mg/kg/d q8 h
SVT or VT	Propranolol	0.5–2 mg/kg/dose q6 h
	Nadolol	0.1–0.25 mg/kg/dose q12 h
	Atenolol	0.5–1 mg/kg/d qd
	Procainamide	20–100 mg/kg/d q4–6 h
	Disopyramide	5–15 mg/kg/d q6 h
	Flecainide	50–200 mg/m²/d or 3–6 mg/kg/d q12 h
	Amiodarone	Loading dose:10–20 mg/kg/day q12 h × 7 d Maintenance: 5–10 mg/kg/dose q d
	Sotalol	2–8 mg/kg/d q12 h
	Propafenone	Adolescent/adult: Immediate release 150–300 mg q8 h Extended release 225 mg q12 h

Abbreviations: IV, intravenous; RT$_3$, reverse T$_3$; SVT, supraventricular tachycardia; TDD, total digitalizing dose; q, every; VT, ventricular tachycardia.

Ectopic Atrial Tachycardia

General information
Ectopic atrial tachycardia (EAT), otherwise known as automatic atrial tachycardia, is caused by catecholamine-sensitive foci with increased automaticity within the atria. It results in inappropriately fast rates and P-wave axes that differ from sinus and are typically low right atrial with a negative P in aVF and positive P in I, or left atrial with a negative P in aVF and a negative P in I, or a positive P in aVF and a negative P in I. Occasionally, when the ectopic focus is near the sinus node, the ECG resembles sinus tachycardia. The rate, at 130 to 250 bpm, is typically not as fast as reentrant tachycardias. Related to its catecholamine sensitivity, EAT typically displays warm-up and cool-down phases, which can help differentiate EAT from other arrhythmias.

Presentation
Ectopic atrial tachycardia is responsible for approximately 18% of SVT in children.[11] Many children with EAT present with signs and symptoms of congestive heart failure from chronically elevated heart rates (usually over 150 bpm); although, when identified earlier, children may report only palpitations or chest pain.

Associated factors and etiology
EAT is believed to be secondary to abnormal foci in the atria. These may be congenital, acquired after a viral infection or after surgery for congenital heart disease.

Evaluation

Chest pain and a mildly elevated heart rate of 100 to 150 bpm, especially if the rate is slightly irregular, should raise concern for EAT and an ECG should be obtained (**Fig. 2**). When the diagnosis is not clear on ECG, Holter monitor or exercise testing can be helpful. On Holter monitoring, particular attention should be paid to the effects of exercise and sleep, as increases in the sinus rate with exercise or decreases in catecholaminergic stimulation during sleep may suppress EAT.

Treatment

Medical treatment initially should focus on slowing conduction through the AV node to control the heart rate or converting the rhythm to sinus, if possible. Some children will have spontaneous resolution of EAT, whereas others require eventual catheter ablation. Chest pain may become a more common complaint when medications are started, as children often begin to notice changes in rate when sinus rhythm is present for a portion of the day, and only periodic episodes of EAT are occurring

Multifocal Atrial Tachycardia

General information

Multifocal atrial tachycardia (MAT), also known as chaotic atrial tachycardia, is characterized by (1) 3 or more P waves of different morphology in a single ECG lead, (2) an isoelectric baseline between P waves (to distinguish it from atrial fibrillation and atrial flutter), and (3) PP and RR intervals of varying lengths.[12,13] Atrial rates can be as fast as 400 bpm and ventricular rates 150 to 250 bpm.[14,15] MAT is technically a supraventricular tachycardia. Unlike most other SVTs in children, the ventricular rate in MAT is highly irregular.

Presentation

More than one-half of children with MAT have no associated medical illness and most present in infancy. In one report of 21 children, the average age at presentation was 1.8 months, with 6 of 21 patients presenting at birth. These children were, therefore, unlikely to exhibit chest pain, but may have exhibited the infant's equivalent symptom,

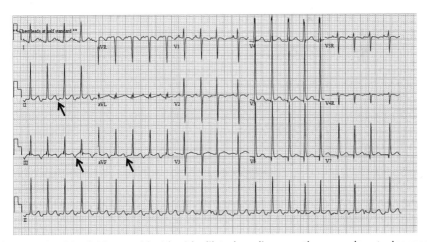

Fig. 2. EAT. ECG of 14-year-old girl with dilated cardiomyopathy secondary to incessant ectopic atrial tachycardia at 140 bpm. Note abnormal P-wave axis of −60 degrees, indicating a low right atrial focus. PR interval is prolonged to 200 msec. LVH and ST-T wave changes are present. Arrows denote ectopic P waves.

irritability. Half of children with MAT are asymptomatic at presentation, yet one-quarter have heart failure.[16,17] There have been case reports of older children presenting with chest pain alone.[12] Most children with MAT experience complete, spontaneous resolution of symptoms. In some reports, mortality has been quite high.[17]

Associated factors and etiology

Multifocal atrial tachycardia is rare in children, representing less than 1% of pediatric SVT, and is less commonly associated with chronic pulmonary disease or other conditions than it is in adults. Only about 100 cases in children have been described in the literature.[12] The exact mechanism of MAT is unknown.

Evaluation

An ECG should be obtained to clarify the diagnosis. When the diagnosis is not clear on ECG, Holter monitor or exercise testing can be helpful. ECHO can be used to evaluate cardiac structure and function.

Treatment

Optimal treatment for MAT remains unclear, although it is often treated similarly to EAT, except that catheter ablation is not effective in MAT. Given the high incidence of spontaneous resolution, and the lack of clear efficacy of treatments in aborting MAT, many cardiologists have proposed that asymptomatic children with MAT undergo close observation alone, although this depends on the underlying cardiac pathology and the physiologic effects of the rate and rhythm.[15]

Atrial Flutter

General information

Atrial flutter (A Flutter) results from a macroreentrant electrical circuit within the atrium. As with other supraventricular arrhythmias, the presence of chest pain depends on the underlying cardiac physiology, the rate of the tachycardia, its sudden onset, and its duration.

Presentation

Atrial flutter in children generally presents with a sensation of an increased heart rate. It is most commonly associated with underlying cardiac pathology, especially postoperative congenital heart disease. With 1:1 AV conduction and very rapid rates, it is not uncommon to present with chest pain, hypotension, and circulatory collapse, especially in those with congenital heart defects and decreased baseline cardiac output.

Associated factors and etiology

The differential of A Flutter includes intra-atrial reentrant tachycardias (IART), a slower macroreentrant atrial arrhythmia most commonly seen after atrial surgery for congenital heart defects. There is a high prevalence of IART, or incisional tachycardia, in children who have had precious cardiac surgeries involving atrial surgery and subsequent scarring, especially for single ventricle complexes (Fontan procedures) and for D-transposition of the great arteries (Senning or Mustard intra-atrial repairs).[18] Within the first postoperative decade, IART occurs in up to 50% of patients who had atriopulmonary Fontan connections for single ventricle physiology, and in up to 30% who had Mustard or Senning procedures. Other predisposing risk factors include sinus node dysfunction and older age at the time of surgery.[19]

Evaluation

Atrial Flutter typically appears as a sawtooth pattern on ECG, especially in leads II, III, aVF (**Fig. 3**). A flutter starts and stops abruptly and has atrial rates of 250 to 300 bpm

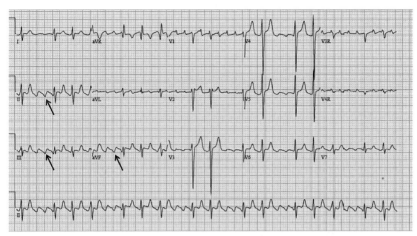

Fig. 3. Atrial flutter. ECG of 12-year-old boy, with an atrial septal defect, showing atrial flutter. Note sawtooth flutter waves, prominent in leads II, III, aVF (*black arrows*). Heart rate is irregular at 100 bpm.

and ventricular rates of 125 to 150 bpm; atrial rates as fast as 400 to 500 bpm in infants with variable AV conduction to the ventricle have been reported. The ventricular rate can vary and will depend on conduction of atrial impulses through the AV node or bypass tract to the ventricles, but is more likely to be more regular than in A Fib. With rapid conduction, A Flutter can be difficult to distinguish from SVT. In such cases, adenosine can be used for diagnostic purposes to unmask the atrial flutter waves by slowing AV nodal conduction. Unlike with reentrant circuits that require AV nodal conduction to sustain the tachycardia (AVRT or AVNRT), adenosine will not interrupt A Flutter.

IART occurs around surgical scars and areas of fixed obstruction. It does not have the sawtooth pattern of A Flutter and has more distinct P waves, generally with an abnormal axis (**Fig. 4**). It also tends to be slower than A Flutter (atrial rate 150 to 250 bpm, though atrial rates can be as higher). ECHO can be used to evaluate function.

Treatment
As with any arrhythmia, treatment of a hemodynamically unstable patient should begin with synchronized cardioversion. For stable patients, medical therapy may be attempted first, including rate control with β-blockers (see **Table 2**). Additionally, catheter ablation has been effective in this population, but more so in those with structurally normal hearts.[20,21]

Atrial Fibrillation

General information
Atrial fibrillation (A Fib), like A Flutter, is an atrial reentrant tachycardia that does not require the AV node to sustain the arrhythmia. In contrast to A Flutter, A Fib involves multiple, smaller, reentrant atrial circuits.

Presentation
Most children with A Fib present with complaints of palpitations, but some children describe their symptoms as pain, especially in association with very rapid heart rates. The irregular nature of this arrhythmia often results in a discomfort that is difficult for children to describe. Patients with A Fib are at increased risk of thromboembolic events, and a small group of children will not present until they develop stroke or

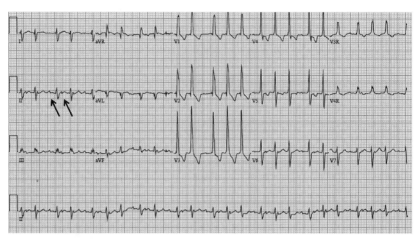

Fig. 4. Intra-atrial reentrant tachycardia. ECG of an 18-year-old, after Mustard intra-atrial repair of D-transposition of the great arteries, showing intra-atrial reentrant tachycardia with more distinct atrial waves (*dark arrows*) than is seen with atrial flutter. Atrial rate is 188 bpm with variable AV conduction. Ventricular rate is 150 bpm. ECG shows right ventricular hypertrophy.

pulmonary embolus, resulting in a different type of chest pain. There is one case report in the pediatric literature of a child who presented with chest pain, who was found to have A Fib and a pulmonary embolus.[13]

Associated factors and etiology

Most children who develop A Fib in developed countries have underlying congenital heart disease and, in particular, a history of cardiac surgery involving the atria. Of note, there is a population of adolescents with structurally normal hearts, who present with idiopathic A Fib, in whom chest pain is the initial complaint. Many of these adolescents do not experience recurrence of symptoms once the rhythm is converted, but those who do may require treatment.[2]

In the developing world, where rheumatic heart disease (RHD) is more prevalent, A Fib frequently develops in association with mitral valve disease and resultant left atrial dilation.[22] Other etiologies of A Fib include cardiomyopathies, whether viral (eg, Coxsackie, echovirus,), metabolic (eg, carnitine deficiency), or genetic (eg, dilated cardiomyopathy, hypertrophic cardiomyopathy); these conditions lead to dilated ventricles and stretched AV valves, resulting in valvar insufficiency and, hence, atrial dilation. Other conditions associated with A Fib include Brugada syndrome, WPW, metabolic abnormalities, ingestions (such as digoxin), hypokalemia, exogenous stimulants (such as psudoephedrine and albuterol), endogenous stimulants (such as those released in the setting of pheochromocytomas), and hyperthyroidism. Less common causes of A Fib in children include cardiac tumors, intra-atrial aneurysms, and other intra-atrial myocardial defects that disrupt the atrial myocardium and predispose to atrial fibrillation.[23]

Evaluation

The evaluation of suspected A Fib should include a careful history, with a past medical and family history and a history of access to medications such as digoxin. Laboratory investigations should include electrolytes, thyroid function tests, and drug levels if ingestion is suspected.

A 12- or 15-lead ECG should be obtained while the child is in the arrhythmia. Although adenosine will not convert A Fib, it can be used to unmask the diagnosis when administered in conjunction with an ECG, as it slows conduction through the AV node, making the rhythm easier to identify. A Fib usually has an abrupt onset and offset, but may be incessant, making symptoms harder to appreciate. On ECG, A Fib frequently is described as an irregularly irregular, narrow complex rhythm. The associated rate is typically 350 to 400 bpm, with variable AV conduction and irregular ventricular rates. As in A Flutter, the ventricular rate depends on conduction through the AV node or a bypass tract to the ventricles. Therefore, the ventricular rate can vary. At high rates, the conduction through the ventricle may be aberrant, resulting in wide QRS complexes (**Fig. 5**). An ECG in sinus rhythm should be obtained to look for signs of associated conditions, such as WPW or Brugada syndrome. An ECHO should be performed to verify cardiac structure and function and to look for evidence of intracardiac thrombi.

Treatment
Treatment of a hemodynamically unstable patient should begin with synchronized cardioversion. For stable patients, medical therapy may be attempted as first-line treatment. Except in patients with WPW, digoxin can be used to control the ventricular rate, by slowing conduction through the AV node. In patients with WPW, both digoxin and verapamil should be avoided, as these may enhance conduction through accessory pathways, while slowing AV nodal conduction, thereby triggering a more rapid ventricular rate in response to A Fib. If medical therapies fail, synchronized cardioversion may be necessary. Use of anticoagulation should follow published guidelines.[24,25]

Junctional Ectopic Tachycardia

General information
Junctional ectopic tachycardia (JET) is an SVT, characterized by a narrow QRS at a rate faster than the sinus rate, usually resulting in AV dissociation, with a slower atrial than ventricular rate. JET is the result of enhanced automatic foci in the AV junction.

Presentation and associated factors and etiology
JET occurs most commonly shortly after open heart surgery, but it can present as a congenital familial arrhythmia, as well. Because these children are usually very

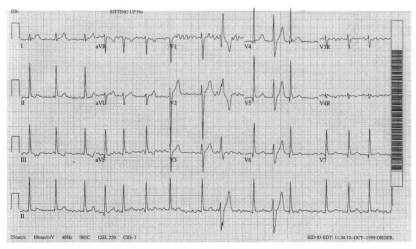

Fig. 5. Atrial fibrillation. ECG of 15-year-old boy, with no known heart disease, and an irregularly irregular rhythm, indicating atrial fibrillation. Note rapid atrial waves of varying rates and morphology and both aberrant and narrow QRS complexes.

young, they may experience chest pain from the rapid rates and coronary insufficiency, but are unable to express this symptom and simply appear irritable and uncomfortable. Postoperative JET is usually limited to the first 48 to 72 hours after surgery and typically resolves with supportive and pharmacologic therapy.

Evaluation

ECG shows a faster junctional than atrial rate, with a narrow QRS, unless aberrant conduction is present (**Fig. 6**). One-to-one retrograde ventriculoatrial conduction can occur. In older children with congenital JET, a Holter monitor can be used to determine if intermittent periods of sinus rhythm occur. ECHO can be used to evaluate function.

Treatment

Cardioversion is not effective with ectopic tachycardias. The initial treatment of JET is pharmacologic. For persistent congenital JET, catheter ablation may be indicated.[26,27]

PREMATURE VENTRICULAR CONTRACTIONS
General Information

Premature ventricular contractions (PVCs) occur commonly in the general population; they are seen in up to one-third of adolescents without and two-thirds of adolescents with structural heart disease.[2]

Presentation

PVCs are often benign and usually are not associated with any serious symptoms. Some children may report feelings of missed or hard beats, "fluttering in the chest," or chest pain or discomfort. Because of the high frequency of PVCs in the general population, they may be one of the most common arrhythmogenic causes of chest pain in children. Chest pain in children with PVCs is usually the result of enhanced diastolic filling related to the extended post extrasystolic pause with a large stroke volume in the contraction after the PVC. On the other hand, the presence of PVCs in association

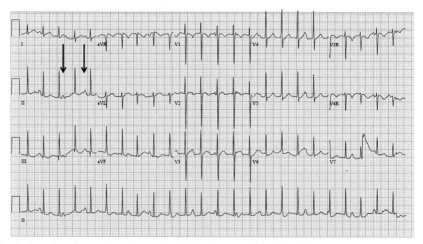

Fig. 6. Junctional ectopic tachycardia. ECG of 5-year-old girl with junctional ectopic tachycardia. Arrows denote P waves with atrial rate of 100 bpm. Narrow QRS complexes originating from the AV junction occur at rate of 144 bpm. There is AV dissociation with a faster junctional than atrial rate.

with chest pain could indicate a more serious, underlying, cardiac condition. Frequent PVCs or runs of PVCs, ventricular tachycardia, can cause ischemia by decreasing cardiac output. Long-term follow-up of children with PVCs demonstrates 37% to 65% regression in patients with structurally normal hearts. Sudden death is rare in patients with PVCs in the absence of underlying cardiac conditions.[28]

Associated Factors and Etiology

In children with structurally normal hearts, PVCs that represent less than 20% of the rhythm usually do not affect cardiac function. PVCs that represent greater than 30% of the rhythm can result in ventricular dysfunction and are more likely to result in chest pain. For children with underlying structural or functional heart disease or primary electrical heart conditions, PVCs may portend more ominous rhythms, such as VT and ventricular fibrillation (VF), especially if the PVCs are complex, or an underlying repolarization abnormality, such as long QT syndrome or cathecholaminergic polymorphic VT (CPVT), is present. However, even asymptomatic PVCs may be associated with a malignant underlying condition.[2,6]

Evaluation

An ECG should be performed to confirm the diagnosis of PVCs. Acute causes such as electrolyte abnormalities, stimulant use, or drug ingestions should be investigated. If PVCs are frequent, coupled or complex, or associated with VT, especially in children with underlying cardiac disease, 24-hour Holter monitoring should be performed to determine the extent of the abnormality. For patients with concerning 24-hour Holter monitoring, exercise stress testing, echocardiogram, MRI, CT angiography or cardiac catheterization and electrophysiological study should be considered in a stepwise fashion. Suppression of PVCs with exercise is generally considered a positive sign. Increased PVC frequency during exercise is concerning. Particular attention should also be paid to the corrected QT interval, especially in the recovery phase after exercise, as frequent PVCs can be associated with long QT syndrome (LQTS), and PVCs in these patients are more likely to fall on the T-waves and, thereby, trigger torsades de pointes or VF.[2,6]

Treatment

In the absence of structural or functional heart disease, it is generally not necessary to treat isolated PVCs. Treatment of complex PVCs may be necessary in patients with physiologic or symptomatic concerns. Additionally, underlying conditions, such as metabolic or electrolyte abnormalities, should be corrected. PVCs that represent the potential for initiating more serious ventricular arrhythmias may need to be treated, but caution is advised, as studies have shown that eliminating PVCs does not decrease the risk of sudden death and may increase the risk in some cases, as was shown in the Cardiac Arrhythmia Suppression Trial.[29]

Assurance that the sensation of chest pain caused by the PVC does not indicate a serious heart condition may relieve anxiety and be the only treatment that is needed.

VENTRICULAR TACHYCARDIA
General Information

Ventricular tachycardia (VT) is a wide complex tachycardia that may be associated with chest pain in children, especially if the rate is fast and if there is underlying cardiac dysfunction.

Presentation

Although up to two-thirds of children with structurally normal hearts and VT are asymptomatic at diagnosis, children with structural heart disease and VT are typically symptomatic.[30,31] In both populations, VT may present with chest or abdominal pain, palpitations, dizziness, syncope, dyspnea, shortness of breath, diaphoresis, exercise intolerance and easy fatigability, or signs and symptoms of heart failure. Chest pain is particularly common in children with structural heart disease and VT.

Associated Factors and Etiology

Although VT is uncommon in children with structurally normal hearts, it is typically seen in 2 settings: right ventricular outflow tract VT and left ventricular fascicular VT. Both present most commonly in adolescence. The first symptom in these children is often chest pain associated with a sensation of a rapid heart rate. VT, in a structurally normal heart, tends to be paroxysmal, and therefore may present as intermittent episodes of chest pain. Initially, the blood pressure falls, which can initiate pain, as myocardial ischemia may occur.

With an increasing number of children surviving correction of complex congenital cardiac disease, VT frequency is increasing.[32] Children with a history of ventriculotomy, ventricular patches (eg, repair of tetralogy of Fallot, ventricular septal defect (VSD), or AV canal defects), or resection of subpulmonic or subaortic obstruction are most susceptible to VT and also are most likely to develop myocardial ischemia and chest pain in the setting of VT. Children with early postoperative VT are more likely to develop recurrent episodes in the late post-operative period. New-onset VT in the very late postoperative period may herald the presence of a new hemodynamic lesion.[32]

Factors associated with chest pain and VT, after congenital heart surgery, include decreased cardiac function, abnormal coronary arteries, older age, and longer postoperative interval. Children with ventricular dysfunction without a history of surgery are at risk of VT.[18] Polymorphic VT, especially in association with LQTS, is particularly likely to present with chest pain, as this very rapid rhythm can significantly impact cardiac output, with resultant myocardial ischemia.[2]

Evaluation

An ECG will generally identify the presence of VT, defined as 3 or more complexes arising from the ventricles. In VT, AV dissociation is common, although some children, especially the very young, will display 1:1 retrograde ventriculoatrial conduction (**Fig. 7**). In children, the normal width of the QRS complex is age specific, and a wide QRS complex in infants and young children, as seen in VT, may be as narrow as 80 msec. The rate of VT in children may vary from 120 to 300 bpm. The presence, on prior cardiac monitoring, of PVCs with similar morphology is further suggestive of the diagnosis of VT. Although VT can look like SVT with bundle branch aberrancy or A Flutter with aberrancy, a practitioner should assume that a wide complex tachycardia is VT until proven otherwise, as failure to rapidly identify and treat VT can result in cardiovascular collapse and death.

The underlying acute (electrolyte or drug ingestion) condition should be sought, as reversal of acute conditions can often result in resolution of VT. Additionally, chronic contributing conditions should be investigated.

Treatment

As VT can rapidly deteriorate into ventricular fibrillation or a cardiac arrest, even asymptomatic children with rapid VT should be treated immediately. If ventricular fibrillation

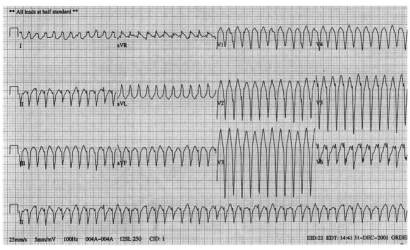

Fig. 7. Ventricular tachycardia. ECG of 16-year-old boy, with repaired tetralogy of Fallot, showing a wide complex tachycardia from the ventricle at 273 bpm. VT pattern is left bundle branch block, suggesting origin of the VT from the right ventricle.

occurs, defibrillation should be used. Treatment of a hemodynamically compromised patient in VT should start with synchronized cardioversion starting at 0.5 J/kg and doubling to 4.0 J/kg. Defibrillation should start at 2 J/kg and doubling to 4 J/kg. Underlying acute conditions, such as electrolyte abnormalities, should be corrected when possible. Acute and chronic medications are shown in **Tables 2** and **3**. Catheter ablation has been used successfully in some patients, as have implantable cardioverter defibrillators. Stable patients with postoperative VT, especially post tetralogy of Fallot (TOF) repair, commonly have VT amenable to ablation.[33,34]

BRADYCARDIAS

Bradycardias result from either sinus or AV nodal dysfunction and can lead to chest pain of cardiac origin.

Sinus Node Dysfunction

General information
Sinus node dysfunction (SND), also known as sick sinus syndrome (SSS), is a failure of the sinus node to generate action potentials and manifests as inappropriately slow atrial rates, including sinus bradycardia, sinus arrest, sinus node exit block, or asystole. Episodic atrial tachyarrhythmias (tachycardia-bradycardia syndrome) also may be seen.

Presentation
Slow heart rates can produce symptoms of chest pain in children, particularly if they are of sudden onset, as with asystole, sinus pause, or exit block. Although SND is significantly more common in adults, it should be considered in children presenting with chest pain, fatigue, exercise intolerance, palpitations, dizziness, syncope, and heart failure, especially if the heart rate is slower than expected for age. Some children may report no symptoms and the diagnosis may be made incidentally, when an ECG is obtained for another reason.

Toddlers can present with a history consistent with breath-holding spells, in which mild noxious or vagal stimuli, such as hair combing or scolding, result in syncope.

These children will often clutch their chest as if in pain before passing out. In some of these children, sinus arrest has been described to be as long as 20 seconds. This may be the result of a hypervagal response, but could be the additive effect of excessive vagal tone and an underlying abnormal sinus node. Although breath-holding spells are a significantly more common etiology of syncope in toddlers than is sinus node dysfunction, an evaluation of syncope in a child, even with a history consistent with breath holding, warrants an ECG and ECG monitoring during symptoms.[2]

Associated Factors and Etiology

In children, sinus node dysfunction occurs most commonly in the setting of trauma to the sinus node or the sinus node artery (typically after cardiac surgery), inflammatory or infiltrative diseases, and structural abnormalities (such as absence of the right superior vena cava [SVC] with persistent left SVC or heterotaxy syndromes). Pediatric studies from the 1970s reported that 80% of patients with SND had a history of previous cardiac surgery for congenital heart disease, especially surgery involving the atria.[35–38] Recently, increasing attention has focused on familial sick sinus syndrome, a genetic form of the disease, resulting from mutations in a variety of ion channels. Most of the gene mutations identified to date show autosomal dominant inheritance, with incomplete penetrance, although a few are autosomal recessive.[39]

Evaluation

A diagnosis of SND typically can be made on ECG and/or 24-hour Holter monitor. An ECHO should be performed to rule out structural heart disease and evaluate ventricular function. If the child is old enough, exercise testing can be performed to evaluate chronotropic competence.

Treatment

The primary treatment for most children with symptomatic sinus node dysfunction is a lifelong implantable pacemaker. In patients with sinus node dysfunction secondary to arrhythmias, such as A Fib or A Flutter, resolution has sometimes been observed with ablation of the primary arrhythmia.[40] Treatment may not be necessary for asymptomatic children with normal heart size and function, although these children should be monitored closely.[2] Medical treatment can be attempted in some children and others will require pacemakers. For details, see **Table 4**.

Atrioventricular Conduction Blocks

General information

In complete heart block, there is complete disruption of AV conduction with resultant slow junctional or ventricular escape rhythms. The defect most commonly originates in the AV node, but may involve the bundle of His. AV conduction block occurs infrequently in children, but it may be associated with chest pain, especially when intermittent or sudden in onset.

In children, complete heart block (3° AV block) is the most common cause of significant bradycardia that does not resolve with stimulation; sinus bradycardia, often seen in sleeping children, resolves promptly upon waking.[2] Congenital complete heart block (CCHB) is estimated to occur in 1 in 15,000 to 20,000 live births, although its incidence in all pregnancies is higher, as it is associated with significant in utero mortality.[41]

Presentation

Fetuses and neonates with CCHB typically present with slow heart rates, heart failure, or hydrops. Older children are frequently asymptomatic, although they can present

Table 4
Acute pharmacologic treatment of bradycardia

Initial Treatment

Agent	Dosage
Atropine	0.02–0.04 mg/kg IV
Isoproterenol	0.01–2 μg/kg/min IV
Secondary Treatments	
Caffeine citrate	Loading oral dose: 20–30 mg/kg Maintenance: 5–6 mg/kg/d <6 wk: 4 mg/kg/d 6 wk to 6 mo: 10 mg/kg/d 6 mo to 1 y: 12–18 mg/kg/d 1–9 y: 20–24 mg/kg/d
Theophylline	9–12 y and adolescent and adult daily smokers: 16 mg/kg/d 12–16 y nonsmokers: 13 mg/kg/d >16 year nonsmokers: 10 mg/kg/d (max 900 mg/d) Cardiac decompensation, cor pulmonale, and/or liver dysfunction: 5 mg/kg/d (max 400 mg/d)

Abbreviation: IV, intravenous.

with signs or symptoms of heart failure or cardiac ischemia, including exercise intolerance or chest pain. Of note, a subset of children may present with dizziness or syncope. Children most likely to develop symptoms of chest pain are those with compromised myocardial function, such as those with underlying structural or functional cardiac abnormalities or those with neuromuscular disorders. The small subset of children with CCHB who develop dilated cardiomyopathy are more likely to experience chest pain.[42]

Associated factors and etiology
Etiology of 3° AV block can be congenital or acquired and most commonly includes autoimmune (eg, lupus) and neuromuscular disorders (eg, Emery-Dreifuss muscular dystrophy, Kearns-Sayre syndrome, and myotonic dystrophy), postoperative trauma to the AV node or conduction system, and infections (eg, Lyme myocarditis), as well as familial, autosomal dominant, idiopathic heart block. The vast majority of children with congenital complete heart block develop this condition in utero, or as neonates. Those with acquired complete heart block present in childhood or after surgery for congenital heart disease.

Antiphospholipid antibody syndrome, the result in a fetus of a maternal autoimmune condition, is the most common cause of congenital heart block. Of note, although antiphospholipid antibody syndrome typically results in heart block between 16 and 24 weeks of gestation, with a high associated morbidity and mortality, other manifestations include late-onset ectopy or ischemia and associated chest pain, and should be considered in the differential of any child with chest pain and a slow heart rate. In addition, although antiphospholipid antibody syndrome classically occurs in the setting of maternal lupus, it has been described in other connective tissue disorders, such as Sjogren. Also of note, although mothers will have autoantibodies (anti-Ro/SS-A and anti-La/SS-B), over half of mothers have no signs of active disease.[42]

Structural heart disease has been described in one-fourth to one-third of patients with congenital CHB.[2] Although the incidence of surgically induced heart block has declined steadily since the early surgical era (from 10% to 1%–2% of all cardiac surgery),[43] patients with L-looped ventricles or those undergoing procedures aimed at decreasing left ventricular outflow tract obstruction are still at risk. Other procedures that place patients at risk include mitral valve replacement as well as repair of VSDs (1%),[43] complete AV canal (up to 7%),[44] and L-TGA (over 20%).[45] Although most heart block develops during surgery or in the immediate postoperative period, it has been reported to occur as late as 14 years postoperatively.[44]

Lyme carditis typically presents 3 to 10 weeks after initial infection and is associated with varying degrees of AV block, as well as junctional rhythms and asystolic pauses.[46] In adults with Lyme disease, 4% to 10% are estimated to have cardiac involvement,[47] and up to 50% of patients with cardiac involvement develop complete heart block.[48] Cardiac manifestations appear to be much less common in children, with only 1% developing Lyme carditis in the largest prospective pediatric study to date (2 of 201 patients).[49] Chest pain is a common complaint in these patients, both with and without arrhythmias.

Evaluation

All children suspected of CHB should have an ECG. Heart rates (ventricular rates) in children with CHB usually range from 40 to 100 bpm, depending on the child's age, and show more rapid atrial than ventricular rates (**Fig. 8**). All children with first-, second-, or third-degree AV block should undergo Holter monitoring to correlate symptoms with rhythm, determine the slowest heart rate, longest pause, QRS duration, and QTc interval, as well as to evaluate periods of complete block or ventricular arrhythmias. In older children, exercise stress testing should be used to determine the extent of ventricular ectopy and chronotropic incompetence.

An ECG should be obtained if Lyme carditis or other associated inflammatory condition is suspected.

Treatment

Treatment of children with heart block depends on the type of block, severity of the symptoms, age of the child, and etiology. Asymptomatic older children can often be followed with observation. Pacemakers in children are generally placed for very low heart rates or long pauses. Fatigue, or other cardiac symptoms, including chest

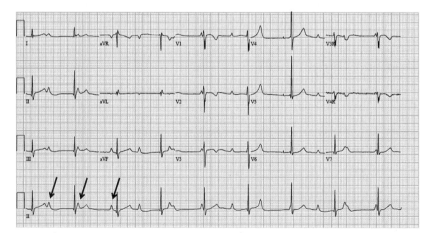

Fig. 8. Congenital complete heart block. ECG of 12-year-old girl with congenital complete heart block. Atrial rate is 70 bpm and faster than ventricular rate of 50 bpm. The QRS complex is narrow, suggesting it originates from high in the AV junction. Arrows denote P waves.

pain, especially during exercise, also can be indications for a pacemaker, as they can be indicative of myocardial ischemia from inadequate cardiac output. In a longitudinal study of 102 patients with congenital CHB followed over 30 years, 90% of patients required pacemakers and there was a 20% incidence of SCD. Poor prognostic signs included prolonged QTc interval and mitral regurgitation.[50] Treatment guidelines for Lyme carditis recommend antibiotics and, possibly, steroids in the case of heart block.[51–54] Some of the patients with acquired heart block, such as Lyme carditis, have significantly better prognosis and will less often require pacemaker implantation.

CHEST PAIN ASSOCIATED WITH OTHER INFECTIOUS AND INFLAMMATORY CONDITIONS
Rheumatic Heart Disease and Associated Arrhythmias

Although chest pain associated with rheumatic heart disease (RHD) is usually seen in the setting of decreased coronary perfusion from aortic regurgitation or stenosis, it can also result from A Fib in association with mitral valve disease or, occasionally, aortic valve disease. The presence of A Fib in the setting of RHD and mitral insufficiency (MI) or mitral stenosis (MS) is common, as the result of left atrial dilation from valvar obstruction secondary to inflammatory and fibrotic changes from the rheumatic process. Chest pain results from the dramatic drop in cardiac output, which may be up to 30% when A Fib starts. Patients with MS or MS and MI are more likely to experience A Fib than those with isolated MI. A Fib is an uncommon complication of isolated aortic stenosis (AS) or aortic regurgitation (AR) in RHD, but its associated drop in cardiac output can result in chest pain or more severe consequences. Of note, chest pain associated with RHD and AS is associated with an estimated 5-year survival after presentation with chest pain, and chest pain associated with RHD and AR is associated with a 10% mortality per year.[22]

Myocarditis

Chest pain is a common presenting symptoms in children with myocarditis and may be associated with serious arrhythmias, either complete heart block or ventricular tachycardia.[55] The presentation of myocarditis, whether infectious or infiltrative in etiology, is often nonspecific and may range from mild flu-like symptoms and chest or abdominal pain to fulminant heart failure, shock, and cardiovascular collapse.

Pediatric chest pain, especially in the setting of fever, respiratory distress, lethargy, new murmur or abnormal heart sounds, hepatomegaly, and tachy- or bradycardia, should prompt consideration of this diagnosis. Although the classic ECG findings associated with myocarditis include tachycardia and ST-segment elevation or depression, similar to that seen in myocardial infarction, these findings are less than 50% sensitive for myocarditis.[56] Other findings include heart block, EAT, JET, bundle branch block, and atrial or ventricular arrhythmias, all of which may make chest pain more likely to occur.

The most common etiology of myocarditis in the developed world is viral (especially Coxsackie, parvo B-19, and human herpes virus-6), but in the developing world decreased access to vaccines and the increased incidence of diseases such as HIV and tuberculosis dramatically increase the incidence of myocarditis from these conditions. Other etiologies include drug reactions, heavy metal ingestions, and auto-immune and other systemic diseases. As mortality associated with pediatric myocarditis has been reported to be as high as 25%, prompt recognition of this condition is essential. Treatment should be aimed improving cardiac output and treating arrhythmias. No evidence exists for the use of antiviral drugs, anti-inflammatory agents, or steroids, although some evidence supports the use of intravenous immune globulin (IVIG) in children. Most of the arrhythmias will abate in 4 to 6 weeks, but temporary or implantable pacemakers or implantable cardioverter defibrillators (ICDs) may be indicated if the arrhythmias are refractory to medical therapy or persistent.[56] Persistently low cardiac output after pacemaker implantation and late-onset VT are poor prognostic signs, as are syncope, right ventricular systolic dysfunction, elevated pulmonary artery pressure, and advanced New York Heart Association (NYHA) functional class.[56,57]

SUMMARY

While cardiac causes of chest pain in children are infrequent, arrhythmias are implicated in most cases. Most of these are caused by supraventricular tachycardias or PVCs, and are self-limited, but more ominous rhythms, such as VT or bradycardias can manifest as chest pain. Investigation of all children with chest pain should include detailed history and physical examination and a 12- or 15-lead ECG if arrhythmia is suspected. In some cases ECHO, 24-hour Holter monitoring, exercise stress testing, or other cardiac evaluations may be indicated. Children with abnormal cardiac examination, abnormal ECG, or abnormal personal or family cardiac history should be referred to a pediatric cardiologist for further evaluation and management. Children with a history of cardiac disease or cardiac surgery should receive special attention when they complain of symptoms of chest pain, as they are particularly at risk for life-threatening arrhythmias and more commonly experience chest pain in association with their arrhythmias.

REFERENCES

1. Salerno JC, Seslar SP. Supraventricular tachycardia. Arch Pediatr Adolesc Med 2009;163:268–74.
2. Vetter VL, Rhodes LA. Evaluation and management of arrhythmias. In: Saksena S, Dorian P, Camm J, editors. Electrophysiologic disorders of the heart. Philadelphia: Elsevier; 2005. p. 533–66.
3. Fyfe DA, Moodie DS. Chest pain in pediatric patients presenting to a cardiac clinic. Clin Pediatr (Phila) 1984;23:321–4.
4. Kaden GG, Shenker IR, Gootman N. Chest pain in adolescents. J Adolesc Health 1991;12:251–5.
5. Anderson BR, John AS. Syncope. Netter's pediatrics. Philadelphia: Elsevier; 2010.
6. Doniger SJ, Sharieff GQ. Pediatric dysrhythmias. Pediatr Clin North Am 2006;53: 85–105, vi.
7. Vos P, Pulles-Heintzberger CF, Delhaas T. Supraventricular tachycardia: an incidental diagnosis in infants and difficult to prove in children. Acta Paediatr 2003;92:1058–61.
8. Perry JC, Garson A Jr. Supraventricular tachycardia due to Wolff-Parkinson-White syndrome in children: early disappearance and late recurrence. J Am Coll Cardiol 1990;16:1215–20.
9. Garson A, Bricker JT, McNamara DG. The science and practice of pediatric cardiology. Philadelphia: Lea and Febiger; 1990.
10. Bardy GH, Packer DL, German LD, et al. Preexcited reciprocating tachycardia in patients with Wolff-Parkinson-White syndrome: incidence and mechanisms. Circulation 1984;70:377–91.

11. Gillette PC, Garson A Jr. Electrophysiologic and pharmacologic characteristics of automatic ectopic atrial tachycardia. Circulation 1977;56:571–5.
12. Hsieh MY, Lee PC, Hwang B, et al. Multifocal atrial tachycardia in 2 children. J Chin Med Assoc 2006;69:439–43.
13. Szwast A, Hanna B, Shah M. Atrial fibrillation and pulmonary embolism. Pediatr Emerg Care 2007;23:826–8.
14. Bradley DJ, Fischbach PS, Law IH, et al. The clinical course of multifocal atrial tachycardia in infants and children. J Am Coll Cardiol 2001;38:401–8.
15. Zuckerman GB, Conway EE Jr, Singh J, et al. Multifocal atrial tachycardia in a child presenting with chest pain. Pediatr Emerg Care 1993;9:348–50.
16. Bevilacqua LM, Rhee EK, Epstein MR, et al. Focal ablation of chaotic atrial rhythm in an infant with cardiomyopathy. J Cardiovasc Electrophysiol 2000;11:577–81.
17. Epstein ML, Kiel EA, Victorica BE. Cardiac decompensation following verapamil therapy in infants with supraventricular tachycardia. Pediatrics 1985;75:737–40.
18. Walsh EP. Interventional electrophysiology in patients with congenital heart disease. Circulation 2007;115:3224–34.
19. Puley G, Siu S, Connelly M, et al. Arrhythmia and survival in patients >18 years of age after the mustard procedure for complete transposition of the great arteries. Am J Cardiol 1999;83:1080–4.
20. Kalman JM, VanHare GF, Olgin JE, et al. Ablation of 'incisional' reentrant atrial tachycardia complicating surgery for congenital heart disease. Use of entrainment to define a critical isthmus of conduction. Circulation 1996;93:502–12.
21. Triedman JK, Saul JP, Weindling SN, et al. Radiofrequency ablation of intra-atrial reentrant tachycardia after surgical palliation of congenital heart disease. Circulation 1995;91:707–14.
22. Rheumatic fever and rheumatic heart disease. Geneva (Switzerland): World Health Organization; 2004. World Health Organization Technical Report Series 923.
23. Zachary CH, Cyran SE. Spontaneous-onset atrial fibrillation in a toddler with review of mechanisms and etiologies. Clin Pediatr (Phila) 2000;39:453–9.
24. Singer DE, Albers GW, Dalen JE, et al. Antithrombotic therapy in atrial fibrillation: American College of Chest Physicians evidence-based clinical practice guidelines (8th edition). Chest 2008;133:546S–92S.
25. Fuster V, Ryden LE, Cannom DS, et al. ACC/AHA/ESC 2006 guidelines for the management of patients with atrial fibrillation: a report of the American College of Cardiology/American Heart Association task force on practice guidelines and the European Society of Cardiology committee for practice guidelines (writing committee to revise the 2001 guidelines for the management of patients with atrial fibrillation): developed in collaboration with the European Heart Rhythm Association and the Heart Rhythm Society. Circulation 2006;114:e257–354.
26. Collins KK, Van Hare GF, Kertesz NJ, et al. Pediatric nonpost-operative junctional ectopic tachycardia medical management and interventional therapies. J Am Coll Cardiol 2009;53:690–7.
27. Rychik J, Marchlinski FE, Sweeten TL, et al. Transcatheter radiofrequency ablation for congenital junctional ectopic tachycardia in infancy. Pediatr Cardiol 1997;18:447–50.
28. Tsuji A, Nagashima M, Hasegawa S, et al. Long-term follow-up of idiopathic ventricular arrhythmias in otherwise normal children. Jpn Circ J 1995;59:654–62.
29. Ruskin JN. The cardiac arrhythmia suppression trial (CAST). N Engl J Med 1989;321:386–8.
30. Deal BJ, Miller SM, Scagliotti D, et al. Ventricular tachycardia in a young population without overt heart disease. Circulation 1986;73:1111–8.

31. Fulton DR, Chung KJ, Tabakin BS, et al. Ventricular tachycardia in children without heart disease. Am J Cardiol 1985;55:1328–31.
32. Vetter VL. Ventricular arrhythmias in pediatric patients with and without congenital heart disease. In: Horowitz LN, editor. Current management of arrhythmias. Philadelphia: BD Decker; 1991. p. 208–20.
33. Morwood JG, Triedman JK, Berul CI, et al. Radiofrequency catheter ablation of ventricular tachycardia in children and young adults with congenital heart disease. Heart Rhythm 2004;1:301–8.
34. Horowitz LN, Vetter VL, Harken AH, et al. Electrophysiologic characteristics of sustained ventricular tachycardia occurring after repair of tetralogy of Fallot. Am J Cardiol 1980;46:446–52.
35. Kugler JD, Gillette PC, Mullins CE, et al. Sinoatrial conduction in children: an index of sinoatrial node function. Circulation 1979;59:1266–76.
36. Radford DJ, Izukawa T. Sick sinus syndrome. Symptomatic cases in children. Arch Dis Child 1975;50:879–85.
37. Yabek SM, Swensson RE, Jarmakani JM. Electrocardiographic recognition of sinus node dysfunction in children and young adults. Circulation 1977;56:235–9.
38. Yabek SM, Jarmakani JM. Sinus node dysfunction in children, adolescents, and young adults. Pediatrics 1978;61:593–8.
39. Benson DW, Wang DW, Dyment M, et al. Congenital sick sinus syndrome caused by recessive mutations in the cardiac sodium channel gene (SCN5A). J Clin Invest 2003;112:1019–28.
40. Hocini M, Sanders P, Deisenhofer I, et al. Reverse remodeling of sinus node function after catheter ablation of atrial fibrillation in patients with prolonged sinus pauses. Circulation 2003;108:1172–5.
41. Jaeggi ET, Friedberg MK. Diagnosis and management of fetal bradyarrhythmias. Pacing Clin Electrophysiol 2008;31(Suppl 1):S50–3.
42. Jayaprasad N, Johnson F, Venugopal K. Congenital complete heart block and maternal connective tissue disease. Int J Cardiol 2006;112:153–8.
43. Gross GJ, Chiu CC, Hamilton RM, et al. Natural history of postoperative heart block in congenital heart disease: implications for pacing intervention. Heart Rhythm 2006;3:601–4.
44. Moss AJ, Klyman G, Emmanouilides GC. Late onset complete heart block. Newly recognized sequela of cardiac surgery. Am J Cardiol 1972;30:884–7.
45. Deal BJ, Mavroudis C, Backer CL. Arrhythmia management in the Fontan patient. Pediatr Cardiol 2007;28:448–56.
46. Silver E, Pass RH, Kaufman S, et al. Complete heart block due to Lyme carditis in two pediatric patients and a review of the literature. Congenit Heart Dis 2007;2:338–41.
47. Cox J, Krajden M. Cardiovascular manifestations of Lyme disease. Am Heart J 1991;122:1449–55.
48. van der Linde MR. Lyme carditis: clinical characteristics of 105 cases. Scand J Infect Dis Suppl 1991;77:81–4.
49. Gerber MA, Shapiro ED, Burke GS, et al. Lyme disease in children in Southeastern Connecticut. Pediatric Lyme Disease Study Group. N Engl J Med 1996;335:1270–4.
50. Michaelsson M, Jonzon A, Riesenfeld T. Isolated congenital complete atrioventricular block in adult life. A prospective study. Circulation 1995;92:442–9.
51. McAlister HF, Klementowicz PT, Andrews C, et al. Lyme carditis: an important cause of reversible heart block. Ann Intern Med 1989;110:339–45.
52. Sigal LH. Early disseminated lyme disease: cardiac manifestations. Am J Med 1995;98:25S–8S.

53. Steere AC, Batsford WP, Weinberg M, et al. Lyme carditis: cardiac abnormalities of lyme disease. Ann Intern Med 1980;93:8–16.
54. Wormser GP, Nadelman RB, Dattwyler RJ, et al. Practice guidelines for the treatment of lyme disease. The Infectious Diseases Society of America. Clin Infect Dis 2000;31(Suppl 1):1–14.
55. Freedman SB, Haladyn JK, Floh A, et al. Pediatric myocarditis: emergency department clinical findings and diagnostic evaluation. Pediatrics 2007;120: 1278–85.
56. Blauwet LA, Cooper LT. Myocarditis. Prog Cardiovasc Dis 2010;52:274–88.
57. Chien SJ, Liang CD, Lin IC, et al. Myocarditis complicated by complete atrioventricular block: nine years' experience in a medical center. Pediatr Neonatol 2008; 49:218–22.

Gastroesophageal Reflux, Eosinophilic Esophagitis, and Foreign Body

Jose M. Garza, MD, Ajay Kaul, MD*

KEYWORDS
- GERD • Foreign body • Chest pain • Pediatrics

Chest pain as a presenting symptom is more common in older children and is usually benign without a life-threatening cause. Infants, toddlers, and children with neurodevelopmental delays (NDD) are often unable to communicate clearly and may therefore present with nonspecific symptoms such as fussiness or other behavioral changes. The causes of chest pain include musculoskeletal, cardiovascular, pulmonary, gastrointestinal (GI), psychogenic, and idiopathic. Only about 0.2% to 0.6% of pediatric emergency room visits are for chest pain[1] and the most common cause (up to 60%) reported in children over 4-years-old is "idiopathic."[2] Prevalence of identified GI diagnosis as a cause of chest pain in children is low (5%–8%).[2,3] Although history and associated symptoms are helpful in revealing the underlying cause for the chest pain, it may often be misleading. As an example, even though epigastric tenderness associated with chest pain is usually indicative of a GI pathology,[4] exertion-associated chest pain does not necessarily rule out a GI cause.[5] It has, therefore, been suggested that children with chest pain be evaluated for upper GI disorders even if associated symptoms may or may not suggest a GI diagnosis.[6] The most consistent symptom of an esophageal disorder is pain localized alongside the course of the esophagus (retrosternal).[7]

In pediatrics, common esophageal causes of chest pain include eosinophilic esophagitis (EoE), gastroesophageal reflux disease (GERD), and motility disorders.[8,9] Accidental ingestion of foreign bodies that are lodged in the esophagus may also present with chest pain. In a study of 19 children, aged 10 to 17 years, complaining of substernal chest pain, 42% had replication of chest pain symptoms with acid infusion and 3 of these 8 patients exhibited abnormal esophageal motility during infusion. All of these patients showed excellent response to acid suppression.[10] This study underscores

The authors have nothing to disclose.
Division of Gastroenterology, Hepatology and Nutrition, Cincinnati Children's Hospital Medical Center, 3333 Burnet Avenue MLC 2010, Cincinnati, OH 45229, USA
* Corresponding author.
E-mail address: ajay.kaul@cchmc.org

Pediatr Clin N Am 57 (2010) 1331–1345
doi:10.1016/j.pcl.2010.09.008
0031-3955/10/$ – see front matter © 2010 Elsevier Inc. All rights reserved.

the fact that acid contact with the esophageal mucosa and abnormal esophageal motility can both cause chest pain.

GERD

Gastroesophageal reflux (GER) is a physiologic phenomenon that occurs at all ages but more frequently in infants. When this retrograde movement of gastric contents into the esophagus causes troublesome symptoms or complications it is referred to as GERD. The refluxed material may be air (belch), liquid, solid, or mixed; and, depending on the pH, may be acid (pH ≤ 4) or nonacid. The relative proportion of acid and nonacid reflux episodes was not known until the advent of the combined pH-impedance technology. This was mainly because the conventional pH probe study only measured episodes that were acid. We now know that nonacid reflux episodes are at least as frequent as acid episodes and are capable of producing symptoms as well.

The lower esophageal sphincter (LES) is the most important physiologic antireflux barrier. The LES is a high-pressure zone maintained by two muscular systems that help keep gastric contents from refluxing into the esophagus. The first is the circular (smooth) muscle layer of the lower end of the esophagus primarily innervated by the intrinsic enteric nervous system. The second is the sling (skeletal) muscle of the diaphragmatic crura that envelops this area and is supplied by the phrenic nerve as well as inhibitory (nitrenergic) motor fibers from the myenteric neurons. The LES is normally situated in the abdominal cavity below the diaphragm and the relative higher pressure in the intra-abdominal cavity over the intrathoracic pressure adds to the sphincter mechanism of the LES. Displacement of the LES into the thoracic cavity in a patient with hiatal hernia therefore disrupts proper functioning of the LES and predisposes to GERD.

Once the refluxed material enters the esophagus, the bolus causes distension of the wall and stimulates the receptors which induce a neurally mediated peristaltic contraction that moves the refluxate back into the stomach. This secondary peristalsis is often supplemented by a swallow-induced primary peristaltic wave that helps clear the esophagus. These clearance or "stripping" waves are an important mechanism for preventing damage to the esophageal mucosa from prolonged contact with the refluxed material. Another physiologic barrier to reflux-induced esophageal damage is reflex swallowing of alkaline saliva in response to a GER episode that helps neutralize acid content of the refluxate. GER-induced swallowing as well as clearance peristaltic waves are inhibited during sleep such that increased nocturnal reflux episodes tend to be more harmful to the mucosal lining.

The physiologic basis for most GER events is a phenomenon referred to as transient lower esophageal sphincter relaxation (TLESR).[11] This brief relaxation of the LES can be triggered by distension of the gastric fundus and is mediated through the vagus nerve.[11] TLESR can result in reflux of air (belch), liquid, solid, or mixed gastric contents into the esophagus. In infants, reflux episodes occur more often and are likely due to frequent feeds that distend the fundus causing more TLESR events. Anatomy of the stomach and gastroesophageal junction and the more frequent recumbent posture also predispose infants to more reflux episodes. When the refluxed material enters the short esophagus of an infant, it usually travels the entire length up to the pharynx and presents as regurgitation or vomiting. Full-column reflux episodes, and GER episodes in general, decrease as the child grows owing to esophageal lengthening and transition of the anatomy of the stomach and gastroesophageal junction to a more adult-like configuration.

The classic symptoms of GERD include heartburn, regurgitation, and retrosternal pain. Extraesophageal symptoms attributed to GERD include cough, hoarseness, back arching, asthma, sinusitis otitis media, apnea, bradycardia, apparent life-threatening events, and dental erosions. Symptoms of GERD, however, vary by age and the description of intensity, localization, and severity may be unreliable until the age of at least 8 years, and sometimes even later, especially in children with NDD.[12] Distinguishing physiologic reflux from GERD when symptoms become "troublesome" remains challenging in younger children and those with NDD as they may not present with the typical symptoms of GERD nor manifest any objective evidence of its complication.[12] As an example, excessive crying in infants and toddlers may be misdiagnosed as GERD and treated with acid suppression agents without resolution of the troublesome symptom. The alarm symptoms that are indicative of a complication of GERD include weight loss or poor weight gain, dysphagia, bleeding, anemia, choking, and feeding difficulties.[13] Children presenting with these symptoms warrant further evaluation. Risk factors for severe GERD include history of central nervous system (CNS) impairment, esophageal atresia or tracheoesophageal fistula repair, chronic lung diseases, and diaphragmatic or hiatal hernia.[12]

Dysphagia may be the sole presenting symptom of reflux esophagitis in children even in the absence of a typical history suggestive of GER.[14] Dysphagia has been reported in more than 30% of adults with GERD.[15] The swallowing difficulty in these adult patients with reflux esophagitis was felt not to be due to abnormal motility of the striated muscle of the proximal esophagus but more likely from inflammation of the distal esophagus. Distal esophageal mucosal injury occurs in GERD because acid clearance is slower in this region, placing it at an increased risk of developing esophagitis.[16]

Even though the typical symptoms are present in 82%–97% of subjects with endoscopically proven esophagitis, their positive and negative predictive values are low and therefore are not recommended for screening purposes. Symptom scores in adults with GERD correlated with the number of reflux episodes but not with the total acid exposure time.[17] Studies in adult patients with GERD have reported that LES pressure and esophageal acid exposure time are poor predictors for disease severity, but hiatal hernia was shown to exert a much stronger influence on the severity of erosive reflux disease.[18]

It is well documented that GER decreases threshold for perception of visceral pain in the esophagus.[17] Somatic pain hypersensitivity after tissue injury has two important properties, first it manifests as allodynia or hyperalgesia, and second it is diffuse, present not only at the site of injury but also surrounding healthy tissue.[19] For example it has been shown that acid infusion to the lower esophagus induces a decrease in pain threshold in the lower and upper esophagus as well as in the anterior chest wall due to a change in sensory processing within the CNS. Healthy individuals can develop persistent visceral (esophageal) hypersensitivity as a result of peripheral and central sensitization after acid or alkaline injury to the esophagus, such that physiologic GER (acid or nonacid), or even eating or drinking can be sufficient to induce pain referred to the chest.[19]

Infants with crying and feeding disorders are perceived as more vulnerable by their parents and depending upon parental perceptions, experience, coping skills, and psychosocial conditions, are often brought to medical attention. A study of infants seen in clinic for a complaint of crying and fussiness reported that they had more feeding difficulties, were less responsive to treatment, and had more maternal stress.[20] Up to 70% of infants have physiologic regurgitation (spit-ups) that resolves without intervention in 95% of them by 12-months-of-age.[12] When given a history of "vomiting" it is important to differentiate between regurgitation and vomiting because the latter is more likely to be pathologic and may need to be evaluated more urgently. Unlike vomiting, regurgitation has no CNS emetic reflex, retrograde intestinal contractions, nausea, or retching. In infants, however, because of a short esophagus, most reflux episodes tend to project as "vomiting" and are commonly reported as such by parents. A history of regurgitation was found to be neither necessary nor sufficient for a diagnosis of GERD owing to its lack of sensitivity and specificity.[12]

When compared with older children, those less than 5-years-old with GERD tend to present more often with food refusal, regurgitation, vomiting, and abdominal pain.[21] Young children with a history of vomiting after feeding (GERD or other reasons) may have difficulty in accepting feeds, despite having no alteration of oral and pharyngeal phases of swallowing.[22] The proposed hypothesis to explain this is that initial acid exposure of the mucosal chemoreceptors and nerve endings in the esophagus triggers afferent signals to the spinal nerves that are transmitted to the brain which perceives the sensation as pain or discomfort. The neurochemical alterations induced in this pathway by repeated reflux episodes appear to persist even after the initial noxious stimulus (vomiting, GERD) resolves and leaves the child with a hypersensitivity to any bolus movement along the esophagus, including swallowing food. Peripheral and central sensitization are believed to be important mechanisms for this ongoing heightened perception of esophageal sensation (visceral hypersensitivity)[23] resulting in food refusal.

Older children are able to give an appropriate history of heartburn and regurgitation thereby making the diagnosis of GERD easier. A community pediatric practice survey showed that 5.2% of children aged 10 to 17 were able to report a burning or painful feeling in the middle of the chest, 8.2% reported regurgitation, 5% reported epigastric pain, and 3.6% actually reported odynophagia.[24] In adolescents, the underlying pathophysiology and symptom presentation of GERD are similar to adults. The predominant symptoms of GERD in children ages 6 to 17 years was reported to be regurgitation or vomiting, cough and epigastric pain, or heartburn.[19] In another study, 18% of children with GERD reportedly presented with retrosternal pain.[25] For unclear reasons, nonerosive reflux disease is more common in symptomatic children with GERD,[26] but erosive esophagitis is reported in more than one-third of pediatric-age patients with underlying GERD-promoting disorders.[27] These risk factors that predispose to severe reflux disease include CNS impairment, esophageal atresia, chronic lung disease, hiatal hernia, and congenital diaphragmatic hernia.[12] *Helicobacter pylori* was previously thought to be protective of GERD by causing atrophic gastritis and a decrease in gastric acid secretion, but recent evidence shows a high prevalence of esophagitis in pediatric patients with *H pylori* infection.[28]

Evaluation

An upper GI contrast study is indicated if there is a history of vomiting, dysphagia, or odynophagia. It should not be done to diagnose GERD but to rule out conditions that may mimic GERD such as structural disorders of the upper GI tract.

In younger children and those with neurodevelopmental disabilities presenting with food refusal, a thorough evaluation of the oral, pharyngeal, and esophageal phases of swallowing and a videofluoroscopic study of swallowing (VFSS) should be performed by a speech pathologist.[29] If there is suspicion or evidence of aspiration, a bronchoscopy with bronchoalveolar lavage should be considered and could be combined with an esophagogastroduodenoscopy (EGD).

Multichannel intraluminal impedance (MII) combined with a pH sensor can detect esophageal bolus flow, determine its direction, quantify the number of reflux episodes and characterize them as acid (pH <4) and nonacid (weakly acidic and weakly alkaline). It can also establish proximal extent of the reflux, and provide information on bolus and acid clearance.[30] A pH-MII identifies more reflux events than conventional pH probe study and improves clinical correlation with symptoms.[31] This is important in children who cannot reliably convey the classic GER symptoms or those who have extraesophageal symptoms attributed to GERD.

In our institution, the authors retrospectively reviewed combined pH-MII studies from 186 infants. In 20 studies, a total of 60 episodes of perceived pain-related symptoms (back arching, crying, restlessness, head side-to-side, thrashing, pain, screaming, and fussiness) were reported by the caregiver but only 38% were associated with GER episodes, all of which were nonacid. Therefore, contrary to popular belief, GER does not appear to play a major role in infants perceived to have pain-related symptoms. In addition to being helpful in associating GER with perceived pain episodes and atypical (extraesophageal) symptoms, pH-MII is also indicated in children that report classic symptoms of GER that are refractory to acid suppression with proton pump inhibitors (PPI). In this situation the study can be done while on acid suppression therapy to evaluate the relationship between persistent symptoms and GER.[32] An adult study showed that persistent symptoms on PPI therapy are either associated with nonacid reflux or are not associated with reflux at all.[33] Our infant study was similar in that we also found that nonacid reflux events are as likely as acid reflux events to be associated with a symptom.

The role of EGD is to rule out other causes of esophagitis and heartburn (**Box 1**). It has been reported that no correlation exists between symptoms and endoscopic esophageal findings.[21,34] A recent study reported that children referred to a cardiology clinic for chest pain had positive endoscopic findings if there was epigastric tenderness on physical examination.[4] Erosive esophagitis (**Fig. 1**) has been noted to be more common in males and increases with age. A hiatal hernia (**Fig. 2**) is the only endoscopic observation that predicted the presence of erosive esophagitis,[34] consistent with studies in adults.[18] Although GER symptom frequency and intensity correlate with severity of mucosal injury, neither will predict the severity in the individual patient. However, when pain is epigastric or mesogastric in location, acid-peptic disorders are high on the differential.[35]

Treatment

Treatment for presumed GERD without prior diagnostic evaluation is not recommended in the infant with feeding refusal because a large variety of disorders, including

---

Box 1
Causes of heartburn

Weakly acid reflux

Weakly alkaline reflux

Gas

Duodeno-gastroesophageal reflux

Eosinophilic esophagitis

Pill esophagitis

Infection

Crohn disease

Functional heart burn or dyspepsia

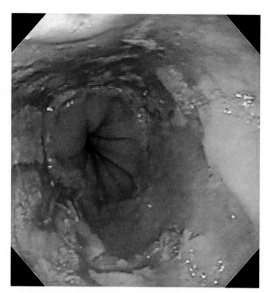

Fig. 1. Distal esophageal peptic erosions in a child with NDD.

behavioral, may contribute to infant-feeding difficulties.[9] One-year follow-up of symptoms of GER during infancy showed no significant difference between case and controls in refusal of feeding, irritability, irritability with feeding, back arching, choking or gagging, and abdominal pain.[36] This study also showed that behavioral feeding problems are common in healthy toddlers (9% reported), which raises doubts concerning the role of GER in causing these symptoms and underscoring a multifactorial cause for feeding disorders. The treatment of infants and toddlers who refuse to eat

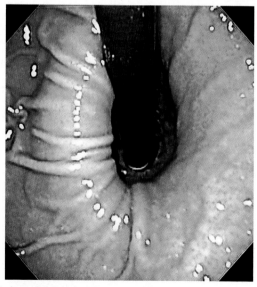

Fig. 2. Hiatal hernia in a child with GERD symptoms.

because of pain resulting from visceral hyperalgesia or reflux esophagitis involves removing the pain associated with eating and making eating a pleasurable experience.[37] Fortunately, a long-term follow-up study of infants with nonorganic cause for refusal to eat comparing with those who did not, showed no increase in disturbing eating attitudes, decrease in body mass index, or less positive self perception in adolescence.[38] In the authors' unpublished data comparing acid reflux episodes in 186 infants on ranitidine, lansoprazole, or no medications, using combined pH-MII technology, there was a statistically significant decrease in the number of acid reflux events in infants who were on PPI compared with those on ranitidine or no medications; however, the total number of reflux episodes were no different in the three groups.

In the older child with typical reflux symptoms suggestive of GERD, an empiric trial of PPI is justified for up to 4 weeks. If symptoms do not resolve, a referral for further testing should be made. However, improvement of heartburn following treatment does not confirm a diagnosis of GERD because symptoms may improve spontaneously or respond to a placebo. When a decision is made to treat chest pain or other symptoms of GERD, a PPI is the treatment of choice. PPI currently approved for use in children in the United States include omeprazole, lansoprazole, and esomeprazole. PPI are recommended as initial therapy in children with documented erosive esophagitis for at least 3 months. Pantoprazole has been proven effective in reducing endoscopically proven GERD in children.[39] Duodenogastroesophageal reflux may sometimes play a role in the pathophysiology of PPI refractory GERD and esophagitis, a fiberoptic spectrophotometric probe that measures bilirubin concentration is required to detect duodenogastroesophageal reflux.[40]

EOE

In children, GERD had been regarded as the most common organic cause for esophagus-related chest pain,[8] but EoE is being increasingly recognized to be a more common cause of dysphagia and odynophagia than GERD.[9] EoE is a clinicopathologic diagnosis that involves a localized eosinophilic inflammation of the esophagus, it is more prevalent in young white males but it can occur at any age and in either sex.[41]

The most frequent symptoms of EoE are nonspecific and may mimic GERD. They include dysphagia, pain, and vomiting.[42] Presentation varies with age. Abdominal pain and vomiting are usually present at diagnoses in preschool and school-aged children; and dysphagia, food impaction, and chest pain in adolescents.[43] Feeding disorders have also been reported as a presenting feature of EoE in infants and toddlers.[44] About 25% of patients with EoE reportedly complain of chest pain at diagnosis. Dysphagia (68%) is the most common symptom followed by emesis (62%), abdominal pain (57%), and heartburn (45%).[45] Children who have pain associated with EoE report chest, epigastric, or abdominal pain. Some have been evaluated for episodic crushing substernal pain that raise concerns for heart disease; however, on further evaluation with endoscopy were found to have EoE.[42]

Evaluation

Children presenting with any of the described symptoms of GERD not responding to PPI therapy should undergo an EGD to rule out EoE, the typical endoscopic features of EoE include mucosal thickening, furrowing (**Fig. 3**), trachealization (**Fig. 4**), and pinpoint or diffuse white exudates (see **Fig. 3**). Biopsies are required to establish the diagnosis. Histologic diagnosis is confirmed by the presence of 15 or more eosinophils per high-powered field isolated to the esophagus and associated with the

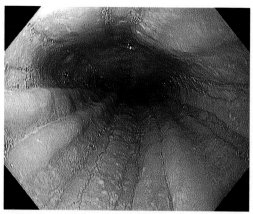

Fig. 3. Scattered exudates, thickening, and furrowing of esophageal mucosa in a child with EoE.

characteristic clinical symptoms. A 6 to 8 week trial of acid-suppression therapy is required before performing a diagnostic upper endoscopy to confirm the diagnosis of EoE[41] as GERD can have similar histologic features. Sometimes an upper GI contrast study done in a child with chest pain or dysphagia my reveal an esophageal narrowing or stricture as a feature of EoE.

Treatment

Treatment options include nutritional management, pharmacologic therapy, and dilatation of esophageal strictures.

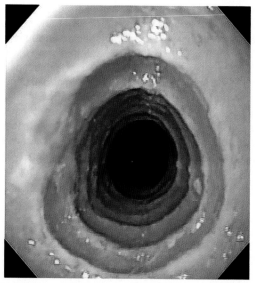

Fig. 4. Trachealization of the esophageal mucosa in a child with EoE presenting with chest pain and food impaction.

Nutritional management

As most EoE is induced by food allergens, identifying specific allergenic foods by skin or patch testing is often the initial step. If elimination of these foods or a panel of foods that most commonly cause EoE (milk, soy, egg, wheat, shellfish, fish, tree nuts, and peanuts)[46] does not resolve EoE then a trial of an elemental diet with sequential reintroduction of foods (beginning with least allergenic and endoscopic surveillance after a certain number of foods) is recommended.

Pharmacologic therapy

Currently, topical (swallowed) corticosteroids are the best pharmacologic option for patients who have EoE. They improve clinical symptoms and the underlying inflammation similar to results gained with systemic steroids.[47] The use of PPI therapy provides symptomatic relief of any symptoms caused by GERD and is recommended as cotherapy. EoE is a chronic condition and needs long-term monitoring by an interdisciplinary team consisting of a gastroenterologist, allergist and dietician.

FOREIGN BODY

Ingestion of small objects remain among the most common causes of injury and fatality to preschool children.[48] Foreign body ingestions occur commonly in children, with the maximum incidence among those under 5-years-of-age (9 months–3 years), they cause serious morbidity in less than 1% of all patients, but 1500 deaths per year in the United States are attributed to ingested foreign bodies.[49] Accidental ingestions are common in children with neurodevelopmental delays and intentional ingestions in those with psychiatric conditions. The incidence of latter appears to be increasing in adolescents.

Children can swallow a wide variety of foreign bodies and the most common reported by the US Federal Bureau of Investigation are coins. Diagnosis of foreign body ingestion can be challenging as quite often the act of ingestion is not witnessed and the child is unable to give a history of ingestion. Additionally, not all foreign bodies are radiopaque (**Fig. 5**) and therefore not visible on radiograph.[50] A long history of dysphagia and chest pain does not rule out foreign body ingestion.[50,51] A recent example at the authors' institution highlighted this fact. A healthy 4-year-old male

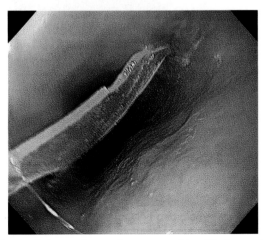

Fig. 5. Plastic foreign body in esophagus that was not identified on a chest radiograph.

Asthma and Pneumonia

Lorin R. Browne, DO*, Marc H. Gorelick, MD, MSCE

KEYWORDS

- Asthma • Pneumonia • Chest pain in children
- Pulmonary pathologies

Data from the 2007 National Hospital Ambulatory Medical Care Survey (NHAMCS) show that chest pain is a presenting complaint in 1.7% of emergency department (ED) visits for children, representing nearly 500,000 annual visits in the United States.[1] Most children with a complaint of chest pain are diagnosed with nonspecific chest pain or pain of musculoskeletal origin (**Table 1**). Asthma and lower respiratory infections are the most common specific diagnoses, ranging from 4.0% to 26.0% of cases from single-center studies[2–7] and 8.7% each in the nationally representative NHAMCS survey. Respiratory causes of chest pain appear to be even more common in children younger than 12 years, although in a study of young adults (13–35 years) in an ED, 11% had respiratory infection as the cause.[8] Even among children referred to a cardiologist for evaluation, respiratory causes are among the most common specific diagnoses. In one study, 73% of children seen in a cardiology clinic for chest pain had reversible decreases in pulmonary function after exercise, suggesting a diagnosis of exercise-induced asthma (EIA).[9]

ASTHMA
Pathophysiology

In children with acute asthma, chest pain is a common symptom, occurring in 13% of patients in one study.[10] Acute asthma is a multifactorial process that includes both bronchospasm and airways inflammation, both of which may cause a sensation of pain attributable to stimulation of nociceptors in the bronchi.[11] Bronchoconstriction also causes a feeling of chest tightness, which may be interpreted or reported as pain by children. Frequent or deep cough in a child with an acute asthma exacerbation may lead to soreness of the muscles of the chest wall. Rarely (0.2%–0.3% of cases), children with acute asthma may develop pneumomediastinum (**Fig. 1**).[10,12] Those children with asthma and sickle cell disease have an increased incidence of acute chest syndrome owing to local pulmonary hypoxia, sickling, and tissue ischemia or infarction (**Box 1**).

Department of Pediatric Emergency Medicine, Children's Hospital of Wisconsin, Medical College of Wisconsin, Suite 550, 999 North 92nd Street, Milwaukee, WI 53226, USA
* Corresponding author.
E-mail address: lbrowne@mcw.edu

Pediatr Clin N Am 57 (2010) 1347–1356
doi:10.1016/j.pcl.2010.09.002
0031-3955/10/$ – see front matter © 2010 Elsevier Inc. All rights reserved.

Table 1
Causes of pediatric chest pain reported in the literature

Study	Setting	Number of Children	Reported Causes of Chest Pain
Selbst et al,[2] 1988	Emergency department (ED)	407	Idiopathic 21% Musculoskeletal 24% Respiratory 21% Cough 10% Asthma 7% Pneumonia 4%
Rowe et al,[3] 1990	ED	336	Idiopathic 12% Musculoskeletal 28% Respiratory 19%
Massin et al,[4] 2004	ED Cardiology clinic	168 69	Musculoskeletal 64% Respiratory 13% Musculoskeletal 89% Respiratory (asthma) 4%
Evangelista et al,[5] 2008	Cardiology clinic	50	Musculoskeletal 76% Respiratory (asthma) 12%
Lin et al,[6] 2008	ED	103	Idiopathic 59% Musculoskeletal 7% Pulmonary 24% Asthma 1% Lower respiratory infection 16%
Danduran et al,[7] 2008	Cardiology clinic	263	Asthma 26%
National Hospital Ambulatory Medical Care Survey,[1] 2007	ED	150	Pulmonary 17.4% Asthma 8.7% Lower respiratory infection 8.7%

Evaluation

Asthma is common: although a past history of asthma may be highly suggestive of this as the cause of chest pain, children with asthma can also have any of a number of other conditions causing their chest pain, and a careful evaluation is required in all cases. Conversely, children may have chest pain as their initial presentation of asthma. Indeed, some authors have proposed the existence of a "chest-pain variant asthma" in which this is the only or most prominent symptom.[11] Unfortunately, there is no diagnostic test for asthma that can be readily applied in the ED; therefore, the evaluation is largely clinical. In a child without a known diagnosis of asthma, several historical features may be suggestive of reactive airways disease. These include prior history of wheezing, history of other atopic disease (eg, eczema), family history of asthma or atopic disease, chronic cough (especially nocturnal), and cough or shortness of breath with exercise. Although asthma-associated chest pain may have various characteristics, a description of tightness is also suggestive, as are occurrence or worsening of the pain with exertion and coexisting cough.

The child with chest pain owing to asthma may have overt signs of airway inflammation and bronchospasm, or the examination may be relatively unremarkable. Examine for signs of obstruction to inflow (inspiratory wheezing, accessory muscle use, retractions, nasal flaring), obstruction to outflow (expiratory wheezing, prolonged expiratory phase), atelectasis (diminished aeration, grunting, crackles), or alveolar hypoventilation

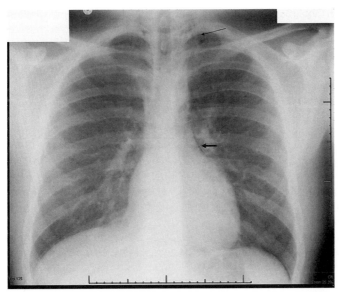

Fig. 1. Pneumomediastinum in a child with asthma. Subcutaneous air is seen in the soft tissues of the neck (*thin arrow*), and a linear lucency appears along the left cardiac border (*heavy arrow*), indicating air between the heart and the mediastinal pleura.

(tachypnea). Look also for signs of atopic disease such as eczematous changes of the skin, rhinitis, and allergic shiners. Subcutaneous crepitus in the neck and Hamman sign (crunching heart sounds) may indicate the presence of pneumomediastinum.

Pulse oximetry may be useful. Although a normal oxygen saturation does not exclude the presence of asthma, hypoxemia may be seen as a result of ventilation-perfusion mismatch from bronchospasm or atelectasis. Peak expiratory flow rate (PEFR) may be a particularly useful adjunct in a child old enough to be taught the maneuver (typically 8 years or older). PEFR less than 70% of predicted with good effort is strongly suggestive of bronchoconstriction. Having the child perform PEFR before and after exercise may demonstrate a decrease in children with exercise-induced asthma.

Chest radiography is not diagnostic of asthma and is often normal, but may provide helpful clues. In the context of an acute exacerbation, radiographic findings may include hyperinflation, atelectasis, and peribronchial thickening owing to airway inflammation. A chest radiograph is not indicated for all children with chest pain attributable to asthma. If the pain resolves after treatment with bronchodilators, the pain may have been related to overuse of chest wall muscles, and no diagnostic studies

---

Box 1
Etiology of chest pain in children with asthma

1. Bronchospasm and airways inflammation stimulate nociceptors in the bronchi

2. Bronchoconstriction causes feeling of "chest tightness"

3. Frequent cough leads to soreness/overuse of chest wall muscles (inflammation of nerves, muscles, costochondral junctions)

4. Pneumomediastinum or pneumothorax

5. Acute chest syndrome (children with sickle cell disease)

are needed. Obtain confirmatory radiographs in a child with known asthma and chest pain in whom pneumomediastinum or pneumothorax is suspected based on physical examination, and in a child with coexisting sickle cell disease to evaluate for acute chest syndrome.

Management

Not surprisingly, management of chest pain associated with asthma is best approached by treating the underlying exacerbation. In cases where asthma is suspected as the cause, a therapeutic trial of an inhaled bronchodilator may provide a diagnostic clue as well as symptomatic relief. Although most children with asthma and chest pain will respond to bronchodilator therapy, in some cases the pain is more related to inflammation; in those children, systemic corticosteroids will produce more pain relief.[11]

If the chest pain in an asthmatic child is a result of thoracic muscle overuse or strain from coughing, administer analgesics such as acetaminophen or ibuprofen.

Pneumomediastinum does not typically require specific treatment (see another article elsewhere in this issue for further exploration of this topic). The subcutaneous air will resorb spontaneously, although resolution may be hastened by providing supplemental oxygen. Similarly, a small nontension pneumothorax may be treated expectantly, whereas larger (>20%) pneumothoraces should generally be evacuated by placing a chest tube. Tension pneumothorax in asthma is rare, but if it occurs it must be evacuated emergently. Similarly, place a chest tube in any patient with pneumothorax if the asthma exacerbation is severe enough that positive-pressure ventilation is required.

For children with sickle cell disease and asthma, administer supplemental oxygen even if oxygen saturation by pulse oximetry is normal, as this may help prevent sickling caused by localized pulmonary hypoxia.

Admission to the hospital for treatment and observation is not generally needed for the child with asthma solely on the basis of chest pain. Admission is recommended for those children with asthma and chest pain with inadequate response to standard ED asthma therapy, as indicated by persistent moderately severe symptoms, peak expiratory flow rate less than 50% of predicted, or hypoxia.

PNEUMONIA
Pathophysiology

Pneumonia is an infection of the lower respiratory tract defined by fever, acute respiratory symptoms, and tachypnea or radiologic evidence of parenchymal infiltrates. It is the leading cause of morbidity among children worldwide, accounting for an estimated 1.9 million deaths in children younger than 5 annually.[13,14] Although the mortality is reduced outside of underdeveloped nations, at an approximate rate of 36 cases per 1000 per year, pneumonia causes significant morbidity in developed countries.[15–17] Pneumonia frequently begins as colonization of the nasopharynx with subsequent infection of the lower respiratory tract and can be caused by bacteria, viruses, atypical organisms, or fungi.

Chest pain associated with acute respiratory infections can be produced through several mechanisms. Direct tracheobronchial irritation and pain travels from the lungs through vagal afferent nerve fibers to the cervical spinal column and can be manifested as a dull, aching, or sharp pain usually felt in the anterior chest or neck.[18] In addition, prolonged and severe coughing causes stress and strain to the chest wall, producing inflammation of the associated nerves, muscles, and costochondral junctions.[18–21] Pain associated with coughing travels through intercostal nerves and can be a constant ache or a sharp pain worse with coughing or deep inspiration. It is typically localized to the lateral chest wall, but may also cause diffuse chest discomfort.[19,20] Pleuritis, or painful inflammation of the pleura, may also be associated with pneumonia. Pleuritic chest pain typically occurs during inspiration when inflamed areas of the pleura rub against one another and is typically sharp, severe, and well localized.[6,18,19] Finally, parapneumonic effusions can complicate bacterial pneumonia and can contribute to the causes of chest pain. This pain is characteristically sharp and dramatically worse with deep inspiration.[19] As the pathophysiology of chest pain in pneumonia is largely associated with symptoms of infection, the pain generally recedes with improvement of cough, tachypnea, and respiratory distress (**Box 2**).[20]

Evaluation

Pneumonia should be suspected as an etiology of chest pain in children presenting with respiratory symptoms. Associated fever and cough are hallmark symptoms of typical bacterial pneumonia.[22] Chills, abdominal pain, and mucous production are also commonly seen with pneumonia.[23] The combination of fever, cyanosis, and at least one other sign of respiratory distress is highly predictive of pyogenic pneumonia.[24] Atypical pneumonias, such as those caused by *Mycoplasma pneumoniae or Chlamydia pneumoniae,* are often accompanied by less severe symptoms of a more gradual onset. These symptoms may include headache, malaise, and low-grade fever.[22] Clinical presentation of children with pneumonia can vary considerably from those who are acutely ill to those who look reasonably well, partly because of the etiologic organism and the age of the child.[23]

The physical evaluation of a patient with suspected pneumonia should include the patient's temperature, pulse and respiratory rate, and pulse oximetry reading. The child's overall demeanor, degree of hydration, color, and the presence of cyanosis should also be assessed. Tachypnea, nasal flaring, chest wall retractions, grunting, and other signs of respiratory distress are suggestive of lower respiratory tract infection. Tachypnea is the most sensitive and the most specific of all physical findings associated with pneumonia. An increased respiratory rate is found twice as often in children with radiographically proven pneumonia than in those children without positive radiographs. Lung examination will often reveal crackles, focal decreased breath sounds, bronchial breath sounds, or dullness to percussion. Observed hypoxemia in a child with complaints of chest pain is concerning for lower respiratory tract etiology. New-onset wheezing may be heard with viral or atypical infections, but are not commonly associated with pyogenic bacterial pneumonia. Similarly, rhonchi, or coarse airway sounds associated with secretions in the large airways, are not necessarily indicative of pneumonia.[22,23]

There is little role for ancillary testing in the well-appearing child with auscultatory findings consistent with pneumonia who is eligible for ambulatory pharmacotherapy.[24]

Box 2
Etiology of chest pain in children with pneumonia

1. Direct tracheobronchial irritation (pain travels from lungs through vagal afferent nerve fibers to cervical spinal column)

2. Severe cough leads to soreness/overuse of chest wall muscles (inflammation of nerves, muscles, costochondral junctions)

3. Inflammation of the pleura is possible (causes pain with inspiration)

4. Parapneumonic effusions are possible (cause pain with inspiration)

Although white blood cell counts and C-reactive protein levels have been shown to be higher in children with bacterial pneumonia, these results showed such significant variability that clinical application is unreliable and have shown little value in differentiating bacterial pneumonia from pneumonia caused by other agents.[23,24] Blood cultures are positive in children with pneumonia no more than 10% of the time and their use is not recommended in outpatient management.[25–28] In children hospitalized with more severe, resistant, or unusual forms of pneumonia, blood cultures may be helpful and may provide a possible opportunity for identification of a causative organism.[23,29–31] Other methods of identifying etiologic organisms are available and include sputum examination, antigen detection testing, and polymerase chain reaction (PCR)-based respiratory infection testing. These ancillary tests are associated with difficulty obtaining an adequate sample, poor testing performance, and high cost, respectively, limiting their use in pediatrics.[23]

Ancillary radiographs in the diagnosis of uncomplicated, ambulatory pneumonia does not appear to modify outcomes and the British Thoracic Society guidelines for pneumonia do not recommend its use in children older than 2 months.[32,33] In daily practice, however, chest radiographs are commonly used to confirm the clinical diagnosis of pneumonia, characterize the severity of the disease, and assess for complications such as effusion or empyema (**Figs. 2** and **3**).[34] Chest radiographs can be beneficial and are recommended in children who are in respiratory distress, ill-appearing, requiring hospitalization, or with physical findings concerning for pleural effusion.[22] This final use of chest radiographs may be especially important in febrile

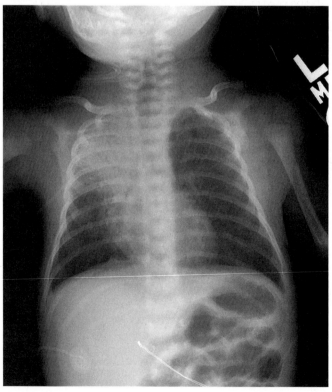

Fig. 2. Lobar pneumonia. Complete consolidation of the right upper lobe is seen in a 19-day-old infant who presented with apnea and lethargy.

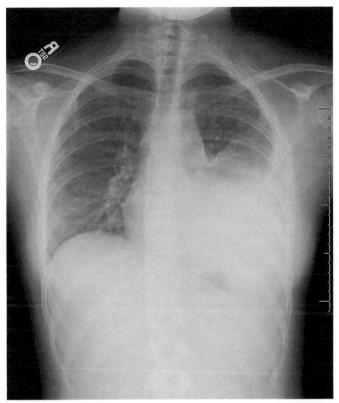

Fig. 3. Parapneumonic effusion in an adolescent female presenting with fever, cough, and chest pain. In addition to the consolidated left lower lobe, note the inability to distinguish the left hemidiaphragm indicating the presence of extrapulmonary fluid. A lateral decubitus radiograph of the chest may reveal a layered appearance to the pleural fluid.

children presenting with chest pain and clinical concern for bacterial pneumonia.[35] Although radiograph findings can guide management in the ill child and may provide clues to the causative organism, they lack sufficient specificity to be considered diagnostic for specific etiologic agents.[23]

Management

The initial management of a child with pneumonia must include rapid cardiopulmonary stabilization. Cardiorespiratory support is essential in the toxic or distressed child and may include the administration of supplemental oxygen, intubation or other advanced airway techniques, intravenous fluid administration, or the use of vasopressor medications. Additional therapies may be instituted concurrently, but should not supplant stabilizing interventions.[36]

Acute pneumonia-associated chest pain can typically be alleviated with over-the-counter analgesia medication such as acetaminophen or ibuprofen. In the acutely ill or distressed child, intravenous narcotic pain medication can be used to treat severe pain; however, an anti-inflammatory medication such as ketorolac is generally favored because of its lack of respiratory depression. Anti-inflammatory medication is especially effective in relieving pleuritic chest pain or musculoskeletal pain associated with coughing.[37] The underlying strategy for treatment of pneumonia-associated chest pain, however, is effective treatment of the causative infection and its associated painful complications (ie, effusion or empyema). The mainstay of therapy for bacterial pneumonia is the administration of antimicrobials.[17,22,27,38,39] Over-the-counter cough medications are not indicated. The specifics of pneumonia management should be based on the age and overall state of the child and the suspected causative organism. Children with clinical concern for bacterial pneumonia who do not appear ill, are without signs of respiratory distress or hypoxemia, and who are maintaining adequate hydration may be treated successfully with outpatient, oral antibiotics. Hospital admission for treatment and observation is appropriate for children who are younger than 3 months old, toxic in appearance, have signs of significant respiratory distress or hypoxemia, are incapable of maintaining adequate fluid intake, or who have serious concomitant chronic conditions.[22,32]

Antibacterial selection is ideally based on an identified organism, but identification of the organism in children is unlikely and empiric therapy is often mandatory.[23] As viral infections are the most common cause of pneumonia in children between the ages of 3 months and 5 years, antibacterials are not needed in the only mildly ill infant or young child who has diffuse findings on lung examination. For children in this age group who are suspected of having bacterial pneumonia, however, empiric treatment for *Streptococcus pneumoniae* is indicated.[22] *S pneumoniae* is the predominant bacterial cause of pneumonia across all pediatric age groups causing approximately 73% of bacterial infections.[7] Oral beta-lactam penicillin antibiotics such as amoxicillin or amoxicillin/clavulanic acid have a low failure rate and are the recommended first-line medications for outpatient therapy.[15,17,23,40,41] *S pneumoniae* resistance to first-line antibacterials is a growing concern. In vitro penicillin and ceftriaxone resistance rates have been shown to be approximately 6% and 2%, respectively.[17] Despite this, in vivo resistance is uncommon and clinical amoxicillin treatment failures are seen in fewer than 3% of children.[27,41]

The high prevalence of pneumonia caused by atypical organisms such as *Mycoplasma pneumoniae* and *Chlamydia pneumoniae* in preschool- and school-age children has recently been noted.[15,22,40,41] When an atypical pneumonia is suspected, a macrolide antibiotic such as azithromycin becomes the drug of choice. Because of the poor response of *S pneumoniae* to macrolide antibiotics and to the significant complications associated with undertreating *S pneumoniae* infection, combination therapy with a beta-lactam and a macrolide antibiotic may be the most prudent course in children where the exact etiology remains unclear.[22]

Patients requiring hospitalization should be treated with an intravenous penicillin antibiotic or a third-generation cephalosporin. Vancomycin is active against *S pneumoniae*, but should be reserved for those who fail to improve on standard antibacterial therapy. In children admitted to the hospital, an intravenous macrolide antibiotic may be added in cases where atypical organisms are suspected.[15,40]

SUMMARY

Chest pain remains a common complaint among children seeking care in the United States. Asthma and lower respiratory tract infections such as pneumonia can be significant causes of chest pain. Children with chest pain caused by either of these pulmonary etiologies generally present with associated respiratory symptoms, including cough, wheezing, tachypnea, respiratory distress, and/or fever. Although analgesic medications can improve chest pain associated with pulmonary pathologies, the mainstay of therapy is to treat the underling etiology; this includes bronchodilator and/or steroid medications in children with asthma and appropriate antibacterial administration in children with suspicions of bacterial pneumonia. The chest pain generally resolves along with the resolution of other respiratory symptoms.

REFERENCES

1. Data obtained from National Center for Health Statistics. Available at: http://www.cdc.gov/nchs/ahcd.htm. Accessed March 4, 2010.
2. Selbst SM, Ruddy RM, Clark BJ, et al. Pediatric chest pain: a prospective study. Pediatrics 1998;82:319–23.
3. Rowe BH, Dulberg CS, Peterson RG, et al. Characteristics of children presenting with chest pain to a pediatric emergency department. Can Med Assoc J 1990; 143:388–94.
4. Massin MM, Bourgignont A, Coremans C, et al. Chest pain in pediatric patients presenting to an emergency department or to a cardiac clinic. Clin Pediatr (Phila) 2004;43:231–8.
5. Evangelista JK, Parsons M, Renneburg AK. Chest pain in children: diagnosis through history and physical examination. J Pediatr Health Care 2000;14:3–8.
6. Lin C-H, Lin W-C, Ho Y-J, et al. Children with chest pain visiting the emergency department. Pediatr Neonatol 2008;49:26–9.
7. Danduran MJ, Earing MG, Sheridan DC, et al. Chest pain: characteristics of children/adolescents. Pediatr Cardiol 2008;29:775–81.
8. Luke LC, Cusack S, Smith H, et al. Non-traumatic chest pain in young adults: a medical audit. Arch Emerg Med 1990;7:183–8.
9. Wiens L, Portnoy J, Sabath R, et al. Chest pain in otherwise healthy children and adolescents is frequently caused by exercise-induced asthma. Pediatrics 1992;90:350–3.
10. Stack AM, Caputo GL. Pneumomediastinum in childhood asthma. Pediatr Emerg Care 1996;12:98–101.
11. Taniguchi H, Kanbara K, Hoshino K, et al. Chest pain relieved with a bronchodilator or other asthma drugs. Allergol Int 2009;58:421–7.
12. Damore DT, Dayan PS. Medical causes of pneumomediastinum in children. Clin Pediatr (Phila) 2001;40:87–91.
13. Wardlaw T, Salama P, Johansson EW, et al. Pneumonia: the leading killer of children. Lancet 2006;368:1048–50.
14. Williams BG, Gouws E, Boschi-Pinto C, et al. Estimates of world-wide distribution of child deaths from acute respiratory infections. Lancet Infect Dis 2002;2:25–32.
15. Ranganathan S, Sonnappa S. Pneumonia and other respiratory infections. Pediatr Clin North Am 2009;56:135–56.
16. Jokinen C, Heiskanen L, Juvonen H, et al. Incidence of community-acquired pneumonia in the population of four municipalities in eastern Finland. Am J Epidemiol 1993;137:977–88.
17. McCracken GH Jr. Etiology and treatment of pneumonia. Pediatr Infect Dis J 2000;19:373–7.
18. Byer RL. Pain-chest. In: Fleisher GR, Ludwig S, editors. Textbook of pediatric emergency medicine. 6th edition. Philadelphia: Lippincott Williams & Wilkins; 2010. p. 435.
19. Leung AK, Robson WL, Cho H. Chest pain in children. Can Fam Physician 1996; 42:1156–64.
20. Kliegman RM, Greenbaum LA, Lye PS, editors. Practical strategies in pediatric diagnosis and therapy. Philadelphia: Elsevier Saunders; 2004. p. 154.

21. Selbst SM. Consultation with the specialist: chest pain in children. Pediatr Rev 1997;18:169–73.
22. Durbin WJ, Stille C. Pneumonia. Pediatr Rev 2008;29:147–60.
23. Lichenstein R, Suggs A, Campbell J. Pediatric pneumonia. Emerg Med Clin North Am 2003;21:437–51.
24. Espositoi S, Bosis S, Cavagna R, et al. Characteristics of streptococcus pneumoniae and atypical bacterial infections in children 2–5 years of age with community-acquired pneumonia. Clin Infect Dis 2002;35(11):1345–52.
25. Chiou CCC, Yu VL. Severe pneumococcal pneumonia: new strategies for management. Curr Opin Crit Care 2006;12:470–6.
26. Claesson BA, Trollfors B, Brolin I, et al. Etiology of community-acquired pneumonia in children based on antibody responses to bacterial and viral antigens. Pediatr Infect Dis J 1989;8(12):856–62.
27. Hickey RW, Bowman MJ, Smith GA. Utility of blood cultures in pediatric patients found to have pneumonia in the emergency department. Ann Emerg Med 1996;27(6):721–5.
28. Cincinnati Children's Hospital Medical Center (2005, 22 December). Community-acquired pneumonia in children 60 days through 17 years of age. Available at: http://www.cincinnatichildrens.org/assets/0/78/1067/2709/2777/2793/9199/1633ae60-cbd1-4fbd-bba4-cb687fbb1d42.pdf. Accessed May 15, 2010.
29. Jadavji T, Law B, Lebel MH, et al. A practical guide for the diagnosis and treatment of pediatric pneumonias. Can Med Assoc J 1997;156:S703–11.
30. British Thoracic Society Standards of Care Committee. British Thoracic Society guidelines for the management of community-acquired pneumonia in childhood. Thorax 2002;57:i1–24.
31. Ruuskanen O, Mertsola J. Childhood community-acquired pneumonia. Semin Respir Infect 1999;14:163–72.
32. Lynch T, Platt R, Gouin S, et al. Can we predict which children with clinically suspected pneumonia will have the presence of focal infiltrates on chest radiographs? Pediatrics 2004;113:e186–9.
33. Swingler GH, Hussey GD, Zawarenstein M. Randomised controlled trial of clinical outcome after chest radiograph in ambulatory acute lower-respiratory infection in children. Lancet 1998;351:404–8.
34. Katz DS, Leung AN. Radiology of pneumonia. Clin Chest Med 1999;20:549–62.
35. Cherian T, Mulholland EK, Carlin JB, et al. Standardized interpretation of paediatric chest radiographs for the diagnosis of pneumonia in epidemiological studies. Bull World Health Organ 2005;83:353–9.
36. Fleisher GR, Ludwig S, Henretig FM, editors. Textbook of pediatric emergency medicine. 5th edition. Philadelphia: Lippincott Williams & Wilkins; 2006. p. 3 (see also page 81).
37. Kass SM, Williams PM, Reamy BV. Pleurisy. Am Fam Physician 2007;75:1357–64.
38. Korppi M. Community-acquired pneumonia in children. Pediatr Drugs 2000;5:821–32.
39. Chetty K, Thomson AH. Management of community-acquired pneumonia in children. Paediatr Drugs 2007;9:401–11.
40. Andrews J, Nadjm B, Gant V, et al. Community-acquired pneumonia. Curr Opin Pulm Med 2003;9:175–80.
41. Fontoura MS, Araújo-Neto CA, Andrade SC, et al. Clinical failure among children with nonsevere community-acquired pneumonia treated with amoxicillin. Expert Opin Pharmacother 2010;11(9):1451–8.

Pneumothorax, Pneumomediastinum, and Pulmonary Embolism

Nakia N. Johnson, MD, Alexander Toledo, DO, PharmD,
Erin E. Endom, MD*

KEYWORDS

- Pneumothorax • Pneumomediastinum • Pulmonary embolism
- Pediatrics

This article discusses pneumothorax (PTX), pneumomediastinum, and pulmonary embolism (PE); including incidence, presentation, diagnosis, and management of each.

PNEUMOTHORAX

Pneumothorax (PTX) is defined as the presence of gas in the potential space between the visceral and parietal pleura. It can be classified into two causal categories.

The first, spontaneous PTX, occurs in the absence of trauma. These pneumothoraces (PTXs) can be further broken down into primary and secondary classifications. A primary spontaneous PTX occurs in a patient with either no or subclinical underlying lung disease. Often attributed to ruptured apical blebs, primary spontaneous PTX is often associated with smoking in adults, but can also be seen in healthy children. A secondary spontaneous PTX occurs as a complication of a chronic or acute underlying pulmonary disease process.

The second, traumatic PTX, occurs via blunt or penetrating mechanisms. Rib fractures may or may not be present. Traumatic PTX takes place when air enters the pleural space from pulmonary, esophageal, chest wall, or tracheobronchial tree injuries.[1] Iatrogenic PTX is an important subset that can occur secondary to medical procedures such as thoracentesis, central venous cannulation, and mechanical ventilation.

The most concerning adverse outcome of traumatic and iatrogenic PTX is progression to a tension PTX. This occurs when the lung or airway defect acts as a one-way

Section of Emergency Medicine, Department of Pediatrics, Baylor College of Medicine, Texas Children's Hospital, 6621 Fannin, Suite A-210, Houston, TX 77030, USA
* Corresponding author.
E-mail address: eendom@bcm.tmc.edu

Pediatr Clin N Am 57 (2010) 1357–1383
doi:10.1016/j.pcl.2010.09.009
0031-3955/10/$ – see front matter © 2010 Elsevier Inc. All rights reserved.

valve, allowing air to flow into the pleural cavity without a means of escape. As the volume of air increases, the pressure leads to vascular compromise of the heart and great vessels. The circulatory system decompensates from mechanical impingement on blood flow and hypoxia due to respiratory compromise. Tension PTX in the absence of trauma is relatively rare and is associated with spontaneous PTX in 1% to 3% of cases.[2]

Incidence, Risk Factors, and Mortality

In the United States the incidence of spontaneous PTX is approximately 7.4 to 18 cases per 100,000 boys and 1.2 to 6 cases per 100,000 girls, with a male-to-female ratio of about 2:1.[3] This ratio appears to be reversed, however, below the age of 9 years.[4] Mean age at presentation has been reported to be 14 to 15.9 years, with one pediatric cohort reporting mean age at diagnosis of 13.8 years.[5,6] It appears to present most typically in tall, thin males with low body mass index. Mortality is considered low in children.[3]

Although the incidence of secondary PTX in children is not well described, those with asthma and cystic fibrosis are considered at particular risk.[7,8] The probability of PTX is thought to increase as the lung function decreases, and the mortality is considered higher because of decreased reserve of the ill lung.[9] Infectious causes such as *Pneumocystis jirovecii* pneumonia in immune disorders and necrotizing pneumonias (anaerobic gram-negative or staphylococcal) are associated with a higher incidence of PTX.[9] Individuals with underlying connective tissue disease, such as Marfan syndrome, Ehlers-Danlos, and ankylosing spondylitis, are also at higher risk.[10]

In the setting of thoracic trauma, PTX occurs in one-third of pediatric cases, with the majority of these having associated intrathoracic and extrathoracic injuries, and only one-third occurring in isolation.[11] In a review of 1533 victims of thoracic trauma listed in the National Pediatric Trauma Registry database, the incidence of isolated PTX in blunt and penetrating trauma was similar, 24% (306:1288) and 23% (52:230) respectively. Of note, PTX not complicated by hemothorax was present in 30% (58:228) of blunt and 0% (0:228) of penetrating trauma patients who died in this series.[12]

Iatrogenic PTX is an unfortunate consequence of medical procedures. A recent review found that 57% of the procedures that lead to PTX at a teaching hospital were performed under emergent conditions. The most frequent procedure types were central venous catheterization (43.8% of iatrogenic PTX), thoracentesis (20.1%), and barotrauma due to mechanical ventilation (9.1%).[13] The internal jugular and subclavian approaches to central venous access are considered to have the highest risk of PTX.[14] A systematic review reported an overall incidence of PTX resulting from thoracentesis of 6%, with 34.1% of these requiring chest tube insertion.[15] The introduction of real-time ultrasound guidance has been shown to reduce the incidence of PTX for both central venous access and thoracentesis in adults.[16,17] A recent meta-analysis of the pediatric literature of ultrasound-guided central venous access, however, failed to show any statistical difference in adverse outcomes.[18]

Presentation, Physical Examination Findings, and Differential Diagnosis

Children with spontaneous PTX typically present with a sudden onset of unilateral thoracic pain and dyspnea while at rest. Valsalva maneuvers such as lifting or straining have also been implicated.[5] In a chart review, 100% of patients presented with chest pain and 42% with dyspnea.[6] Children presenting after 24 hours may have little to no pain.[10] Patients with secondary spontaneous PTX can present in greater cardiopulmonary distress. Vital signs may include tachycardia, tachypnea with hypoxia, and hypotension in the most severe cases. Physical examination findings depend on the size of the PTX; many small air collections are undetected, whereas findings in large PTXs often include decreased breath sounds, vocal fremitus, and hyperresonance to percussion on the affected side.

Traumatic PTX has a wide spectrum of presentation. As in primary PTX, vital signs and symptomatology will depend on the size of the PTX. Physical examination findings that can differentiate tension PTX from simple traumatic PTX include neck vein distension, tracheal deviation away from the affected side, and cyanosis. Patients often present in moderate to severe distress, and tachycardia, hypotension, and oxygen desaturation are also seen.

Diagnostic Imaging

The plain radiograph, or chest x-ray (CXR), is the primary radiographic test to screen for PTX. Diagnosis is made by visualization of the visceral pleural margin, with the absence of lung markings peripheral to the pleural line. The sensitivity of CXR in the detection of PTX has been reported as high as 80%.[19] When clinically feasible, an upright CXR is the procedure of choice for suspected PTX, although a lateral decubitus view may also be diagnostic (**Fig. 1**).[20] Inspiratory and expiratory views are reported to be equally sensitive in detection of PTXs,[21] so the routine use of expiratory views for detection of PTX is not recommended.[22] In many patients, especially those presenting with multiple trauma, an upright CXR cannot be performed. Supine anteroposterior (AP) CXR is unreliable at detecting PTX, with a sensitivity of 36% to 48% in some studies.[23–25] Some may exhibit the deep sulcus sign (**Fig. 2**), which represents lucency of the lateral costophrenic angle extending toward the hypochondrium and giving the deepened lateral costophrenic angle a sharp, angular appearance.[26] Unfortunately, CXRs frequently underestimate the size of PTXs.[27]

The introduction and increased availability of CT scam has changed the ability of physicians to evaluate for PTX. Because it is the most sensitive and specific modality in the clinical setting, chest CT scan has become the reference standard for the diagnosis of PTX.[25] Traumatic PTXs not detected on supine AP CXR but seen on CT scan are a fairly recent phenomenon approximated to be present in 5% of all injured patients.[28] In a pediatric cohort of blunt trauma patients the incidence was found to

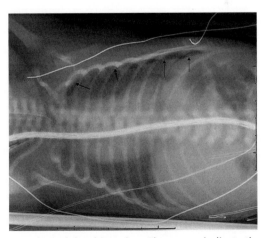

Fig. 1. Pneumothorax on lateral decubitus view. The arrows indicate the pleura; lung markings are absent distally. (*Courtesy of* Dr Rajesh Krishnamurthy of the Diagnostic Imaging Department of Texas Children's Hospital and Baylor College of Medicine, Houston, TX.)

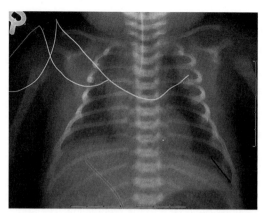

Fig. 2. Deep sulcus sign on left in supine anteroposterior radiograph. (*Courtesy of* Dr Rajesh Krishnamurthy of the Diagnostic Imaging Department of Texas Children's Hospital and Baylor College of Medicine, Houston, TX.)

be 3.7%.[29] Referred to in the trauma literature as "occult PTXs," their clinical relevance is a subject of debate as management guidelines have not been clearly delineated.[28] The literature describing the benefit of chest CT scan in the evaluation of primary and secondary PTX also appears to be unclear.[22,30] The increased sensitivity of CT scan, however, has been used to predict the risk of recurrence and to justify and plan surgical intervention.[3]

With the increased use and acceptance of the Focused Assessment with Sonography in Trauma (FAST) examination, ultrasound has become more readily available at the bedside. Techniques for detecting PTXs using ultrasound and its efficacy have been reported.[25,31] A recent literature review reported a sensitivity between 86% to 98% and specificity between 97% to 100%.[23] When compared with the sensitivity of supine CXR between 28% to 75% in this series, it appears the ultrasound will play a major role in evaluation of traumatic PTX in the near future.

Management

Initial treatment of the child with PTX should include prompt administration of oxygen, intravenous access, and placement on oximetry and cardiac monitors. Patients with suspected tension PTX and significant respiratory distress require immediate and aggressive intervention even before a CXR is obtained. A large-bore needle or intravenous catheter should be inserted on the ipsilateral side at the second intercostal space at the midclavicular line (**Fig. 3**A, B). If the needle fails to evacuate enough air to stabilize the patient, emergent thoracostomy will be required. There is no evidence that a chest tube with a larger diameter will be more effective in the treatment of any PTX than a smaller size (**Table 1**).

Pigtail catheters are smaller bore catheters inserted using the Seldinger technique. These catheters have been shown to offer a safe and effective alternative to larger bore chest tubes in children.[32] It must be remembered that tube thoracostomy is not a benign procedure, with an adverse event rate as high as 21%.[33] Complications of tube thoracostomy include injuries to thoracic or abdominal organs, empyema, bleeding, re-expansion pulmonary edema, pain, chest tube occlusion, and residual pneumothorax.[34]

Eighty percent of PTXs of less than 15% have no persistent air leak, and the rate of recurrence in such patients managed with observation alone is lower than in those

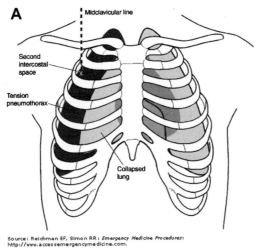

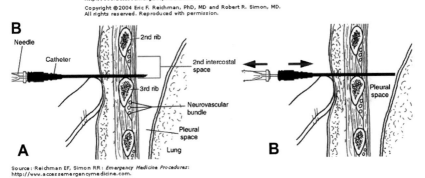

Fig. 3. (*A*) Needle thoracostomy. (*B*) Needle thoracostomy. (*From* Emergency medicine procedures. Reichman EF, Simon RR, editors. 2004; with permission. Available at: www.accessemergencymedicine.com.)

Table 1	
Chest tube size by patient weight	
Weight, kg	**Chest Tube Size, French**
3–5	10–12
6–9	12–16
10–11	16–20
12–14	20–22
15–18	22–24
19–22	24–28
23–30	24–32
>32	32–40

Data from Bliss D, Silen M. Pediatric thoracic trauma. Crit Care Med 2002;30(Suppl 11):S409–15.

treated with chest tubes.[35] The asymptomatic patient with primary PTX of less than 15% may be observed for 3 to 6 hours, and then discharged home with close follow-up if a repeat CXR shows no progression of the PTX. Patients with poor social situations or unreliable follow-up should be admitted.[29]

In the setting of primary (spontaneous) PTX, symptomatic patients and patients with PTX of 15% or greater should be admitted. Mildly symptomatic patients may be observed with or without the administration of high-flow oxygen via a nonrebreather mask.[22,29] Oxygen may increase the rate of PTX reabsorption, with a fourfold effect demonstrated in the presence of PTX greater than 30%.[5] The duration of therapy is dependent on resolution of symptoms and reabsorption of the PTX, usually between 1.25% and 2.2% of hemithoracic volume every 24 hours.[36–38] There is no evidence that invasive intervention improves the associated chest pain, which is more appropriately managed with analgesia.[39]

Larger and more significantly symptomatic primary PTXs should undergo re-expansion.[29] Simple needle aspiration is recommended as first-line therapy by the British Thoracic Society,[22] whereas the American College of Chest Physicians guidelines consider simple aspiration to be "appropriate rarely in any clinical circumstance" and recommend tube thoracostomy as primary management.[29]

Admission should be strongly considered in all cases of secondary spontaneous PTX. Hemodynamically stable patients with small secondary PTX may be observed as inpatients without invasive intervention. Clinically unstable patients, patients with respiratory distress, and patients with large PTXs should undergo tube thoracostomy.[22,29] Patients with persistent air leaks or recurrent PTX should be referred for surgical intervention such as video-assisted thoracoscopy.[22]

All patients with traumatic PTX should be considered to be at risk for cardiopulmonary decompensation and should be admitted. Penetrating PTXs and large blunt trauma PTXs are treated with tube thoracostomy. As stated previously, treatment of the small occult PTX remains controversial. Concern exists that these PTXs can expand, especially in the ventilated patient, leading to tension PTX.[24] The available literature for children and adults, however, appears to support the position that these patients may be safely observed regardless of mechanical ventilation and rarely require tube thoracostomy.[28,30,40]

PNEUMOMEDIASTINUM

Pneumomediastinum is defined as air in the mediastinum and should be included in the differential diagnosis of acute chest pain. The anatomic borders of the mediastinum are as follows: superior, thoracic inlet; inferior, diaphragm; posterior, thoracic spine; and anterior, sternum (**Fig. 4**). Pneumomediastinum may affect any or all of these spaces.

Classification of pneumomediastinum stems from its cause. Secondary or acquired pneumomediastinum generally occurs as a result of thoracic or abdominal surgery, foreign body ingestion, cardiac catheterization, or endotracheal intubation and mechanical ventilation.[41–46] Other medical procedures predisposing to mediastinal emphysema include dental, endotracheobronchial and endoesophageal procedures. Severe cases may result from trauma to the chest or neck with disruption of the tracheobronchial tree.[45,47]

Spontaneous pneumomediastinum occurs in the absence of the above causes, and often occurs as a result of infections or asthma.[48–51] Asthma is the most common underlying condition, with up to 35% of cases associated with asthma and other obstructive pulmonary diseases.[52,53] Infectious causes include bronchiolitis,

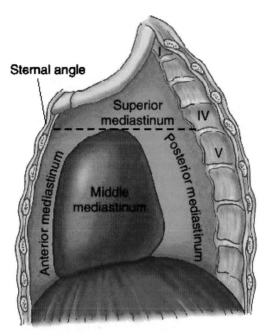

Fig. 4. Anatomic borders of the mediastinum. Roman numerals I, IV and V indicate the corresponding thoracic vertebrae. (*From* WA Newman Dorland WAN, Dorland's medical dictionary for health consumers, Elsevier 2007; with permission.)

bronchitis, viral pneumonia, and retropharyngeal abscesses. Valsalva maneuvers such as coughing, screaming, deep breathing with physical activity, or vomiting are frequent causes of spontaneous pneumomediastinum.[48,50] Diabetic ketoacidosis has been associated with the development of spontaneous pneumomediastinum,[48] possibly as a result of associated vomiting.[54] Inhaled drug use is another important risk factor for developing this condition.[51]

The most common mechanism resulting in pneumomediastinum is thought to be alveolar rupture, resulting in tracking of free air toward the hilum of the affected lung, into the mediastinum and upwards into the subcutaneous space of the upper chest and neck. Rupture or perforation of the esophagus or large airways can also result in the characteristic clinical picture.

Incidence

Whereas its true incidence is unknown, it has been reported in an estimated 1 per 14,000 individuals between 14 and 29 years of age.[51] The incidence has a bimodal peak, occurring more frequently in children between 6 months and 3 to 4 years of age and in adolescents,[48,51,53] and in 1 per 20,000 patients presenting to emergency departments with exacerbations of asthma.[53] Tall, thin adolescent boys are more commonly affected.[51]

Presentation

Patients typically complain of retrosternal chest pain that increases with respirations, dyspnea, and neck pain. The history may reveal the presence of sore throat, coughing or vomiting, low-grade fevers, dysphagia, and dysphonia.[7,55,56] A history of risk factors and predisposing conditions may also be elicited. Physical examination findings include subcutaneous emphysema (air in the subcutaneous tissues of the chest and neck), often with visible neck edema; palpable crepitus is diagnostic. Precordial crepitus auscultated during systole (Hamman's sign) indicates the presence of subcutaneous emphysema and is pathognomonic for pneumomediastinum. Patients may also present with torticollis as a result of cervical subcutaneous air.

The differential diagnosis for pneumomediastinum includes pericarditis and pneumothorax, both of which present with dyspnea and chest pain; however, respiratory distress in PTX is often more pronounced than in pneumomediastinum. Hamman's sign, neck edema, and torticollis are not usually seen in pneumothorax. Pericarditis differs from pneumomediastinum and PTX in that the severity of chest pain sometimes varies with position (increased pain when supine and decreased in a seated position while leaning forward). Auscultation may reveal a friction rub, a finding distinct to pericarditis.[57]

Diagnosis

Plain radiographs remain the gold standard for diagnosing pneumomediastinum. Anterior and lateral views of the chest including the neck are usually sufficient to demonstrate typical findings.[51,56] The anterior view may reveal a continuous diaphragm sign, which is a lucency that extends between the pericardium and diaphragm. A vertical line of lucency surrounding the left side of the trachea, heart, and aortic arch may also be visualized on the anterior view (**Fig. 5**). The spinnaker sail sign, superior and lateral elevation of the thymus, is often seen in infants.[58] Lateral views may demonstrate retrocardiac, pericardiac, periaortic, and peritracheal lucency. PTX may coexist with pneumomediastinum.

High-resolution chest CT scan is not routinely necessary to diagnose pneumomediastinum, but is recommended when history and physical examination raise clinical suspicion of esophageal perforation. Boerhaave's syndrome, which is esophageal rupture resulting from forceful vomiting, is the most common cause of esophageal

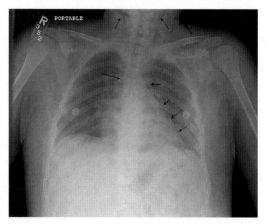

Fig. 5. Pneumomediastinum on posteroanterior chest radiograph. Arrows indicate air bilaterally in the soft tissue of the neck, surrounding the right side of the thoracic vertebrae, and outlining the left cardiac border. (*Courtesy of* Matthew Urban and Scott Dorfman, MD, of the Diagnostic Imaging Department of Texas Children's Hospital and Baylor College of Medicine, Houston, TX.)

perforation.[55] The diagnosis is strongly indicated by the presence of Mackler's triad: (1) history of violent vomiting, (2) chest pain, and (3) subcutaneous emphysema on examination. Perforation of the esophagus may also result from ingestion of a foreign body (**Fig. 6**A, B).[56,59] Barium swallow or esophagoscopy, though not indicated to diagnose pneumomediastinum, should also be obtained in this instance to identify disruption of the esophageal wall. It is preferable to obtain both studies as contrast studies may not indicate the diagnosis alone.[51]

Management of pneumomediastinum primarily consists of supportive care, including rest, pain control, cough suppression, and avoidance of Valsalva and other aggravating factors. Most cases will resolve without sequelae over 3 to 15 days.[53,60] Most cases may be managed in the outpatient setting. Admission criteria include hypoxia, significant respiratory distress, esophageal perforation, and severity

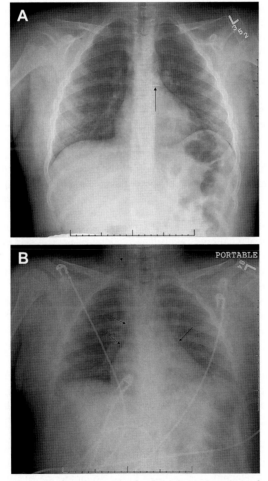

Fig. 6. (*A*) Posteroanterior chest radiograph of a child demonstrating a foreign body (*arrow*) in the left mainstem bronchus. (*B*) Posteroanterior chest radiograph after removal of the foreign body from the left mainstem bronchus visualized above, demonstrating pneumomediastinum. Arrows indicate the extent of air in the soft tissues of the neck and outlining the left and right cardiac borders. (*Courtesy of* Dr Rajesh Krishnamurthy of the Diagnostic Imaging Department of Texas Children's Hospital and Baylor College of Medicine, Houston, TX.)

requiring surgical intervention. Definitive treatment consists of treating the underlying cause. In the instance of marked hypoxia or respiratory distress requiring mechanical ventilation, a collar mediastinotomy (release incisions made in the infraclavicular region) should be performed.[56,61]

Complications of pneumomediastinum are rare and include laryngeal compression, pseudotamponade, mediastinitis in the setting of esophageal perforation, and tension pneumomediastinum or pneumothorax.[51] These complications generally require surgical management. Pneumomediastinum is rarely fatal. A few case reports demonstrate increased mortality in children with serious chronic pulmonary disease and in a group of children in a developing country with measles.[51,62]

PULMONARY EMBOLISM

Although pulmonary embolism (PE) occurs rarely in children as compared with adults, its incidence has increased in recent years, with a current documentable incidence of between 0.86 and 5.3 cases per 10,000 hospital admissions.[63,64] This increase is expected to continue for a number of reasons, including increased survival of children with previously fatal disease conditions that increase PE risk, and increased use of central venous catheters, a known risk factor for PE development. The true incidence is almost certainly much greater than reported for a number of reasons, including lower index of suspicion on the part of physicians treating children, lower reliability of screening algorithms in children than in adults,[65] and masking of symptoms by other ongoing disease processes. In a recent literature review, 12 of 20 (60%) of children with massive PE died suddenly, with diagnosis made only at autopsy.[66]

Despite these factors, PE remains much less common in children than in adults. Possible protective mechanisms in children may include reduced capacity to generate thrombin and increased antithrombic potential of blood vessel walls compared with adults.[63] PE incidence in children is bimodal, with peaks in infancy and in adolescence.

PE severity can be roughly divided into three groups. In the first, the PE is small and well tolerated clinically, without hemodynamic instability. The second group consists of patients with sufficient obstruction of flow in the pulmonary arterial bed to produce pulmonary hypertension and right ventricular strain from afterload, but without systemic hypotension. The third group involves massive PE, which has been defined as PE associated with systemic hypotension, shock, syncope, or cardiac arrest,[66–68] or as obstruction equivalent to loss of flow to two or more lobar arteries resulting in acute right heart failure and cardiogenic shock.[69]

Risk Factors

Ninety-five percent of venous thromboembolic events (VTE) in children are associated with serious medical conditions such as cancer, surgery or trauma, congenital heart disease, and collagen vascular disease.[70] Virchow's triad delineates three types of risk factors for VTE: alterations in blood flow, endothelial injury, and hypercoagulability (**Table 2**).

The development of deep vein thrombosis (DVT) is influenced by these factors and can result in PE, either by embolization or by direct extension through the inferior or superior vena cava. Recent studies have found an incidence of DVT in 55% to 72% of pediatric patients with documented PE.[64,71]

One of the most frequent VTE-PE risk factors in children is the presence of a central venous catheter (CVC),[64,72] particularly when the CVC is infected.[73,74] The presence of malignancy is also a significant factor separately from its common association with CVCs, due to both inherent hypercoagulability state and embolization or direct

Table 2 Virchow's triad of risk factors for PE		
Alterations in Blood Flow (Venous Stasis)	**Vascular Endothelial Injury**	**Thrombophilic (Hypercoagulable) States**
Immobilization	Central venous catheters	Cancer or chemotherapy
Surgery	Trauma	Nephrotic syndrome
Venous malformations	Infection	Genetic disorders (protein C, S, antithrombin deficiencies)
Blood flow obstruction (May-Thurner syndrome)	—	Estrogen
—	—	Acquired disorders (lupus)

Data from Refs.[63,92,108]

extension of tumor material; the latter has been shown in one study to cause 40% of PEs in children.[66] Other risk factors include congenital heart disease and cardiac surgery, especially involving right heart bypass surgery such as the Fontan procedure,[63] other recent surgery, and immobilization.

Sepsis and other forms of infection are also risk factors for PE, particularly septic PEs arising from localized infections. These may include suppurative otitis media,[74] pyomyositis and other soft tissue infections,[74–77] osteomyelitis,[74,78] and Lemierre syndrome (jugular venous thrombosis associated with anaerobic infection of the head and neck).[79] The most frequent causative organism is *Staphylococcus aureus*,[74–78] except in the case of Lemierre syndrome, which is commonly caused by *Fusobacterium necrophorum* or is polymicrobial.[79]

Thrombophilia (hypercoagulability) has a large number of causes, both genetic and acquired; they may be present in combination, further increasing the risk of VTE-PE (**Table 3**).

A 2008 study found factors causing thrombophilia in 14 of 40 (35%) of patients with PE who were evaluated for thrombophilia.[64] Vascular malformations, especially of the lower limb, and syndromes associated with these such as Klippel-Trenaunay and Proteus syndromes predispose to clot formation and PE as well.[80,81]

Trauma is well established as a risk factor for hypercoagulability and PE in adults. While pediatric data is limited, children seem to be at much lower risk.[82–85] Pediatric trauma patients at increased risk include those with high Injury Severity Scores, thoracic or spinal injuries, or CVCs.[86]

Nonthrombotic PEs may include tumor embolism from myxomata in the right side of the heart, or from other types of tumor; fat embolism following severe trauma to long bones or adipose tissue; and foreign materials such as catheters, guide wires, or endovascular occlusive materials used to embolize arteriovenous malformations.[63,87]

Idiopathic PE (no clinical or laboratory risk factors identified) is rare in children, with an incidence between 0% and 4%.[63,88,89]

Pathophysiology

While the most common origin of PE in adults is in the deep veins of the lower extremities, PE in children may also arise from the upper extremity veins, the right side of the heart, and the pelvic or renal veins.[90] PE produces obstruction of blood flow through the affected pulmonary vasculature. Combined with ongoing ventilation of these segments, this leads to an increase in alveolar dead space, ventilation-perfusion mismatch, hypoxemia, and hypercarbia. In severe cases, the increase in pulmonary arterial resistance can lead to right heart failure.

Table 3
Causes of thrombophilia

Genetic	Acquired
Protein S deficiency	Antiphospholipid antibodies in antiphospholipid syndrome, including lupus anticoagulant in systemic lupus erythematosus (SLE); cause prolonged activated PTT
Protein C deficiency or resistance	Anticardiolipin antibodies
Antithrombin III deficiency	Anti-β2-glycoprotein-1antibodies
Dysfibrinogenemia	Acquired antithrombin, protein C, protein S abnormalities
Plasminogen deficiency	Elevated factor VIII in systemic inflammatory states such as SLE
Impairment of fibrinolysis	Nephrotic syndrome: induces hypercoagulable state due to urinary losses of antithrombin and free protein S, elevated FVIII levels, elevated fibrinogen and lipoprotein A, reduction in antithrombin, hyperaggregability of platelets
Prothrombin 20210A mutations	Exogenous estrogen therapy (oral contraceptive use)
Lipoprotein (a) elevation	Pregnancy
Factor V Leiden	Diabetes mellitus
Thalassemia (especially following splenectomy)	Hyperlipidemia
Sickle cell disease	—
Hyperhomocystinemia	—

Data from Babyn PS, Gahunia HK, Massicotte P. Pulmonary thromboembolism in children. Eur J Pediatr 1991;150:304–7; Biss TT, Brandão LR, Kahr WH, et al. Clinical features and outcome of pulmonary embolism in children. Br J Haematol 2008;142(5):808–18; Monagle P, Chalmers E, Chan A, et al. Antithrombotic therapy in neonates and children. Chest 2008;133(Suppl 6);887–968S; Bomgaars L, Cassady C, Chase L, et al. Texas Children's Hospital evidence-based outcomes center deep vein thrombosis clinical guideline, 2009.

Presentation

The classic clinical presentation of PE consists of pleuritic chest pain (the most common presenting complaint in adolescents),[91] dyspnea, cough or hemoptysis, or fever; other symptoms include tachycardia and syncope. Severe cases may present with symptoms of acute right heart failure. Massive PE presents with acute onset of dyspnea, diaphoresis, chest or abdominal pain, hypoxemia, hypotension, and often hemoptysis; these symptoms rapidly progress to respiratory failure or cardiopulmonary arrest. Abdominal pain is a rare presenting symptom, and may result from diaphragmatic pleurisy or hepatic congestion.[92] Septic PE often includes symptoms and signs of sepsis such as fever and tachypnea, or a shock-like state with cyanosis and bradycardia.[74]

Physical examination findings may include a pleural friction rub, dullness to percussion over the involved lung segments, hypotension, and arrhythmias. Right heart failure in severe cases may produce rales, hepatomegaly, and edema.

Evaluation and Diagnosis: Laboratory

Initial laboratory testing for suspected PE should include: complete blood count with differential and platelet count; prothrombin time (PT), partial thromboplastin time

(PTT), and International Normalized Ratio (INR); thrombin time; fibrinogen level; and D-dimer. Hepzyme PTT, which determines whether heparin contamination is responsible for prolonged PTT, should also be obtained if indicated. Antithrombin level should be checked in infants less than 6 months of age.[93] Arterial blood gas analysis may reveal hypoxia, hypocapnia, respiratory alkalosis, and a significant a-A CO_2 gradient; however, these findings are neither sensitive nor specific for PE.[94] Girls of childbearing age should be tested for pregnancy.

D-dimer is released during plasmin-mediated proteolysis of fibrin, and is elevated in the bloodstream in acute VTE. An elevated D-dimer is a highly sensitive marker for VTE-PE in adults, but not specific as many other conditions can cause D-dimer elevation, including malignancy, trauma, infection, and surgery.[63,95] However, D-dimer levels appear to be less reliable in children than in adults; children with documented PE have been found to have D-dimer elevations in 50% to 87% of cases.[64,89,96]

The Wells criteria are a set of factors widely used to assess the clinical probability of PE in adults (**Table 4**).[97] These criteria are used in combination with D-dimer levels to determine likelihood of PE.[98] Unfortunately, these criteria are much less reliable in children than in adults, even with modification to account for higher baseline heart rates in children.[96]

Evaluation may be indicated for genetic or acquired conditions causing thrombophilia, potentially including the following: protein C; protein S; antithrombin III; lipid profiles; lipoprotein (a); anticardiolipin IgG and IgM; antiphospholipid antibodies; lupus anticoagulant; anti-β2-glycoprotein-1–IgG and –IgM; homocysteine; factors II, V, VII, VIII, IX, and XI; factor V G1691A (factor V Leiden); or prothrombin G20210A.[88,93] These tests may be available as a single panel depending on lab capacity, and should be obtained before beginning therapy.

Electrocardiographic changes are usually nonspecific and not reliable in children. They may include sinus tachycardia, ST-T segment changes, right axis deviation, or right bundle branch block.[63,99]

Table 4	
Wells simplified probability score for PE	
Clinical signs and symptoms of DVT (leg swelling, pain with palpation of deep veins)	3.0
Alternative diagnosis less likely than PE	3.0
Heart rate >100 1–10 years old: >120 Less than 1 year old: >160	1.5
Immobilization (complete bed rest 3 or more days, or lower extremity cast); or surgery in previous 4 wk	1.5
Previous DVT or PE	1.5
Hemoptysis	1.0
Malignancy (being treated; treated in last 6 mo; or palliative)	1.0

Total score >4: PE likely
Total score < or = 4: PE unlikely

Data from Biss TT, Brandão LR, Kahr WHA, et al. Clinical probability score and D-dimer estimation lack utility in the diagnosis of childhood pulmonary embolism. J Thromb Haemost 2009;7(10):1633–38; and Wells PS, Anderson DR, Rodger M, et al. Excluding pulmonary embolism at the bedside without diagnostic imaging: management of patients with suspected pulmonary embolism presenting to the emergency department by using a simple clinical model and D-dimer. Ann Intern Med 2001;135(2):98–107.

Evaluation and Diagnosis: Radiologic

CXR and CT scan findings are generally nonspecific, including peripheral wedge-shaped parenchymal infiltrates, atelectasis, and pleural effusion (**Fig. 7**)[63]; close to 50% are normal.[71] Chronic PE may produce cardiomegaly (primarily right-sided), enlarged central pulmonary arteries with rapid tapering, and patchy decreased pulmonary vascularity.[63,100] Septic emboli may be seen as patchy infiltrates on plain radiographs. They may be accompanied by empyema, bronchopleural fistula, or pneumothorax.[77]

Echocardiography, either transthoracic or transesophageal, allows direct visualization of clots in the heart and central pulmonary arteries, but is less effective at detecting distal clots.[63]

Radionuclide scintigraphy (ventilation-perfusion or V/Q scan) is historically the primary method of diagnosing PE (**Fig. 8**).[63] The Prospective Investigation of Pulmonary Embolism Diagnosis (PIOPED) study established V/Q interpretation criteria in adults (**Table 5**).[101]

A high-probability scan in the appropriate clinical setting is considered diagnostic of PE. However, V/Q has low specificity; a low-probability V/Q scan is still associated with a 20% chance of PE.[71] Another drawback is that the study is frequently nondiagnostic, with normal and high-probability scans seen in only 25% of adult cases.[63] Other causes of V/Q mismatch include pulmonary artery stenosis, pneumonia, pulmonary tuberculosis, collagen vascular diseases, and sickle cell anemia. The study is difficult to interpret in presence of congenital heart disease, especially with right-to-left shunting. Finally, the validity of PIOPED criteria in children has not been established.[63]

Pulmonary angiography (PA) is the traditional gold standard for diagnosis of PE; it involves injection of contrast medium into the right or left pulmonary artery. Intraluminal filling defects, sudden vessel cutoff, or perfusion defects are diagnostic of PE. PA

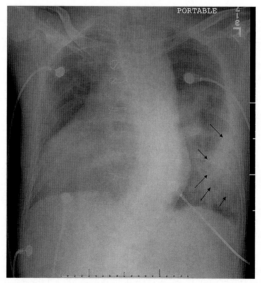

Fig. 7. Wedge-shaped density (outlined by the *arrows*) indicative of PE in a patient with heterotaxy and a Glenn shunt. (*Courtesy of* Dr Rajesh Krishnamurthy of the Diagnostic Imaging Department of Texas Children's Hospital and Baylor College of Medicine, Houston, TX.)

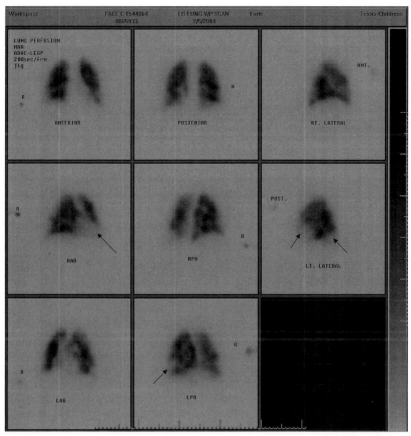

Fig. 8. Pulmonary ventilation-perfusion scan showing multiple areas of decreased perfusion, consistent with a high probability of PE. (*Courtesy of* Dr Rajesh Krishnamurthy of the Diagnostic Imaging Department of Texas Children's Hospital and Baylor College of Medicine, Houston, TX.)

is highly reliable, with nondiagnostic results in only 3% of studies.[102] PA is more invasive than other diagnostic modalities due to the necessity of central venous or arterial access.

Spiral CT pulmonary angiography (CTPA) is being used with increasing frequency in both adults and children for multiple reasons: it permits both direct thrombus visualization and assessment for alternative diagnoses, as the entire chest (mediastinum, lung parenchyma, and pleura) is visualized; inadequate imaging occurs less frequently (0.9%–3.0%)[95]; and it may be combined with CT scan venography of the lower extremities.[63,103] Findings diagnostic or suggestive of PE include intraluminal defects with a sharp interface with contrast and peripheral wedge-shaped parenchymal opacities (**Figs. 9** and **10**).[104] Other findings may include air trapping or mosaic perfusion; right ventricular failure and enlarged pulmonary arteries in severe cases; and extensive collateral vessel development in chronic disease.

Thoracic ultrasound has been shown to compare favorably with CTPA in sensitivity and specificity in adults[105] and in a single, small pediatric study.[106] Two or more typical triangular or rounded pleural-based lesions in the appropriate clinical setting

Table 5	
PIOPED V/Q scan interpretation criteria	
High Probability	≥2 large (>75% of segment) segmental perfusion defects without corresponding ventilation
	1 large segmental perfusion defect and ≥2 moderate (25%–75% of a segment) segmental perfusion defects without matching ventilation or chest radiographic abnormalities
	≥4 moderate segmental perfusion defects without corresponding ventilation or chest radiographic abnormalities
Intermediate Probability	1 moderate to 2 large segmental perfusion defects without corresponding ventilation or radiographic abnormalities
	Corresponding V/Q defects and radiographic parenchymal opacity in lower lung zone
	Single moderate matched V/Q defects with normal radiographic findings
	Corresponding V/Q defects and small pleural effusion
	Difficult to categorize as normal, low or high probability
Low Probability	Multiple matched V/Q defects, regardless of size, with normal radiographic findings
	Corresponding V/Q defects and radiographic parenchymal opacity in upper or middle lung zone
	Corresponding V/Q defects and large pleural effusion
	Any perfusion defect with substantially larger chest radiographic abnormality
	Defects surrounded by normally-perfused lung (stripe sign)
	>3 small segmental perfusion defects (<25% of a segment) with a normal chest radiograph
	Nonsegmental perfusion defects (cardiomegaly, aortic impression, enlarged hila)
Very Low Probability	≤3 small segmental perfusion defects (<25% of a segment) with a normal chest radiograph
Normal	No perfusion defects and perfusion outlines the shape of the lung seen on chest radiographs

Data from Babyn PS, Gahunia HK, Massicotte P. Pulmonary thromboembolism in children. Pediatr Radiol 2005;35(3):258–74.

are considered confirmatory of PE; a single typical lesion with pleural effusion indicates probable PE; and the presence of either multiple small (< 5 mm) subpleural lesions or pleural effusion indicates possible PE.[106]

Magnetic resonance pulmonary angiography (MRPA), unlike CTPA, does not use ionizing radiation. Findings indicating PE include filling defects in the vascular system and an enlarged central pulmonary artery with abnormal tapering proximally to distally (indicating pulmonary hypertension). Drawbacks of MRPA include the fact that it is less sensitive in detecting small or peripheral small PEs, therefore a negative study does not rule out PE; the required prolonged imaging time and intensive monitoring is difficult in severely ill patients; and the study is not readily available in most centers.[63,95]

Babyn and colleagues[63] suggest that in the clinical suspicion of PE in a clinically stable child, documentation of DVT can be substituted for detailed evaluation of the lungs, as the treatment is generally the same. Ultrasonography (US), including gray-scale, color Doppler, and spectral analysis, is the preferred modality for diagnosis

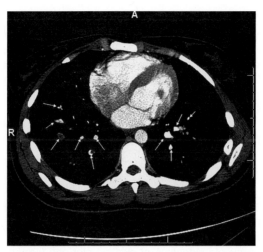

Fig. 9. Multiple subsegmental pulmonary emboli on CT angiogram, indicated by the arrows. (*Courtesy of* Dr Rajesh Krishnamurthy of the Diagnostic Imaging Department of Texas Children's Hospital and Baylor College of Medicine, Houston, TX.)

of lower-extremity DVT as it readily detects echogenic thrombi, presence or absence of flow, and compressibility or noncompressibility of the vein. US is less sensitive than venography, MR venography, or CT scan in detecting thrombi in the pelvic veins and the upper venous system.

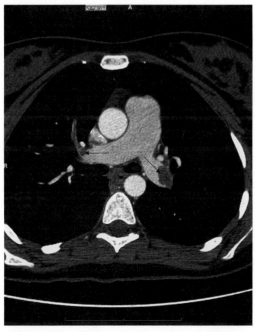

Fig. 10. Arrows indicate PE in both major pulmonary arteries. (*Courtesy of* Dr Rajesh Krishnamurthy of the Diagnostic Imaging Department of Texas Children's Hospital and Baylor College of Medicine, Houston, TX.)

Differential Diagnosis

The differential diagnosis of PE is broad and includes conditions that can cause chest pain, dyspnea, hypoxia, and hemoptysis, such as pneumonia, atelectasis, intrathoracic malignancies, and trauma. Whereas studies in children are limited, a 2009 study of 123 pediatric CTPA studies found that 17% had PE. Of the remainder, 41% of studies were normal; the most common alternative diagnoses identified were pneumonia and atelectasis in 39% each, and pleural effusion in 17%. Also identified on CTPA were malignancies, congenital heart disease, pulmonary hypertension, pericardial effusion, pulmonary nodules, rib fractures, right atrial thrombus, and fat embolism.[107]

Management

Management of PE depends on a number of factors, including size of the clot, severity of symptoms, and any contraindications to the different modes of management; it may involve anticoagulation, thrombolysis, filtering, or thrombectomy.

Anticoagulation prevents extension of existing clot and formation of new clots by inhibiting coagulation enzymes. Unfractionated heparin (UFH) is the traditional treatment standard; its advantages include rapid onset of action, short half-life, and reversibility with protamine. Disadvantages are that it requires continuous intravenous infusion; clinical dose response is unpredictable; adverse effects include osteopenia and heparin-induced thrombocytopenia (HIT); and it requires adequate levels of antithrombin, which is deficient in neonates.[93,108]

Low molecular weight heparin (LMWH) is widely used as a heparin equivalent in both adult and pediatric patients; the most widely used is enoxaparin. Its advantages over UFH include subcutaneous rather than intravenous administration, a longer half-life permitting scheduled rather than continuous dosing, a lower risk of osteopenia and HIT compared with UFH, and self- or parental administration. However, it still requires monitoring via the antiactivated factor X (Xa) assay; protamine is only partially effective as an antidote; HIT is still a known adverse effect; and, like UFH, it requires adequate antithrombin levels.[63,90] Neonates, infants, and young children require higher doses for body weight than older children to achieve therapeutic levels.[70,109] **Table 6** shows UFH and LMWH administration guidelines.

Fondaparinux is a synthetic pentasaccharide with antithrombotic activity mediated through selective antithrombin-mediated inhibition of factor Xa. It is administered subcutaneously for both prophylaxis and treatment of VTE in adults; little pediatric data is available at this time. It may be used in patients with HIT, as its risk of producing HIT in the absence of concomitant or recent heparin or LMWH is low.[110] Other advantages of fondaparinux include predictable pharmacokinetics, obviating the need for frequent dose monitoring, and once-daily dosing. Fondaparinux requires dose reduction and intensive monitoring in renal failure, as it is excreted by the kidneys, and is poorly dialyzable leading to potential accumulation.[111]

Vitamin K is necessary for the function of coagulation factors II, VII, IX, and X. Warfarin, a vitamin K antagonist (VKA), is the only anticoagulant in established use that can be administered orally. It is not used as initial anticoagulation therapy, but rather as long-term therapy and prophylaxis of VTE; it may be started concurrently with or subsequently to heparin or LWMH, with at least a 5-day overlap during which both medications are given. Warfarin dosage is monitored via PT, expressed as an INR. Warfarin therapy is particularly difficult in children because no liquid preparation is available, and because multiple factors can interfere with its metabolism, including concomitant medications, colds and other viral and bacterial infections, many foods,

Table 6
Suggested regimens for anticoagulation in the setting of pulmonary embolism

	Dose	Target Levels	Monitoring	Bleeding Reversal	Notes
UFH	75 U/kg IV over 10 min; then: under 1 year: 28 U/kg/h 1 year or older: 20 U/kg/h	Anti-FXA 0.35–0.7 U/mL	Anti-FXA level 4 h after initiation and any dose changes Platelet level every 3 days until discharge.	Stop infusion. Hematology service consult Protamine sulfate[a]	Administer through dedicated line. Continue for 5–10 d
Enoxaparin (LMWH)	<2 months: 1.7 mg/kg SQ every 12 hours. 2 months or older: 1.0 mg/kg SQ every 12 h.	Anti-FXA 0.5–1.0 U/mL, 4 h following dose	Anti-FXA level 4 h after second dose, and 4 h after any dose changes. Platelet level every 3 days.	Stop enoxaparin. Hematology service consult. Protamine sulfate[b]	Deep SQ injection. Continue x 5–10 d
Warfarin (VKA)	0.2 mg/kg/dose once daily	INR 2.5 (2–3)	INR daily until stable; then twice a week for 1–2 weeks; then every 2–4 weeks. Check with changes in other medications, dietary vitamin K intake, hepatic function, and viral or bacterial illnesses.	Stop warfarin. Hematology service consult. FFP and IV Vitamin K for life-threatening bleeding. Oral Vitamin K for minor bleeding.	Ensure 5-d overlap with UFH/LMWH therapy.

Abbreviations: FFP, fresh frozen plasma; FXA, activated coagulation factor X; SQ, subcutaneous; U, unit; UFH, unfractionated heparin; VKA, vitamin K antagonist.

[a] Protamine sulfate dosage for significant bleeding with UFH therapy, based on the amount of heparin received in the last 2 h and the time since discontinuation of UFH infusion. Protamine should be administered at a concentration of 10mg/mL, at a rate not to exceed 5 mg/min. Maximum dose 50 mg. Obtain partial thromboplastin time 15min after infusion.

[b] Protamine sulfate dosage for significant bleeding with enoxaparin therapy, based on the amount of enoxaparin received and the time since the last injection. Protamine concentration, rate of infusion and maximum dosage are the same as for UFH above.

Data from Monagle P, Chalmers E, Chan A, et al. Antithrombotic therapy in neonates and children. Chest 2008;133(Suppl 6):887–968S; Bomgaars L, Cassady C, Chase L, et al. Texas children's hospital evidence-based outcomes center deep vein thrombosis clinical guideline. 2009.

and lack of enteral intake.[93,112] Additionally, variable dose response and a narrow therapeutic window require frequent INR monitoring. The most common complication of VKA therapy is bleeding; warfarin's long half-life precludes rapid reversal of its effects without the use of antidotes (fresh frozen plasma and vitamin K). Reduced bone density has been documented with use for longer than 1 year. See **Table 6** for warfarin administration guidelines.

Anticoagulation should only be undertaken in consultation with a hematologist (a pediatric hematologist if at all possible). Relative contraindications to anticoagulation include recent trauma, recent or anticipated surgery, and intracranial or gastrointestinal bleeding.[113]

Thrombolysis, or actual clot destruction, is (in combination with heparin or LMWH) the first line of therapy for hemodynamically significant PE in the absence of contraindications.[69] Thrombolytic drugs convert plasminogen to plasmin, which mediates clot lysis. The three major thrombolytics are streptokinase, urokinase, and tissue plasminogen activator (tPA). Although little specific data is available for pediatric use, tPA is considered the agent of choice in children because of its specificity and lower immunoreactivity.[70] Systemic tPA for lysis of PE is administered as a continuous infusion of 0.1 to 0.6 mg/kg/hour for 6 hours; fibrinogen, thrombin clotting time, PT, and activated PTT should be monitored.[70] The major complication of thrombolytic therapy is clinically significant bleeding, including pulmonary, gastrointestinal, and intracranial. Contraindications include the following: active bleeding; recent surgery or other invasive procedure; thrombocytopenia less than 50 to 100,000/μL; hyperfibrinogenemia greater than 100 mg/dL; seizures in the past 48 hours; and the presence of intracranial neoplasm or arteriovenous malformation.[93,114–116] Recent lumbar puncture may be a relative contraindication as well.[114]

Thrombectomy is physical clot removal from the affected blood vessels, either surgically or via catheter. Surgical thrombectomy is technically difficult, especially in infants and smaller children, and has a mortality rate as high as 64%.[69] It is usually reserved for massive or otherwise hemodynamically significant clots when time does not permit anticoagulation alone and when thrombolysis is contraindicated. Catheter-based thrombectomy usually involves one of the following techniques: extraction of the clot with a cup or basket device; mechanical fragmentation of the clot using guide-wires, pigtail catheters or balloons, dispersing the clot into multiple smaller downstream branches and increasing its surface exposure to pharmacologic thrombolytics; or hydrodynamic fragmentation and aspiration.[67,117] Risks include blood vessel perforation or damage; worsening of clinical condition owing to distal fragment embolization; and significant bradycardia, especially with the hydrodynamic method.[67]

IVC filter placement prevents migration or embolization of lower extremity (LE) thrombi into the lungs and central circulation; it may be indicated in patients (more than 10 kg in weight) with documented LE thrombi in whom anticoagulation is contraindicated, unsuccessful, or results in complications. Inferior vena cava (IVC) filtration is well-established in adults; its use in pediatric patients is limited but appears to be successful.[113,118] IVC filters in children are usually temporary or retrievable rather than permanent, owing to the risk of incorporation of the filter into the vessel wall; repositioning of a retrievable filter has been shown to extend its useful life.[119] The most common complication is thrombosis at the filter site. Other complications include malpositioning, pneumothorax, filter migration, infection, and vessel injury with bleeding.[113]

Other adjunctive therapies under investigation, particularly in the setting of massive PE, include inhaled nitric oxide, which decreases pulmonary arterial hypertension and improves perfusion, and emergent extracorporeal life support.[66]

All management decisions should be made in consultation with a hematologist, preferably a pediatric hematologist. Surgical or cardiologic consultations may be necessary as well, especially when surgical or catheter-based thrombectomy or IVC filter placement is considered.

Outcome

Mortality in pediatric patients with PE has been reported to be around 10% to 18%[64,72]; however, these registries must be assumed to be selecting for patients with PE that is not immediately lethal (thus diagnosed only at autopsy, and missed in a significant number of patients), but produces symptoms severe and obvious enough to be diagnosed (overcoming the generally low index of suspicion in physicians treating children).

In a 1994 study, data from the Canadian Registry of Venous Thromboembolic Complications (CRVTE) study showed that most deaths in children with DVT-PE were related to underlying disease processes; mortality directly related to DVT-PE was 2.2%.[120] A second study published in 1998, focusing on a subgroup of children with PE and CVC, found that 9 of 57 total deaths (16%) were directly attributable to VTE; 7 of these 9 resulted from massive PE, while the other two were due to obstructive intracardiac thrombosis.[121]

A subsequent study of data collected by the Canadian Childhood Thrombophilia Registry also showed 2.2% mortality rate directly attributable to DVD/PE; all deaths in this study were in children with central venous lines.[122]

Children appear to have a better outcome than adults; this is possibly related to less chronic lung disease, greater pulmonary reserve, less cardiopulmonary disease, and decreased thrombogenic capability.[71,103]

REFERENCES

1. McDevitt BE, Foltin GL, Cooper A. Thoracic trauma. In: Baren JL, Rothrock SG, Brennan JA, et al, editors. Pediatric emergency medicine. Philadelphia: Saunders/Elsevier; 2008. p. 210–24.
2. Weissberg D, Refaely Y. Pneumothorax: experience with 1,199 patients. Chest 2000;117(5):1279–85.
3. Shaw KS, Prasil P, Nguyen LT, et al. Pediatric spontaneous pneumothorax. Semin Pediatr Surg 2003;12(1):55–61.
4. Poenaru D, Yazbeck S, Murphy S. Primary spontaneous pneumothorax in children. J Pediatr Surg 1994;29(9):1183–5.
5. Robinson PD, Cooper P, Ranganathan SC. Evidence-based management of paediatric primary spontaneous pneumothorax. Paediatr Respir Rev 2009; 10(3):110–7.
6. Wilcox DT, Glick PL, Karananoukia HL, et al. Spontaneous pneumothorax: a single-institution, 12-year experience in patients under 16 years of age. J Pediatr Surg 1995;30(10):1452–4.
7. Damore DT, Dayan PS. Medical causes of pneumomediastinum in children. Clin Pediatr (Phila) 2001;40(2):87–91.
8. Hafen GM, Ukoumunne OC, Robinson PJ. Pneumothorax in cystic fibrosis: a retrospective case series. Arch Dis Child 2006;91(11):924–5.
9. Sahn SA, Heffner JE. Spontaneous pneumothorax. N Engl J Med 2000;342(12): 868–74.
10. Posner K, Needleman JP. Pneumothorax. Pediatr Rev 2008;29(2):69–70.

11. Bliss D, Silen M. Pediatric thoracic trauma. Crit Care Med 2002;30(Suppl 11): S409–15.
12. Cooper A, Barlow B, DiScala C, et al. Mortality and truncal injury: the pediatric perspective. J Pediatr Surg 1994;29(1):33–8.
13. Celik B, Sahin E, Nadir A, et al. Iatrogenic pneumothorax: etiology, incidence and risk factors. Thorac Cardiovasc Surg 2009;57(5):286–90.
14. Askegard-Giesmann JR, Caniano DA, Kenney BD. Rare but serious complications of central line insertion. Semin Pediatr Surg 2009;18(2):73–83.
15. Gordon CE, Feller-Kopman D, Balk EM, et al. Pneumothorax following thoracentesis: a systematic review and meta-analysis. Arch Intern Med 2010;170(4):332–9.
16. Kumar A, Chuan A. Ultrasound guided vascular access: efficacy and safety. Best Pract Res Clin Anaesthesiol 2009;23(3):299–311.
17. Duncan DR, Morgenthaler TI, Ryu JH, et al. Reducing iatrogenic risk in thoracentesis: establishing best practice via experiential training in a zero-risk environment. Chest 2009;135(5):1315–20.
18. Sigaut S, Skhiri A, Stany I, et al. Ultrasound guided internal jugular vein access in children and infant: a meta-analysis of published studies. Paediatr Anaesth 2009;19(12):1199–206.
19. Harrigan RA, DeAngelis MA. Evaluation and management of patients with chest syndromes. In: Mattu A, Goyal D, editors. Emergency medicine: avoiding the pitfalls and improving the outcomes. Malden (MA): Blackwell Publishing/BMJ Books; 2007. p. 12–3.
20. Beres RA, Goodman LR. Pneumothorax: detection with upright versus decubitus radiography. Radiology 1993;186(1):19–22.
21. Seow A, Kazerooni EA, Pernicano PG, et al. Comparison of upright inspiratory and expiratory chest radiographs for detecting pneumothoraces. AJR Am J Roentgenol 1996;166(2):313–6.
22. Henry M, Arnold T, Harvey J. BTS guidelines for the management of spontaneous pneumothorax. Thorax 2003;58(Suppl 2):ii39–52.
23. Wilkerson RG, Stone MB. Sensitivity of bedside ultrasound and supine anteroposterior chest radiographs for the identification of pneumothorax after blunt trauma. Acad Emerg Med 2010;17(1):11–7.
24. Tocino IM, Miller MH, Frederick PR, et al. CT detection of occult pneumothorax in head trauma. AJR Am J Roentgenol 1984;143(5):987–90.
25. Rowan KR, Kirkpatrick AW, Liu D, et al. Traumatic pneumothorax detection with thoracic US: correlation with chest radiograph and CT—initial experience. Radiology 2002;225(1):210–4.
26. Kong A. The deep sulcus sign. Radiology 2003;228(2):415–6.
27. Sudwarts G, Foler D. Best evidence topic report. Does plain radiography predict pneumothorax size? Emerg Med J 2007;24(1):49.
28. Ball CG, Kirkpatrick AW, Feliciano DV. The occult pneumothorax: what have we learned? Can J Surg 2009;52(5):E173–9.
29. Baumann MH, Strange C, Heffner JE, et al. Management of spontaneous pneumothorax: an American College Of Chest Physicians Delphi consensus statement. Chest 2001;119(2):590–602.
30. Holmes JF, Brant WE, Bogren HG, et al. Prevalence and importance of pneumothoraces visualized on abdominal computed tomographic scan in children with blunt trauma. J Trauma 2001;50(3):516–20.
31. Blaivas M, Lyon M, Duggal S. A prospective comparison of supine chest radiography and bedside ultrasound for the diagnosis of traumatic pneumothorax. Acad Emerg Med 2005;12(9):844–9.

32. Dull KE, Fleisher GR. Pigtail catheters versus large-bore chest tubes for pneumothoraces in children treated in the emergency department. Pediatr Emerg Care 2002;18(4):265–7.
33. Etoch SW, Bar-Natan MF, Miller FB, et al. Tube thoracostomy. Factors related to complications. Arch Surg 1995;130(5):521–5.
34. Joseph KT. Chapter 28: Tube thoracostomy. In: Reichman E, Simon RR, editors. Emergency medicine procedures. New York (NY): McGraw-Hill. Chapter 28. Available at: http://www.accessemergencymedicine.com/content.aspx?aID=48871. Accessed May 21, 2010.
35. O'Rourke JP, Yee ES. Civilian spontaneous pneumothorax. Treatment options and long term results. Chest 1989;96(6):1302–6.
36. Flint K, Al-Hillawi AH, Johnson NM. Conservative management of spontaneous pneumothorax. Lancet 1984;1(8378):687–9.
37. Kircher LT, Swartzel RL. Spontaneous pneumothorax and its treatment. J Am Med Assoc 1954;155(1):24–9.
38. Kelly AM, Loy J, Tsang AY, et al. Estimating the rate of re-expansion of spontaneous pneumothorax by a formula derived from computed tomography volumetry studies. Emerg Med J 2006;23(10):780–2.
39. Macduff A, Arnold T, Harvey J. 2009. Pneumothorax guide-lines revision – draft. Available at: http://www.brit-thoracic.org.uk/Portals/0/Clinical%20Information/Pleural%20Disease/Draft%20guidelines/BTS%20Guideline%20Pneumothorax%2029%20July%202009%20(2).pdf. Accessed July 15, 2010.
40. Brasel KJ, Stafford RE, Weigelt JA, et al. Treatment of occult pneumothoraces from blunt trauma. J Trauma 1999;46(6):987–90.
41. Findlay CA, Morrissey S, Paton JY. Subcutaneous emphysema secondary to foreign-body aspiration. Pediatr Pulmonol 2003;36(1):81–2.
42. Ötgün İ, Fakioğlu E, Arda İS, et al. Subcutaneous emphysema and pneumomediastinum due to foreign body aspiration. Eur J Pediatr Surg 2008;18(2):129–30.
43. Okada T, Sasaki F, Todo S. Perforation of the piriform recessus by a swallowed glass splinter presenting as pneumomediastinum in a child. Pediatr Surg Int 2004;20(8):643–5.
44. Chang MY, Chang ML, Wu CT. Esophageal perforation caused by fish vertebra ingestion in a seven-month-old infant demanded surgical intervention: a case report. World J Gastroenterol 2006;12(44):7213–5.
45. Marathe US, Tran LAP. Pediatric neck trauma causing massive subcutaneous emphysema. J Trauma 2006;61(2):440–3.
46. Peña MT, Aujla PK, Choi SS, et al. Acute airway distress from endotracheal intubation injury in the pediatric aerodigestive tract. Otolaryngol Head Neck Surg 2004;130(5):575–8.
47. Cay A, İmamoğlu M, Sarihan H, et al. Tracheobronchial rupture due to blunt trauma in children: report of two cases. Eur J Pediatr Surg 2002;12(6):419–22.
48. Lee CY, Wu CC, Lin CY. Etiologies of spontaneous pneumomediastinum in children of different ages. Pediatr Neonatol 2009;50(5):190–5.
49. Küükosmanoğlu O, Karako B, Yilmaz M, et al. Pneumomediastinum and pneumopericardium: unusual and rare complications of asthma in a 4 years old girl. Allergol Immunopathol (Madr) 2001;29(1):28–30.
50. Chiu CY, Wong KS, Yao TC, et al. Asthmatic versus non-asthmatic spontaneous pneumomediastinum in children. Asian Pac J Allergy Immunol 2005;23(1):19–22.
51. Chalumeau M, Le Clainche L, Sayeg N, et al. Spontaneous pneumomediastinum in children. Pediatr Pulmonol 2001;31(1):67–75.

52. Bullaro FM, Bartoletti SC. Spontaneous pneumomediastinum in children. Pediatr Emerg Care 2007;23(1):28–30.
53. Giuliani S, Franklin A, Pierce J, et al. Massive subcutaneous emphysema, pneumomediastinum, and pneumopericardium in children. J Pediatr Surg 2010; 45(3):647–9.
54. Stevens MS, Mullis TC, Carron JD. Spontaneous tracheal rupture caused by vomiting. Am J Otolaryngol 2010;31(4):276–8.
55. Chen IC, Tseng CM, Hsu JH, et al. Spontaneous pneumomediastinum in adolescents and children. Kaohsiung J Med Sci 2010;26(2):84–8.
56. Nounla J, Tröbs RB, Bennek J, et al. Idiopathic spontaneous pneumomediastinum: an uncommon emergency in children. J Pediatr Surg 2004;39(1): E23–4.
57. Inaba A, Horeczko T. Cardiac disorders. In: Marx JA, Hockberger R, Walls R, editors. Rosen's emergency medicine. 7th edition. Philadelphia: Elsevier; 2009. p. 1054–9.
58. Lawal TA, Glüer S, Reismann M, et al. Spontaneous neonatal pneumomediastinum: the "spinnaker sail" sign. Eur J Pediatr Surg 2009;19(1):50–2.
59. Gardikis S, Tsalkidis A, Limas C, et al. Spontaneous pneumomediastinum: is a chest X-ray sufficient? Minerva Pediatr 2003;55(3):293–6.
60. Cicak B, Verona E, Mihatov-Stefanović I, et al. Spontaneous pneumomediastinum in a healthy adolescent. Acta Clin Croat 2009;48(4):461–7.
61. Verteegh FGA, Broeders AJM. Spontaneous pneumomediastinum in children. Eur J Pediatr 1991;150:304–7.
62. Yellin A, Gapany-Gapanavicius M, Lieberman Y. Spontaneous pneumomediastinum: is it a rare cause of chest pain? Thorax 1983;38(5):383–5.
63. Babyn PS, Gahunia HK, Massicotte P. Pulmonary thromboembolism in children. Pediatr Radiol 2005;35(3):258–74.
64. Biss TT, Brandão LR, Kahr WH, et al. Clinical features and outcome of pulmonary embolism in children. Br J Haematol 2008;142(5):808–18.
65. Parker RI. Thrombosis in the pediatric population. Crit Care Med 2010;38(Suppl 2): S71–5.
66. Baird JS, Killinger JS, Kalkbrenner KJ, et al. Massive pulmonary embolism in children. J Pediatr 2010;156(1):148–51.
67. Todoran TM, Sobieszczyk P. Catheter-based therapies for massive pulmonary embolism. Prog Cardiovasc Dis 2010;52(5):429–37.
68. Obayashi MT, Tanabe Y, Yagi H, et al. Tokyo CCU Network Scientific Committee. Latest management and outcomes of major pulmonary embolism in the cardiovascular disease early transport system: Tokyo CCU network. Circ J 2010;74(2): 289–93.
69. Sur JP, Garg RK, Jolly N. Rheolytic percutaneous thrombectomy for acute pulmonary embolism in a pediatric patient. Catheter Cardiovasc Interv 2007; 70(3):450–3.
70. Monagle P, Chalmers E, Chan A, et al. Antithrombotic therapy in neonates and children. Chest 2008;133(Suppl 6):887–968S.
71. Victoria T, Mong A, Altes T, et al. Evaluation of pulmonary embolism in a pediatric population with high clinical suspicion. Pediatr Radiol 2009;39(1):35–41.
72. Van Ommen CH, Peters M. Acute pulmonary embolism in childhood. Thromb Res 2006;118(1):13–25.
73. van Rooden CJ, Schippers EF, Barge RM, et al. Infectious complications of central venous catheters increase the risk of catheter-related thrombosis in hematology patients: a prospective study. J Clin Oncol 2005;23(12):2655–60.

74. Wong KS, Lin TY, Huang YC, et al. Clinical and radiographic spectrum of septic pulmonary embolism. Arch Dis Child 2002;87(4):312–5.
75. Yuksel H, Yilmaz O, Orguc S, et al. A pediatric case of pyomyositis presenting with septic pulmonary emboli. Joint Bone Spine 2007;74(5):491–4.
76. Romeo S, Sunshine S. Pyomyositis in a 5-year-old child. Arch Fam Med 2000; 9(7):653–6.
77. Celebi S, Hacimustafaoglu M, Demirkaya M. Septic pulmonary embolism in a child. Indian Pediatr 2008;45(5):415–7.
78. Yüksel H, Özgüven AA, Akil I, et al. Septic pulmonary emboli presenting with deep venous thrombosis secondary to acute osteomyelitis. Pediatr Int 2004; 46(5):621–3.
79. Goldenberg NA, Knapp-Clevenger R, Hays T, et al. Lemierre's and Lemierre's-like syndromes in children: survival and thromboembolic outcomes. Pediatrics 2005;116(4):e543–8.
80. Huiras EE, Barnes CJ, Eichenfield LF, et al. Pulmonary thromboembolism associated with Klippel-Trenaunay syndrome. Pediatrics 2005;116(4):e596–600.
81. Slavotinek AM, Vacha SJ, Peters KF, et al. Sudden death caused by pulmonary thromboembolism in Proteus syndrome. Clin Genet 2000;58(5):386–9.
82. Azu MC, McCormack JE, Scriven RJ, et al. Venous thromboembolic events in pediatric trauma patients: is prophylaxis necessary? J Trauma 2005;59(6): 1345–9.
83. Vavilala MS, Nathens AB, Jurkovich GJ, et al. Risk factors for venous thromboembolism in pediatric trauma. J Trauma 2002;52(5):922–7.
84. Grandas OH, Klar M, Goldman MH, et al. Deep venous thrombosis in the pediatric trauma population: an unusual event: report of three cases. Am Surg 2000; 66(3):273–6.
85. Truitt AK, Sorrells DL, Halvorson E, et al. Pulmonary embolism: which pediatric trauma patients are at risk? J Pediatr Surg 2005;40(1):124–7.
86. Cyr C, Michon B, Petterson G, et al. Venous thromboembolism after severe injury in children. Acta Haematol 2006;115(3-4):198–200.
87. De Luca D, Piastra M, Pietrini D, et al. "Glue lung": pulmonary microembolism caused by the glue used during interventional radiology. Arch Dis Child 2008; 93(3):263.
88. Tavil B, Kuskonmaz B, Kiper N, et al. Pulmonary thromboembolism in childhood: a single-center experience from Turkey. Heart Lung 2009;38(1):56–65.
89. Rajpurkar M, Warrier I, Chitlur M, et al. Pulmonary embolism—experience at a single children's hospital. Thromb Res 2007;119(6):699–703.
90. Johnson AS, Bolte RG. Pulmonary embolism in the pediatric patient. Pediatr Emerg Care 2004;20(8):555–60.
91. Bernstein D, Coupey S, Schonberg K. Pulmonary embolism in adolescents. Am J Dis Child 1986;140(7):667–71.
92. Sethuraman U, Siadat M, Lepak-Hitch CA, et al. Pulmonary embolism presenting as acute abdomen in a child and adult. Am J Emerg Med 2009;27(4): 514.e1–5.
93. Bomgaars L, Cassady C, Chase L, et al. Texas Children's Hospital evidence-based outcomes center deep vein thrombosis clinical guideline. 2009.
94. Rodger MA, Carrier M, Jones GN, et al. Diagnostic value of arterial blood gas measurement in suspected pulmonary embolism. Am J Respir Crit Care Med 2000;162(2):2105–8.
95. Huisman MV, Klok FA. Diagnostic management of clinically suspected acute pulmonary embolism. J Thromb Haemost 2009;7(Suppl 1):312–7.

96. Biss TT, Brandão LR, Kahr WHA, et al. Clinical probability score and D-dimer estimation lack utility in the diagnosis of childhood pulmonary embolism. J Thromb Haemost 2009;7(10):1633–8.

97. Wells PS, Anderson DR, Rodger M, et al. Excluding pulmonary embolism at the bedside without diagnostic imaging: management of patients with suspected pulmonary embolism presenting to the emergency department by using a simple clinical model and D-dimer. Ann Intern Med 2001;135(2):98–107.

98. Pasha SM, Klok FA, Snoep JD, et al. Safety of excluding acute pulmonary embolism based on an unlikely clinical probability by the Wells rule and normal D-dimer concentration: a meta-analysis. Thromb Res 2010;125(4):e123–7.

99. Sandoval JA, Sheehan MP, Stonerock CE, et al. Incidence, risk factors, and treatment patterns for deep venous thrombosis in hospitalized children: an increasing population at risk. J Vasc Surg 2008;47(4):837–43.

100. Woodruff WW 3rd, Merten DF, Wagner ML, et al. Chronic pulmonary embolism in children. Radiology 1986;159(2):511–4.

101. Worsley DF, Alavi A. Comprehensive analysis of the results of the PIOPED study. J Nucl Med 1995;36(12):2380–7.

102. Stein PD, Athanasoulis C, Alavi A, et al. Complications and validity of pulmonary angiography in acute pulmonary embolism. Circulation 1992;85(2):462–8.

103. Kritsaneepaiboon S, Lee EY, Zurakowski D, et al. MDCT pulmonary angiography evaluation of pulmonary embolism in children. AJR Am J Roentgenol 2009; 182(5):1246–52.

104. Lee EY, Zurakowski D, Diperna S, et al. Parenchymal and pleural abnormalities in children with and without pulmonary embolism at MDCT pulmonary angiography. Pediatr Radiol 2010;40(2):173–81.

105. Mathis G, Metzler J, Fussenegger D, et al. Sonographic observation of pulmonary infarction and early infarctions by pulmonary embolism. Eur Heart J 1993;14(6):804–8.

106. Kosiak M, Korbus-Kosiak A, Kosiak W, et al. Is chest sonography a breakthrough in diagnosis of pulmonary thromboembolism in children? Pediatr Pulmonol 2008;43(12):1183–7.

107. Lee EY, Kritsaneepaiboon S, Zurakowski D, et al. Beyond the pulmonary arteries: alternative diagnoses in children with MDCT pulmonary angiography negative for pulmonary embolism. AJR Am J Roentgenol 2009;193(3): 888–94.

108. Maurer SH, Wilimas JA, Wang WC, et al. Heparin induced thrombocytopenia and re-thrombosis associated with warfarin and fondaparinux in a child. Pediatr Blood Cancer 2009;53(3):468–71.

109. Ignjatovic V, Najid S, Newall F, et al. Dosing and monitoring of enoxaparin (Low molecular weight heparin) therapy in children. Br J Haematol 2010;149(5): 734–8.

110. Re G, Legnani C. Thrombocytopenia during fondaparinux prophylaxis: HIT or something different? Intern Emerg Med 2010;5(4):361–3.

111. Sharathkumar AA, Crandall C, Lin JJ, et al. Treatment of thrombosis with fondaparinux (Arixtra) in a patient with end-stage renal disease receiving hemodialysis therapy. J Pediatr Hematol Oncol 2007;29(8):581–4.

112. Bauman ME, Black K, Kuhle S, et al. KIDCLOT: the importance of validated educational intervention for optimal long term warfarin management in children. Thromb Res 2009;123(5):707–9.

113. Raffini L, Cahill AM, Hellinger J, et al. A prospective observational study of IVC filters in pediatric patients. Pediatr Blood Cancer 2008;51(4):517–20.

114. Komvilaisak P, Grant R, Weitzman S, et al. Epidural hematoma following tissue plasminogen activator (tPA) therapy for pulmonary embolism in a pediatric patient with stage IV Burkitt's lymphoma: a case report. Thromb Res 2008; 121(5):709–12.
115. Manco-Johnson MJ, Grabowski EF, Hellgreen M, et al. Recommendations for tPA thrombolysis in children. Thromb Haemost 2002;88(1):157–8.
116. Markel A, Manzo RA, Strandness DE Jr. The potential role of thrombolytic therapy in venous thrombosis. Arch Intern Med 1992;152(6):1265–7.
117. Menon SC, Hagler DJ, Cetta F, et al. Rheolytic mechanical thrombectomy for pulmonary artery thrombus in children with complex cyanotic congenital heart disease. Catheter Cardiovasc Interv 2008;71(2):237–43.
118. Cahn MD, Rohrer MJ, Martella MB, et al. Long-term follow-up of Greenfield inferior vena cava filter placement in children. J Vasc Surg 2001;34(5):820–5.
119. Haider EA, Rosen JC, Torres C, et al. Serial repositioning of a Günther tulip retrievable inferior vena cava filter in a pediatric patient. Pediatr Radiol 2005; 35(11):1135–8.
120. Andrew M, David M, Adams M, et al. Venous thromboembolic complications (VTE) in children: first analyses of the Canadian registry of VTE. Blood 1994; 83(5):1251–7.
121. Massicotte MP, Dix D, Monagle P, et al. Central venous catheter related thrombosis in children: analysis of the Canadian Registry of Venous Thromboembolic Complications. J Pediatr 1998;133(6):770–6.
122. Monagle P, Adams M, Mahoney M, et al. Outcome of pediatric thromboembolic disease: a report from the Canadian Childhood Thrombophilia Registry. Pediatr Res 2000;47(6):763–6.

Musculoskeletal Causes of Pediatric Chest Pain

Mary Beth F. Son, MD*, Robert P. Sundel, MD

KEYWORDS

- Pediatric chest pain • Musculoskeletal causes
- Anterior chest wall • Costochondritis
- Precordial catch syndrome

OVERVIEW

Chest pain is one of the most common reasons for a child to urgently visit a pediatrician or the emergency department. Various disorders may cause chest pain in children and adolescents, including cardiac, gastrointestinal, respiratory, psychogenic, and idiopathic conditions. Overall, however, musculoskeletal causes are the most common of the identified causes of pediatric chest pain, accounting for 15%[1] to 31%[2] of cases brought to medical attention. Cardiac causes, which are of greatest concern to patients and families, are among the least common of the potential causes.[1–3]

Although most cases of pediatric chest pain turn out to be benign, significant functional impairment may nonetheless occur in children with noncardiac discomfort.[4] In 2 separate prospective studies, approximately 30% to 40% of children missed school as a result of chest pain.[1,2] Perhaps of even greater concern is that, in one study, nearly 70% of adolescents with chest pain restricted their physical activities.[1,2] Likely related to this finding is that noncardiac chest pain may be part of a broader picture of increased sensitivity to physiologic arousal.[5,6] Lipsitz and colleagues[7] found that nearly 60% of children with noncardiac chest pain met criteria for an anxiety disorder several years after their initial presentation.

In view of all of these factors, and given the significant medical, emotional, and societal burden of chest pain, it is important that physicians be well versed in the causes and treatment of pediatric chest pain. This article outlines the differential diagnosis of chest pain based on anatomic and functional considerations. Using this approach, caregivers should be able to convey appropriate reassurances to patients and families in a convincingly knowledgeable and confident manner.

The authors have nothing to disclose.
Division of Immunology, Harvard Medical School, Children's Hospital Boston, 300 Longwood Avenue, Boston, MA 02115, USA
* Corresponding author.
E-mail address: marybeth.son@childrens.harvard.edu

Pediatr Clin N Am 57 (2010) 1385–1395
doi:10.1016/j.pcl.2010.09.011
0031-3955/10/$ – see front matter © 2010 Elsevier Inc. All rights reserved.

pediatric.theclinics.com

HISTORY AND PHYSICAL EXAMINATION

A focused musculoskeletal history and physical examination will often allow for the rapid determination of the cause of a child's chest pain. In the absence of an obvious explanation such as known trauma, it is helpful to start the evaluation by categorizing the type of pain or discomfort according to the nature of onset (acute vs chronic), and whether or not the chest is the only region involved. Thus, the examination should not be overly focused: a case of spondyloarthritis causing costochondritis and chest pain may only be evident after the examination also reveals Achilles tendinitis and sacroiliac tenderness. Most normally active children will have a history of trauma during the preceding 24 hours. However, unless the trauma is significant (typically a football injury, automobile accident, or bicycle fall), it is more likely to have unmasked preexisting pathology than it is to have caused a problem in the resilient tissues of a child's chest.

Key elements of the history that can help identify the cause of pain include (1) timing of the pain; (2) nature of the pain with regard to alleviating and exacerbating factors, particularly effects of activity; and (3) character of the pain, such as dull, sharp, radiating, or burning. In small or nonverbal children who are not able to articulate the specifics of their symptoms, observations made by the parents and other caregivers substitute for the patient's description.

Similarly, the physical examination is crucial in delineating the source of a child's chest pain. It is important to disrobe a child adequately to allow a complete examination, usually requiring the use of a hospital gown. The examination should begin with inspection, looking in particular for areas of right-left asymmetry. Active and passive motion of all parts of the chest, arms, and head allows for isolation of various anatomic structures and localization of the pain. Only then should the chest be palpated, because this is likely to be the most uncomfortable and frightening part of the examination for children. Palpation must be forceful enough to elicit at least some discomfort; overly gentle handling may not distinguish between normal and abnormal areas. Careful palpation will also allow for the identification of particular sites of bony discomfort or disruption, soft tissue injury, and neuropathic hypersensitivity.

Mechanical Derangement

Pain caused by injury or overuse typically increases with activity. Children typically feel well in the morning when they awaken. The more active they are, the more uncomfortable they become. Rest and ice tend to alleviate mechanical symptoms, rather than the activity and heat that are typically salubrious in arthritis. Because they are generally immobile while asleep, children are generally not awakened from sleep by mechanical pains.

Inflammatory Pain

Pain caused by arthritis and other chronic inflammatory disorders is typically improved, not worsened, by use; the mirror image of mechanical pain. The single most characteristic feature of discomfort related to inflammatory processes is the classic morning stiffness of arthritis. Difficulties are also often reported after naps or other periods of inactivity such as long car rides or sitting in classes at school (the so-called theater sign). However, children with arthritis typically feel better after a warm bath or several minutes of activity. Accordingly, a child with arthritis may suffer from joint stiffness in the morning, but may be comfortable exercising strenuously later in the day. It is atypical for inflammatory arthritis to awaken children from sleep. Cold, damp weather, or swimming in cool water tend to be more difficult for children with arthritis, whereas warm weather generally relieves symptoms.

Bony Pain

Pain originating in the osseous compartment tends to be constant, and does not change significantly with activity. Bone pain raises concerns for infection, trauma, and also for malignancy. Although inflammatory and mechanical pains do not usually awaken children at night, bony pain may do so, particularly when related to primary or metastatic tumors.

Neuropathic Pain

Nerve pain tends to be worst at bedtime, when the usual distractions of daily activities disappear. In children old enough to describe the sensation, neuropathic pain typically has a burning or shooting character. It is also commonly associated with allodynia, painful hypersensitivity of overlying normal soft tissues. Although joints may be involved, neuropathic pain generally also encompasses extra-articular areas, and can follow a dermatomal distribution. Activity does not have a significant effect on neuropathic pain.

THE SKELETON AND JOINTS OF THE ANTERIOR CHEST WALL

The chest wall consists of the skeleton, which includes the joints, the muscles, the nerves, the vessels, and the skin. Abnormalities in any of the layers of the chest wall can be associated with chest pain in children and adolescents (**Table 1**). Musculoskeletal causes of chest pain are suggested by a history of trauma to the chest wall, or findings of reproducible pain with palpation on physical examination. However, such features are not consistently found.[8]

ANATOMIC CONSIDERATIONS

The bony components of the chest wall consist of 12 ribs, the sternum, and the clavicles. The first 7 ribs (true ribs) are attached to the sternum by bars of hyaline

Table 1 Layers of the anterior chest wall with corresponding causes of pediatric chest pain	
Skeleton	Trauma Stress fractures (ribs or sternum) Chest wall deformities Chronic recurrent multifocal osteomyelitis SAPHO syndrome Precordial catch syndrome Hyperalgesia
Joints	Costochondritis Tietze syndrome Spondyloarthropathies (ie, psoriatic arthritis) Hyperalgesia
Muscles	Muscle strains Viral myalgias Muscle contusions Hyperalgesia
Nerves	Slipping rib syndrome Intercostal neuralgia Hyperalgesia
Skin	Herpes zoster Hyperalgesia

cartilage, the so-called costal cartilages (**Fig. 1**). The costochondral joints are cartilaginous joints between the ribs and the costal cartilages, which permit smooth movement as the lungs expand and contract. The sternocostal joints are at the junction of the sternum with the costal cartilages. Like the costochondral joints, the first sternocostal joint is primarily cartilaginous. The remaining sternocostal articulations are synovial joints, with articular surfaces at the junction of the sternum that are covered by the radiate ligaments.

Ribs also vary in form and function. Ribs 8 to 10 are considered false ribs because they do not attach to the sternum directly, but are pivoted to the next higher rib by costal cartilages. Ribs 11 and 12 are floating ribs, attached to the vertebrae posteriorly but not connected with the anterior chest wall (see **Fig. 1**).

SKELETAL SOURCES OF CHEST PAIN

Trauma to the chest wall can produce chest pain by bruising the tissues or, in the most severe cases, disrupting the skeleton with potentially devastating results. The history is typically clear in such cases, and examination may reveal a spectrum of findings from

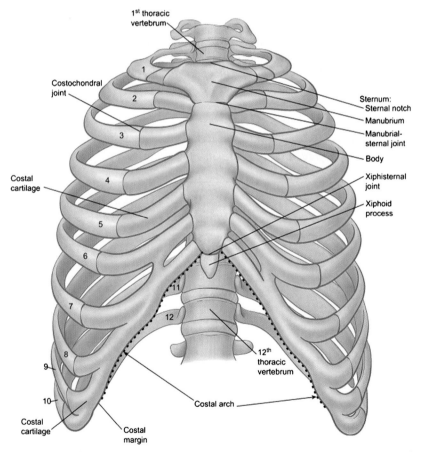

Fig. 1. Skeleton of the anterior chest wall. (*From* Graeber G, Nazim M. The anatomy of the ribs and the sternum and their relationship to chest wall structure and function. Thorac Surg Clin 2007;17:473–89; with permission.)

subtle chest wall tenderness with palpation to rib fractures, flail chest, and crush injuries.

Even in the absence of a recent history of significant trauma, adolescent athletes should be carefully evaluated for stress fractures of the ribs or sternum. Stress fractures are differentiated from acute fractures by the characteristic lack of a history of proximate trauma. The first rib is the most common site of stress rib fractures in athletes, caused by repetitive deformations during contraction of the anterior scalene muscles on the subclavian sulcus of the first rib. Such injuries most commonly occur in baseball, basketball, tennis, and weightlifting.[9] Stress fractures of the remaining ribs are reported most often among rowers and golfers. Stress fractures of the sternum are unusual, but they have been reported in wrestlers who experience a great deal of upper torso stress.[10] Diagnosis is by history, physical examination, plain radiographs of the chest, and nuclear bone scan in some cases. Treatment is largely supportive.

Chest wall deformities, such as pectus carinatum and pectus excavatum, are rarely associated with chest pain in pediatric patients. Pectus excavatum, literally a depression in the sternum, is the most common congenital deformity of the chest wall. It is typically asymptomatic, although the appearance of pectus deformities of any sort are a common source of psychological distress, especially among adolescents.[11] Nonetheless, some patients do develop chest pain. Furthermore, physiologic sequelae, including a restrictive pattern on pulmonary function tests,[12] and electrocardiographic abnormalities[11] including arrthymias,[13] have been reported. Decreased cardiac output caused by compression of the right-sided chambers of the heart by the sternum has also been described.[14] Referral to a pediatric surgeon is recommended for patients with moderate to severe chest wall deformities.

JOINTS OF THE ANTERIOR THORAX

Costochondritis is a common cause of musculoskeletal chest pain, with an incidence between 9%[1] and 14%[2] in pediatric patients presenting with chest pain. It is usually associated with a history of prolonged cough or chest wall strain that irritates the junction of the ribs and the costal cartilages. Patients describe the pain as a unilateral, sharp, stabbing pain located along several costochondral joints. It is typically transient, resolving within seconds or minutes. It may also be pleuritic, causing painful and difficult respirations. The pain is reproducible on examination by palpating the costochondral joints, with the second to the fourth being the most commonly affected. The examination is otherwise unremarkable. Because pain caused by costochondritis is inflammatory, supportive measures and nonsteroidal antiinflammatory drugs (NSAIDs) are generally effective. However, a lack of benefit from such conservative measures should cause the caregiver to reexamine the diagnosis.

INFLAMMATORY CHEST PAIN

Tietze syndrome is a localized form of costochondritis that can affect a single costochondral, costosternal, or sternoclavicular joint.[15,16] As in the more diffuse form of costochondritis, Tietze syndrome may be triggered by an upper respiratory tract infection with cough. An area of active inflammation with swelling, warmth, and tenderness on examination distinguishes this entity from other types of costochondritis. The pain is narrowly localized; the second and third ribs are the most commonly affected areas. Treatment is similar to costochondritis. Recurrence of Tietze syndrome following discontinuation of NSAIDs should precipitate further investigation, because cases of malignant lymphoma have presented as Tietze syndrome in children.[17,18]

As with other synovial joints, the second to the seventh sternocostal joints may be affected by spondyloarthritis. Although this is a rare development in children, it particularly occurs in axial arthropathies such as ankylosing spondylitis.[19,20] Chronic recurrent multifocal osteomyelitis[21] and the synovitis, acne, pustulosis, hyperostosis, and osteitis (SAPHO) syndrome[22] are additional inflammatory conditions that may affect the skeleton of the anterior chest wall. Both have a predilection for the clavicles and present with swelling, warmth, and pain with palpation. Treatment is directed toward the underlying inflammatory process. If NSAIDs are incompletely effective, disease-modifying antirheumatic drugs such as sulfasalazine or methotrexate, and biologic response modifiers such as etanercept or infliximab, are the next-line therapies.

Precordial catch syndrome, or Texidor twinge, was initially described by Miller and Texidor[23] in 1955 in a series of 10 patients, 1 of whom was Miller himself. The pain of precordial catch syndrome develops abruptly and is described as sharp, stabbing, or needlelike. It is exacerbated by inspiration, may occur at rest, but never interferes with sleep. It is transient and typically lasts from 30 seconds to 3 minutes. The pain is well localized, most commonly centered along the left sternal border, right anterior chest, or the flanks, and patients can point to the involved area with 1 or 2 fingers. The cause is unclear, although posited theories include an irritation of the parietal pleura, rib or cartilage injury, or poor posture with resultant nerve impingement.[16,24] Although some investigators have proposed that precordial catch is a clear and distinct syndrome,[24] others argue that it is poorly described and should be categorized with idiopathic causes of pediatric chest pain.[1] Treatment consists of reassurance and clearly explaining the benign and self-limited nature of the pain, despite its intensity. Medications are not indicated.

MUSCULAR PAIN OF THE ANTERIOR CHEST WALL

The major muscle groups of the anterior chest wall include the pectoralis major and minor, intercostal, and rectus abdominis (**Fig. 2**). The primary cause of pain in the muscles of the chest wall is strain caused by overuse, as seen in athletes such as weight lifters and bodybuilders.[16] Less strenuous activities such as carrying heavy backpacks may also lead to muscle strain in students, including overuse of the rectus abdominis muscles.[25] Treatment consists of identifying and addressing the cause of the strain. In addition to rest to allow healing and avoidance of repeated episodes of overuse, supportive measures such as NSAIDs and physical therapy provide analgesia and relief.

Injuries to the intercostal muscles may also be seen in athletes.[9] The pain tends to be worse with maneuvers such as twisting, coughing, or deep inspiration. Diagnosis is based on findings of pain with palpation between the ribs, in contrast to costochondritis in which the pain is palpated along the rib joints. Treatment is rest and NSAIDs.

Patients who have myalgias of the chest wall and a history of fever and malaise may have viral myalgias such as those caused by Coxsackie B virus. These myalgias are seldom isolated to the thorax, and should be apparent with a careful history and physical examination. Therapy is supportive and nonspecific. Trauma to the chest wall can cause painful muscle contusions, the most important of which to consider is myocardial contusion with hemopericardium. The patient's history and physical examination should make this diagnosis readily apparent.

NEUROPATHIC PAIN OF THE CHEST WALL

The intercostal nerves are the anterior, or ventral, divisions of the thoracic spinal nerves, T1 to T11. They run in a bundle alongside the anterior intercostal arteries and veins on the posterior surface of each of the ribs (**Fig. 3**).

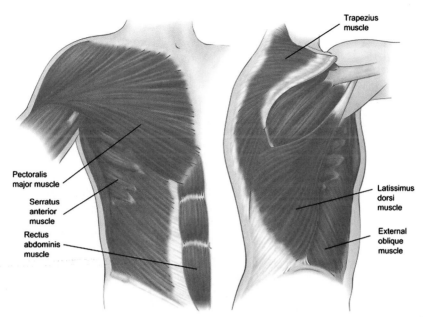

Fig. 2. Muscles of the anterior chest wall. (*From* Miller J. Muscles of the chest wall. Thorac Surg Clin 2007;17(4):463–72; with permission.)

The location of the intercostal nerves may play an important role in the slipping rib syndrome, also called the rib tip syndrome. In 1993, Scott and Scott[26] defined the slipping rib syndrome as pain in the lower chest or upper abdomen. It is associated with physical examination findings of a tender area on the lower costal margin, with reproduction of the pain by pressing on that area.[26] Patients describe the pain as sharp and stabbing. It typically persists for only a few minutes and is followed by a dull ache. Occasionally patients complain of a slipping sensation or a popping sound. The classic physical examination finding in slipping rib syndrome is elicited with the hooking maneuver, whereby the patient lies on the unaffected side. Reproduction of the pain, often with an associated clicking sound, when the examiner hooks his or her fingers beneath the rib cage and pushes anteriorly and superiorly, is diagnostic of the condition.

The cause of slipping rib syndrome has been debated. The most commonly accepted explanation is that the false ribs (ribs 8, 9, and 10) are hypermobile in patients with the syndrome, which leads to slipping of the cartilages superiorly and impingement on an intercostal nerve. Ribs 11 and 12 have also been implicated in the syndrome, but the distribution of the 11th and 12th intercostal nerves is inferior because they also innervate the abdominal peritoneum. Thus, irritation of these nerves is more commonly associated with groin than with chest pain. However, not all investigators agree with nerve impingement as the cause of slipping rib syndrome; alternative theories include psychogenic causes[27] and myofascial pain.[28]

Treatment of slipping rib syndrome varies, but includes avoidance of triggers such as certain postures and movements. Other conservative measures include strapping the ribs and performing local anesthetic nerve blocks. If these measures fail, surgery in the form of excision of the anterior end of the rib and its cartilage has been curative in some reported cases.[29]

Intercostal neuralgia has been described as a cause of pain in patients who have undergone a thoracotomy.[30] As with other types of nerve pain, this condition results

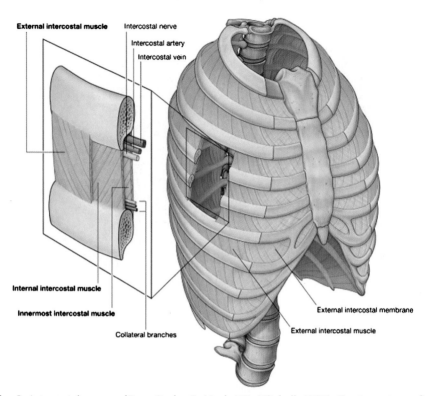

External intercostal muscle   Intercostal nerve

Intercostal artery

Intercostal vein

Internal intercostal muscle

Innermost intercostal muscle

Collateral branches

External intercostal membrane

External intercostal muscle

Fig. 3. Intercostal nerves. (*From* Drake R, Vogl AW, Mitchell AWM. Gray's anatomy for students, 2nd edition. Philadelphia: Elsevier Churchill Livingston, 2005; with permission.)

in sharp or burning pain that may occur at any time of the day or night. This diagnosis needs to be considered in only a specific population. It may take months or years to resolve and, during that time, pain may be ameliorated by analgesics, corticosteroid injections,[31] or neurectomy.[32]

CUTANEOUS CHEST WALL PAIN

The skin of the anterior chest wall may be affected by Herpes zoster. Zoster is caused by the reactivation of latent Varicella zoster virus in spinal dorsal root ganglia. Such reactivation occurs most commonly in immunocompromised individuals, but it also may occur in healthy hosts. Postherpetic neuralgia, frequently seen in the adult population following zoster, is seen much less frequently in the pediatric population.

Patients with zoster may complain of intense pain before the development of a unilateral, vesicular rash, typically in a dermatomal pattern. The thoracic dermatomes are most commonly involved, followed by lumbar dermatomes. Patients describe the pain as burning, throbbing, or stabbing. The lesions are similar to those of chicken pox, the initial manifestation of infection with Varicella zoster virus, classically described as dewdrops on a rose petal.

Treatment of zoster involves antiviral agents as well as pain control. For maximal effect, acyclovir or valacyclovir should be started within 48 to 72 hours of the appearance of the rash. NSAIDs, narcotics, and agents effective against neuropathic pain, such as gabapentin, have been used for pain control as well as to decrease the incidence of postherpetic neuralgia in patients with zoster. Decisions regarding initiating antiviral medications in immunocompromised patients typically should be made in conjunction with an infectious disease specialist.

Any of these types of pain may be described by patients with a hypersensitivity syndrome.[33] Such patients may experience pain in any of the layers of the anterior chest wall, from the muscles and skeleton to the skin. Patients with hyperalgesia have a characteristic history of finding even light touch (such as wearing clothing made of certain materials) unbearably painful. The physical examination is characterized by extreme discomfort and allodynia unaccompanied by objective evidence of disease. Not only may any location on the anterior chest wall be affected, but the pain may be intermittent, migratory, and inconsistent.

Patients with hypersensitivity pain syndromes typically have a variety of additional somatic complaints as well, including myalgias, arthralgias, headaches, and abdominal pain. Unlike children with arthritis or postherpetic neuralgia who want to remain normal and indistinguishable from their peers, pain from hypersensitivity syndromes often disrupts school attendance and other normal functioning.[34]

Expeditious recognition of patients with pain amplification is essential; excessive reliance on diagnostic studies is likely to be both fruitless and counterproductive, often increasing the anxiety level of patient and family alike.[1,2,35] Acknowledging and carefully explaining the concept of nonprotective pain is the first step in reassuring families that supportive measures with physical therapy, cognitive-behavioral interventions, and, in some cases, medications such as amitryptyline or gabapentin, will lead to improvement in symptoms. As with all cases of chest pain, but particularly among children with hypersensitivity syndromes, reassurance is a critical component in the treatment plan. Unacknowledged concerns about chest pain may lead to significant anxiety, disability, and morbidity.[36]

SUMMARY

Acute or chronic chest pain may account for as many as 1 in 7 sick visits to a pediatrician or a pediatric emergency department. Dangerous conditions, from myocardial infarctions to pulmonary emboli, must be excluded, but these account for fewer than 2% of cases of pediatric chest pain. Most children with thoracic discomfort have a more prosaic and benign explanation for their complaints. Knowledge of the anatomy of the chest and the differential diagnosis of various types of chest pain will allow caregivers to diagnose the cause of chest pain efficiently and effectively, and, in turn, will conserve resources and minimize the potential long-term consequences of inadequately or incorrectly categorized chest pain.

REFERENCES

1. Selbst SM, Ruddy RM, Clark BJ, et al. Pediatric chest pain: a prospective study. Pediatrics 1988;82:319–23.
2. Pantell RH, Goodman BW Jr. Adolescent chest pain: a prospective study. Pediatrics 1983;71(6):881–7.
3. Cava JR, Sayger PL. Chest pain in children and adolescents. Pediatr Clin North Am 2004;51(6):1553–68, viii.
4. Goodman BW Jr, Pantell RH. Chest pain in adolescents–functional consequences. West J Med 1984;141(3):342–6.
5. Gilleland J, Blount RL, Campbell RM, et al. Brief report: psychosocial factors and pediatric noncardiac chest pain. J Pediatr Psychol 2009;34(10):1170–4.

6. Lipsitz JD, Masia-Warner C, Apfel H, et al. Anxiety and depressive symptoms and anxiety sensitivity in youngsters with noncardiac chest pain and benign heart murmurs. J Pediatr Psychol 2004;29(8):607–12.

7. Lipsitz JD, Masia C, Apfel H, et al. Noncardiac chest pain and psychopathology in children and adolescents. J Psychosom Res 2005;59(3):185–8.

8. Gokhale J, Selbst SM. Chest pain and chest wall deformity. Pediatr Clin North Am 2009;56(1):49–65, x.

9. Gregory PL, Biswas AC, Batt ME. Musculoskeletal problems of the chest wall in athletes. Sports Med 2002;32(4):235–50.

10. Keating TM. Stress fracture of the sternum in a wrestler. Am J Sports Med 1987; 15(1):92–3.

11. Ellis DG. Chest wall deformities in children. Pediatr Ann 1989;18(3):161–2, 164, 165.

12. Haller JA Jr, Loughlin GM. Cardiorespiratory function is significantly improved following corrective surgery for severe pectus excavatum. Proposed treatment guidelines. J Cardiovasc Surg (Torino) 2000;41(1):125–30.

13. Park JM, Farmer AR. Wolff-Parkinson-White syndrome in children with pectus excavatum. J Pediatr 1988;112(6):926–8.

14. Zhao L, Feinberg MS, Gaides M, et al. Why is exercise capacity reduced in subjects with pectus excavatum? J Pediatr 2000;136(2):163–7.

15. Mukamel M, Kornreich L, Horev G, et al. Tietze's syndrome in children and infants. J Pediatr 1997;131(5):774–5.

16. Reddy SR, Singh HR. Chest pain in children and adolescents. Pediatr Rev 2010; 31(1):e1–9.

17. Fioravanti A, Tofi C, Volterrani L, et al. Malignant lymphoma presenting as Tietze's syndrome. Arthritis Rheum 2002;47(3):229–30.

18. Thongngarm T, Lemos LB, Lawhon N, et al. Malignant tumor with chest wall pain mimicking Tietze's syndrome. Clin Rheumatol 2001;20(4):276–8.

19. Guglielmi G, Cascavilla A, Scalzo G, et al. Imaging of sternocostoclavicular joint in spondyloarthropathies and other rheumatic conditions. Clin Exp Rheumatol 2009;27(3):402–8.

20. Guglielmi G, Scalzo G, Cascavilla A, et al. Imaging of the seronegative anterior chest wall (ACW) syndromes. Clin Rheumatol 2008;27(7):815–21.

21. Girschick HJ, Krauspe R, Tschammler A, et al. Chronic recurrent osteomyelitis with clavicular involvement in children: diagnostic value of different imaging techniques and therapy with non-steroidal anti-inflammatory drugs. Eur J Pediatr 1998;157(1):28–33.

22. Matzaroglou C, Velissaris D, Karageorgos A, et al. SAPHO syndrome diagnosis and treatment: report of five cases and review of the literature. Open Orthop J 2009;3:100–6.

23. Miller AJ, Texidor TA. Precordial catch, a neglected syndrome of precordial pain. J Am Med Assoc 1955;159(14):1364–5.

24. Gumbiner CH. Precordial catch syndrome. South Med J 2003;96(1):38–41.

25. Motmans RR, Tomlow S, Vissers D. Trunk muscle activity in different modes of carrying schoolbags. Ergonomics 2006;49(2):127–38.

26. Scott EM, Scott BB. Painful rib syndrome–a review of 76 cases. Gut 1993;34(7): 1006–8.

27. Smith G. The slipping rib syndrome - editorial comment. Arch Surg 1983;118(11): 1332.

28. Dyer NH. Painful rib syndrome. Gut 1994;35(3):429.

29. Udermann BE, Cavanaugh DG, Gibson MH, et al. Slipping rib syndrome in a collegiate swimmer: a case report. J Athl Train 2005;40(2):120–2.

30. Steegers MA, Snik DM, Verhagen AF, et al. Only half of the chronic pain after thoracic surgery shows a neuropathic component. J Pain 2008;9(10):955–61.
31. Shankar H, Eastwood D. Retrospective comparison of ultrasound and fluoroscopic image guidance for intercostal steroid injections. Pain Pract 2010;10(4):312–7.
32. Williams EH, Williams CG, Rosson GD, et al. Neurectomy for treatment of intercostal neuralgia. Ann Thorac Surg 2008;85(5):1766–70.
33. Clinch J, Eccleston C. Chronic musculoskeletal pain in children: assessment and management. Rheumatology (Oxford) 2009;48(5):466–74.
34. Roth-Isigkeit A, Thyen U, Stoven H, et al. Pain among children and adolescents: restrictions in daily living and triggering factors. Pediatrics 2005;115(2):e152–62.
35. Fyfe DA, Moodie DS. Chest pain in pediatric patients presenting to a cardiac clinic. Clin Pediatr (Phila) 1984;23(6):321–4.
36. Palermo TM. Impact of recurrent and chronic pain on child and family daily functioning: a critical review of the literature. J Dev Behav Pediatr 2000;21(1):58–69.

Miscellaneous Causes of Pediatric Chest Pain

Stephen John Cico, MD*, Carolyn A. Paris, MD, MPH,
George A. Woodward, MD, MBA

KEYWORDS

• Pediatric • Chest • Pain • Precordial catch • Marfan syndrome
• Cocaine

There are many causes of chest pain, both cardiac and noncardiac, and as cardiovascular disease is the primary cause of death in the United States, physicians and parents are often appropriately concerned when a child presents with chest pain. Fortunately, cardiovascular disease is rarely the source of chest pain in the pediatric population. As one of the primary causes of sick visits to primary care and emergency physicians, pediatric chest pain may lead to pediatric cardiologist consultation.[1,2] This article describes some of the miscellaneous etiologies of pediatric chest pain that are important to recognize early and diagnose. Up to 45% of pediatric chest pain cases may elude definitive diagnosis, and these patients are often labeled as having idiopathic chest pain.[3] Serious morbidity or mortality is infrequent. Accurate diagnosis of more obscure causes may help to avoid unnecessary referral and can alleviate the concern and stress families and patients experience when dealing with chest pain.

PRECORDIAL CATCH SYNDROME

Precordial catch syndrome refers to a common cause of pediatric chest pain that was first described in 1955 by Miller and Texidor.[4] It is often referred to as Texidor twinge.[5] The pain is described as a sudden onset, sharp, stabbing, midsternal or precordial chest pain without radiation. Patients generally can point to the area of maximal pain, although the pain or tenderness is often absent at the time of evaluation, because the pain characteristically resolves without intervention. Typical duration of the pain is from 30 seconds to 3 minutes. The pain may be exacerbated by deep breathing, but it is not associated with dyspnea, cough, or other respiratory findings. The most common age of presentation for precordial catch syndrome is 6 to 12 years.

There was no financial support for this publication.
The authors have nothing to disclose.
Division of Emergency Medicine, Department of Pediatrics, Seattle Children's Hospital, University of Washington, M/S B-5520, 4800 Sand Point Way North East, Seattle, WA 98105, USA
* Corresponding author.
E-mail address: stephen.cico@seattlechildrens.org

The pathophysiology of precordial catch syndrome is unknown, although it is hypothesized to originate from the parietal pleura,[5] from rib cartilage, or the chest musculature and boney structures. Like most causes of chest pain, there is a broad differential when encountered in the pediatric patient. Actual diagnosis is made with a thorough history, lack of findings on physical examination, and normal ancillary testing, although electrocardiography and chest radiography are not indicated as part of the initial evaluation of precordial catch syndrome. If history and physical examination alone cannot rule out other causes of chest pain, such as spontaneous pneumothorax, rib fractures, or pericarditis, then ancillary tests may be necessary.[6]

Management and treatment of patients diagnosed with precordial catch syndrome is supportive. Family and patient anxiety may be high surrounding chest pain, particularly if there is a family history of cardiovascular disease. Reassurance is required. Analgesic medications may not be helpful, as the pain is self-limiting and of short duration.

CHEST PAIN ASSOCIATED WITH COCAINE OR METHAMPHETAMINE USE

Illicit drug use is frequent, with an estimated 19.9 million illicit drug users in 2007, which represented 8% of the population over 12 years of age. After marijuana, cocaine was the second most commonly used drug in the United States, accounting for 0.8% of the population over the age of 12, which equates to 2.1 million users. Overall, rates of illicit drug use among 12- to 17-year-olds have decreased in the United States, from 11.6% in 2001 to 9.5% of the population in 2007. A similar decrease was seen in 18- to 25-year-olds, although the use of prescription pain medications has recently been on the rise.[7]

Chest pain associated with both cocaine and methamphetamine use is described in the literature, and it is important for health care workers to remember that people often combine illicit drugs and concomitantly use tobacco, alcohol, or prescription medications. Chest pain associated with cocaine use is often described as tight rather than sharp, is typically confined to the chest and arm, and can be associated with diaphoresis, nausea, vomiting, or dyspnea. The incidence of these symptoms is similar to patients presenting with cardiac chest pain.[8]

The incidence of acute myocardial infarct with cocaine use is as high as 6% in adults.[9,10] However, the incidence with the use of methamphetamine and other illicit drugs is not reliably reported in the literature. Pediatric incidence of acute myocardial infarction due to cocaine use is unknown, although screening for illicit drugs in teenagers with chest pain should be considered.[11] The pathophysiology of chest pain associated with illicit drug use is commonly coronary artery vasospasm, which may or may not be associated with underlying atherosclerotic or congenital cardiac disease, having implications for treatment options. Cocaine acts as a sympathomimetic agent by blocking the reuptake of norepinephrine and dopamine at presynaptic adrenergic terminals, leading to excessive postsynaptic stimulation, thus increasing overall oxygen demand by the heart.[12] Cocaine also leads to premature coronary thrombus formation and is associated with early onset coronary artery disease and premature coronary artery plaque formation.[13]

Adult and pediatric patients are unreliable at self-reporting drug use.[14] Physiologic changes seen on physical examination include elevated systolic and diastolic blood pressures with increased mean arterial pressures compared with noncocaine users presenting with chest pain. Heart rate is increased due to sympathomimetic effects, and patients may exhibit tachypnea and diaphoresis.[10] Electrocardiographic findings consistent with acute coronary ischemia, arrhythmias, or pericarditis may be found, and serum cardiac enzymes may be elevated in patients with chest pain who use cocaine or methamphetamine. Angiography frequently is normal, with no or minimal evidence of atherosclerotic cardiac artery disease.

Treatment of chest pain associated with ischemia induced by cocaine is similar to patients presenting with acute coronary syndrome, and should include antiplatelet drugs such as aspirin and clopidogrel. Beta-blockers should be avoided, as unopposed alpha-adrenergic stimulation can lead to increased coronary artery vasospasm and worsening cardiac circulation and ischemia. Benzodiazepines should be instituted as an early management strategy, because they decrease the central stimulation of cocaine, decrease actual chest pain, and can improve cardiovascular hemodynamics.[15] Nitroglycerine also has been shown to decrease coronary artery vasospasm in patients who have used cocaine and present with evidence of ischemia.[16] Angiography frequently is normal, with no or minimal evidence of atherosclerotic cardiac artery disease. Long-term, ongoing drug treatment may be required for these patients.

AORTIC DISSECTION

Aortic dissection is rare in the pediatric population, with estimates being less than 0.1% of chest pain cases. Aortic dissection, however, can be life threatening if not recognized early and treated aggressively. Aortic dissection can be associated with various pediatric conditions, including trauma, Marfan syndrome, Ehlers-Danloss syndrome, congenital bicuspid aortic valve, coarctation of the aorta, vasculitis, cocaine use, recent cardiac surgery, or aortic cannulation as seen with congenital heart disease.[17] Traumatic aortic dissection accounts for nearly 50% of cases of aortic dissection under the age of 21 years, and Marfan syndrome accounts for roughly 25% of cases.[18] In Marfan syndrome, aortic dissection is associated with aortic root dilatation, and the incidence is increased during pregnancy. Cocaine and other illicit drug use likely contribute to the increased incidence of aortic dissection through various mechanisms, most commonly unchecked hypertension.

An aortic root diameter of greater than 6 cm in adults is associated with the greatest risk of rupture, and intervention is recommended for aortic root diameters of greater than 5.5 cm. In trauma, however, there is usually no dilatation, but rather the force of the impact may disrupt the aortic root.

The pain typically is described as a sudden onset, sharp, "tearing" or "ripping" pain that may be anterior in the chest or radiating to the back. Patients also may present with abdominal pain, depending on the extent of the dissection, and more rarely with syncope or extremity and organ blood flow disruption from the extent of the dissection.[19]

In someone with a recent history of surgery, pneumonia, pulmonary embolism, or complications of surgery should be part of the differential for the cause of chest pain. For a patient with Marfan syndrome, it is important to also consider spontaneous pneumothorax as a cause of chest pain. Patients with congenital heart disease additionally may have disease-specific considerations, pericardial effusions, or infectious etiologies for chest pain.

The diagnostic gold standard for aortic dissection had been aortic angiography; however, in recent years computed tomography (CT), cardiovascular magnetic resonance imaging, and cardiac ultrasound all have been shown to be accurate and less invasive methods for the diagnosis of aortic dissection.[20] Chest radiography may show a widening of mediastinal structures in up to 85% of patients for those with traumatic aortic disruptions or high thoracic aortic dissections. Electrocardiographic findings may suggest left ventricular strain, hypertrophy, cardiac ischemia, nonspecific ST-T wave changes, or even an acute myocardial infarct pattern.[19]

Initial treatment involves controlling both blood pressure and heart rate to minimize the stress on the wall of the aorta while preparing for definitive operative repair. The goal values for adult systolic blood pressure are between 100 and 120 mm Hg, with a heart rate around 60 beats per minute. The goal values for vital signs should be appropriately age-adjusted in the pediatric population. Beta-blockers are the mainstay of therapy, as they also control blood pressure and heart rate, although peripheral vasodilators also can be helpful in decreasing blood pressure and left ventricular contractility forces. Many beta-blockers, such as labetalol, have extremely short half-lives. Sodium nitroprusside is commonly used in pediatric hypertensive crises, but should not be used as monotherapy in acute aortic dissections, because it can raise the peak maximal rate of pressure rise in the left ventricle during contraction, thus potentially expanding or rupturing an aortic dissection.[19]

For patients with underlying medical conditions such as Marfan syndrome, primary prevention with control of hypertension, aortic root dilatation monitoring, and early intervention is the best option. Definitive treatment of acute aneurysms requires prompt recognition, blood pressure and pulse control, and definitive surgical intervention. Despite monitoring and prompt evaluation, acute aortic dissections have a very high mortality rate.

CHEST TUMORS/MALIGNANCY

Primary tumors arising from mediastinal structures are rare, and more commonly occur in the adult population. The average age of presentation for patients with mediastinal tumors is 30 years old.[21,22] The ratio of males to females is roughly 2.8:1. Chest tumors in the pediatric population are likely to be neuroblastoma, lymphoma, or primary neurectodermal tumors (PNET).[22] The location of the tumor (anterior, middle, or posterior) within the mediastinum can suggest possible etiologies. Lymphoma, teratomas, thymomas, and thyroid tumors are more likely in the anterior and middle mediastinum, and neuroblastoma, neurofibroma, sarcoma, and germ cell tumors are more common in the posterior mediastinum.[23]

Patients may present with cough, wheezing, stridor, and anterior chest pain that is characterized by a deep sensation. Chest pain is found in half of all patients who present with a new diagnosis of mediastinal tumor, and it is usually not associated with activity or movement. Respiratory symptoms may be related to activity, and cough is found in over 80% of patients. Less commonly, supraclavicular lymphadenopathy, pleural effusions, symptoms consistent with superior vena cava syndrome, or respiratory distress or failure may be the presenting symptoms.[22,23]

Identification of the mass may be made by chest radiography or CT, but a biopsy is needed to confirm mass type, malignancy status, and treatment options. Fine needle aspiration, percutaneous lymph node biopsy, serum tumor markers, and mediastinoscopy or thoracostomy are all methods of obtaining tissue samples when chest masses have been identified. Individual therapy and outcome depend on the severity of the presentation and etiology of the tumor.

Chest pain with leukemia has been reported and may be due to mediastinal mass, mediastinal lymphadenopathy, focal bony destruction, pathologic fracture, pericarditis, pulmonary infarction from leukemic sludging, or coronary ischemia from direct infiltration of leukemic cells into the coronary arteries. In one case report, a 7-year-old with leukemia presented with vague, reproducible chest pain initially thought to be caused by costochondritis. He had persistent pain, but a rather unremarkable examination, and it is not clear what prompted the clinicians to obtain a complete blood count, which revealed the diagnosis.[24]

HERPES ZOSTER

Herpes zoster of the chest wall, or shingles, is a common cause of adult chest pain and is also well recognized in the pediatric population. The lesions are caused by reactivation of latent varicella zoster virus in the dorsal root or cranial nerve ganglion. It is seen with increasing frequency in the pediatric population among those who are immunosuppressed or immunocompromised, such as those with advanced HIV disease.[25] Herpes zoster occurs in healthy children who have had wild-type infection as well as children who have received the primary herpes zoster vaccination, although the incidence of herpes zoster is lower in vaccinated children. Primary vaccination does not prevent herpes zoster, and the isolate of varicella zoster causing the outbreak can be either wild type, vaccine strain, or mixed.

Patients present with pain that typically precedes rash formation, and the pain can vary in both character and intensity.[26] It often is described as burning, sharp, or aching, and is located unilaterally in a dermatomal pattern. Following the pain, an erythematous macular-turning vesicular rash characterized by crusting lesions can appear and follows the same dermatomal pattern as the pain. More so in children, fever may be associated with the presentation of herpes zoster. Treatment involves the use of antiviral medications such as acyclovir, famciclovir, and valacyclovir. Although this treatment has little impact on the acute course of zoster, it does decrease the incidence of postzoster neuralgia.[27] Postzoster neuralgia is pain associated with an outbreak that lasts for greater than 30 days after the onset of the initial rash, and this pain can be debilitating for patients.[28] Patients with lesions need to be placed in contact isolation for a minimum of 5 days after the onset of skin lesions, as contact with herpes zoster can transmit varicella to unvaccinated or immunocompromised patients. Herpes zoster is most commonly transmitted by direct contact with secretions from the skin lesions, but risk of transmission drops after the lesions have crusted over.[29]

SICKLE CELL DISEASE AND CHEST PAIN

Patients with sickle cell disease (SCD) are subject to a number of circumstances in which they are likely to experience chest pain as a consequence of acute worsening of their chronic hemolytic anemia. Vasoocclusive pain crises occur when sickled red blood cells (RBCs) obstruct blood flow and cause tissue ischemia. While isolated chest pain is not commonly described, individual variation in the location and severity of painful crises makes this a possible cause of chest pain for these patients. Infectious conditions, such as septic arthritis and osteomyelitis, often from encapsulated organisms, are more common in patients with SCD. Isolated costochondral, rib, or sternum involvement is rare, but the diagnosis should be entertained, especially in the setting of fever. Viral infections, particularly parvovirus B19, may result in marrow suppression, leading to hemoglobin drops that precipitate pain crises or congestive heart failure in the patient with SCD. Less commonly, an aplastic crisis may result from the folate deficiency common in SCD. Similar drops in hemoglobin may be seen when abnormal sickle shaped-cells are sequestered in the spleen during a splenic sequestration crisis. Ischemia or referred pain from the rapidly expanding spleen may lead to left-sided pain. Again, isolated chest pain in each of these settings would not be common, but only consideration will identify them.

The most serious and likely cause of isolated chest pain in the patient with SCD is acute chest syndrome. Patients present with a history of pain, frequently with fever, cough or some evidence of respiratory distress. The specific constellation of symptoms at presentation is highly variable and depends on age. Wheezing, cough, and fever are more common in the young, and pain and dyspnea are more often seen in adult patients. Less common symptoms include abdominal pain, rib or sternal pain, neurologic dysfunction, cyanosis, or heart failure. Because no single sign or symptom is pathognomonic for acute chest syndrome, and almost half of patients may present for a different reason such as fever, hypoxia, or pain elsewhere in the body, a high degree of suspicion is necessary to ensure prompt diagnosis of acute chest syndrome. The mean age at first episode of acute chest syndrome is 14 years. Even in the younger pediatric age range, a history of acute chest syndrome is common, and recurrences are frequent. Patients older than 20 years of age diagnosed with acute chest syndrome have a more severe course than those who are younger, including longer hospitalization and more interventions while hospitalized.

The pathophysiology of acute chest syndrome is not well understood. Less than half of cases are found to have a precipitating factor such as infarction, infection, pulmonary fat embolism, or asthma exacerbation.[30,31] When an infectious cause is identified, the most common etiologies are *Chlamydia*, *Mycoplasma*, or viral. Bacterial causes are less commonly identified as precipitating acute chest syndrome. When identified, the bacteria most often associated with acute chest syndrome include *Staphylococcus*, *Streptococcus*, or *Haemophilus influenza*. Infrequent cases have been attributed to *Legionella* and mycobacterium species. Bacterial etiologies are usually identified in fatal cases of acute chest syndrome. Testing may reveal progression of symptoms, including worsening hypoxia, decreasing hemoglobin values, and progressive multilobar chest radiograph infiltrates. Elevation of the white blood cell count is common.

The general management of painful crises in SCD includes cautious and judicious hydration with isotonic solution to ensure euvolemia. Dehydration can contribute to RBC sickling, and overhydration may lead to pulmonary edema and congestive heart failure. Pain should be treated aggressively, most often with acetaminophen (with or without oxycodone), nonsteroidal anti-inflammatory drugs (NSAIDs) (such as ketorolac, if no prior NSAIDs taken), and potentially narcotics (morphine sulfate is most commonly used in the pediatric population). Controlling pain in patients with sickle cell disease prevents the respiratory splinting that is thought to contribute to progression of the vaso-occlusive crisis to acute chest syndrome. Careful monitoring for hypoventilation caused by respiratory drive suppression is important. Because hypoxia is common during acute chest syndrome and can lead to further RBC sickling, oxygen is commonly administered to patients with oxygen saturations less than 90%. The specific treatment of acute chest syndrome includes early consideration of packed red cell transfusion and possible exchange transfusion. Antibiotics (broad-spectrum, including a macrolide) should be administered. Bronchodilators may be appropriate in selected cases.[32]

BREAST SWELLING, MASSES (PREGNANCY, PHYSIOLOGIC)

Patients with breast disorders may present with the complaint of chest pain. Diseases of the breast are uncommon among pediatric patients, but may occur at any age. Boys more frequently complain of unilateral breast swelling and tenderness, especially at the onset of puberty. The breast nodule may be tender to palpation but in the absence of discharge, overlying skin changes, or lymphadenopathy, this may be considered benign and managed with reassurance only. Breast tenderness in teenage females during the menstrual cycle is common. Up to 50% of women experience fibrocystic disease, and pain associated with this condition commonly increases before onset of the menstrual cycle and resolves with the onset of menstruation.[33] Some teenage girls who present with the complaint of breast tenderness are found to be pregnant.

The clinician should consider this possibility when evaluating teenage girls with chest pain or breast tenderness.

Breast lumps in women are most commonly fibroadenomas. Hamartomas and other benign breast tumors are rare but present similarly as a solitary, mobile, and sometimes tender mass. Malignancy potential of both fibroadenomas and hamartomas is extremely low, particularly in younger patients, although patients and their families may find confirmation of nonmalignancy via excision biopsy to be reassuring.[34] Infection and localized abscess of the breast may be seen in the setting of body piercing.[35]

PLEURODYNIA

Pleurodynia is an uncommon cause of severe chest or upper abdominal pain. Also known as Bornholm disease, historically pleurodynia was an epidemic febrile disease of older children and young adults. Today both outbreaks and sporadic cases are occasionally seen. Several coxsackieviruses and echoviruses have been associated with pleurodynia; case reports with other viruses, such as herpes simplex, have been reported as well.[36] Although the pain intensity is variable, abrupt onset of excruciating pain spasms are typical and often lead to profuse sweating and pallor. The pain is often described as stabbing in quality and is thought to be muscular in origin. Its duration may be from minutes to hours (15 to 30 minutes most common), and it is exacerbated by sneezing, coughing, or deep inspiration. Associated symptoms are similar to enteroviral infections and include anorexia, vomiting, sore throat, and headache. While the symptoms are usually short lived (1 to 2 days), the painful episodes are frequently biphasic (rarely may occur more frequently), with repeat pain and fever occurring several days after the initial symptoms have resolved.

Physical examination may reveal tenderness at the site of pain, but the presence of erythema and swelling are uncommon. A pleural friction rub may be auscultated during pain episodes, but it is frequently absent when the pain has diminished. Rapid, shallow, grunting respirations may suggest pneumonia or pleural inflammation. Diagnosis is suspected by clinical history and consideration of season, viral presence in the community, and incubation period. Diagnostic confirmation, when needed, is obtained by polymerase chain reaction (PCR) of infected fluids (sputum, blood, stool, or pleural or spinal fluid), with culture being possible but less helpful clinically because of the time required for growth. Ancillary data most commonly demonstrate an elevated white blood count (frequently caused by polymorphonuclear neutrophils and band forms), an elevated erythrocyte sedimentation rate and C-reactive protein, and a normal chest radiograph.

Treatment is typically supportive, with analgesia for pain and antipyretics for fever. Reassurance and teaching of prevention measures related to the natural history of prolonged excretion in the stool are required to decrease spread of the disease. For severe cases in the young or immunocompromised patient, consideration of immunoglobulin therapy may be warranted. Commercially available immunoglobulin preparations have been shown to contain antibodies to most enteroviruses, and although published data do not support a clear benefit, this may be a useful adjunct to consider.[37]

OTHER CAUSES

Severe chest pain warrants consideration of several other rare entities that may mimic the entities already discussed. *Cervical arthritis* can produce radicular pain that is likely to be focal, severe, and described as sharp.[38] *Cysts of the spinal cord* are uncommon but can cause precordial pain that may mimic pleurodynia.[39] Intraspinal cysts may present with isolated intermittent pain that is difficult to diagnose; chronicity, increasing severity, and neurologic findings such as paresthesia and intermittent spastic weakness may give additional clues to this condition. Symptoms and diagnosis are generally established in the first decade of life. Complete excision is the definitive treatment, but drainage may provide relief of pain. Furthermore, *osteomyelitis of the rib* has been reported as a very rare cause of chest pain.[40] The patient with this rare infection is likely to have fever and reproducible chest pain.

Chest pain is rarely caused by a sprain disorder known as *slipping rib syndrome*. This is caused by trauma to the costal cartilages of the 8th, 9th, and 10th ribs that do not attach to the sternum. Children with slipping rib syndrome complain of pain under the ribs or in the upper abdominal quadrants.[41] They also may report hearing a clicking or popping sound when they lift objects, flex the trunk, or walk. It is believed the pain is caused when one of the ribs hooks under the rib above it and irritates the intercostal nerves. The pain can be duplicated and the syndrome confirmed by performing the hooking maneuver, whereby the affected rib margin is grasped and then pulled anteriorly. The only definitive management is surgical, although most patients are treated satisfactorily with nonopioid analgesics.[41]

Tietze syndrome is another rare condition of unknown etiology that causes sharp or stabbing sternal chest pain. Physical examination of children with this condition may reveal tender, spindle-shaped swelling at the sternochondral junctions, which differentiates this condition from costochondritis. This syndrome is diagnosed clinically and can last for months. Suggested treatments include reassurance, local application of heat, and nonsteroidal anti-inflammatory agents.[42]

Finally, a recent case of a teenager with sudden, severe, midsternal chest pain after multiple episodes of forceful vomiting offered a surprising diagnosis of *Boerhaave syndrome*.[43] The patient's emesis had some brownish material, and he had tachycardia on presentation, but no subcutaneous emphysema was appreciated. A chest radiograph revealed a pneumomediastinum extending into the soft tissues of the neck. A ruptured esophagus was suspected, and a contrast esophagogram confirmed this. Boerhaave syndrome, spontaneous nontraumatic rupture of the esophagus, is different than Mallory-Weiss syndrome, as the former involves transmural rupture, and the latter involves longitudinal tears on the lower esophageal mucosa. A history of vomiting, chest pain, and the finding of subcutaneous emphysema should raise the suspicion of Boerhaave syndrome.

Early recognition and management of the both the common and more obscure causes of pediatric chest pain, which is most often not of cardiac origin, may help to avoid unnecessary referral and can alleviate the concern and stress families and patients experience when dealing with chest pain.

REFERENCES

1. Geggel R. Conditions leading to pediatric cardiology consultation in a tertiary academic hospital. Pediatrics 2004;114:e409–17.
2. Brenner J, Ringel R, Breman M. Cardiologic perspectives of chest pain in childhood: a referral problem? to whom? Pediatr Clin North Am 1994;316:1241–58.
3. Selbst SM. Consultation with the specialist: chest pain in children. Pediatr Rev 1997;18:169.
4. Miller A, Texidor T. "Precordial catch," a neglected syndrome of precoridal pain. JAMA 1955;159:1364–5.
5. Selbst S, Ruddy R. Pediatric chest pain: a prospective study. Pediatrics 1988;82: 319–23.
6. Gumbiner C. Precordial catch syndrome. South Med J 2003;96:38–41.

7. Substance Abuse and Mental Health Services Administration. Results from the 2007 national survey on drug use and health: national findings. Rockville (MD): Office of Applied Studies; 2008.

8. Brown S. Chest pain and cocaine use in 18- to 40-year-old persons: a retrospective study. Appl Nurs Res 1997;10(3):136–42.

9. Bansal D, Eigenbrodt M, Gupta E, et al. Traditional risk factors and acute myocardial infarction in patients hospitalized with cocaine-associated chest pain. Clin Cardiol 2007;30:290–4.

10. Hollander J, Hoffman R, Gennis P, et al. Prospective multicenter evaluation of cocaine-associated chest pain. Cocaine-associated chest pain (CHOCHPA) study. Acad Emerg Med 1994;1:330–9.

11. Woodward GA, Selbst SM. Chest pain secondary to cocaine use. Pediatr Emerg Care 1987;3(3):153–4.

12. McCord J, Jneid H, Hollander J, et al. Management of cocaine-associated chest pain and myocardial infarction: a scientific statement from the American heart association acute cardiac care committee of the council on clinical cardiology. Circulation 2008;117:1897–907.

13. Kolodgie F, Virmani R, Cornhill J, et al. Increase in atherosclerosis and adventitial mast cells in cocaine abusers: an alternative mechanism of cocaine-associated coronary vasospasm and thrombosis. J Am Coll Cardiol 1991;17:1553–60.

14. Lee M, Vivier P, Diercks D. Is the self-report of recent cocaine or methamphetamine use reliable in illicit stimulant drug users who present to the emergency department with chest pain? J Emerg Med 2009;37(2):237–41.

15. Hollander J. The management of cocaine-associated myocardial ischemia. N Engl J Med 1995;333:1267–72.

16. Brogan W 3rd, Lange R, Kim A, et al. Alleviation of cocaine-induced coronary vasoconstriction by nitroglycerine. J Am Coll Cardiol 1991;18:581–6.

17. Gravholt C. Turner syndrome and the heart: cardiovascular complications and treatment strategies. Am J Cardiovasc Drugs 2002;2(6):401–13.

18. Fikar C, Fikar R. Aortic dissection in childhood and adolescence: an analysis of occurances over a 10-year interval in New York state. Clin Cardiol 2009;32(6):E23–6.

19. Ramanath V, Oh J, Sundt T 3rd, et al. Acute aortic syndromes and thoracic aortic aneurysm. Mayo Clin Proc 2009;84(5):465–81.

20. Pennell D. Cardiovascular magnetic resonance. Circulation 2010;121:692–705.

21. Ayadi-Kaddour A, Ismail O, Hassen F, et al. [Benign mature teratomas of the mediastinum]. Rev Mal Respir 2008;25(5):531–8 [in French].

22. Dubashi B, Cyriac S, Tenali S. Clinicopathological analysis and outcome of primary mediastinal malignancies - a report of 01 cases from a single institution. Ann Thorac Med 2009;4(3):140–2.

23. Kennebeck S. Tumors of the mediastinum. Clin Pediatr Emerg Med 2005;6:156–64.

24. Knapp JF, Padalik S, Conner H, et al. Case records of Wright State University: recurrent stabbing chest pain. Pediatr Emerg Care 2002;18(6):460–5.

25. Feder H, Hoss D. Herpes zoster in otherwise healthy children. Pediatr Infect Dis J 2004;23(5):451–7.

26. Katz J, Cooper E, Walther R, et al. Acute pain in herpes zoster and its impact on health-related quality of life. Clin Infect Dis 2004;46(6):342–8.

27. Tyring S, Barbarash R, Nahlik J, et al. Famciclovir for the treatment of acute herpes zoster: effects on acute disease and postherpetic neuralgia. a randomized, double-blind, placebo controlled trial. Ann Intern Med 1995;123(2):89–96.

28. Volpi A, Gatti A, Guisepppe S, et al. Clinical and psychological correlates of acute pain in herpes zoster. J Clin Virol 2007;28:275–9.

29. Straus SE, Ostrove JM, Inchauspe G, et al. Varicella-zoster virus infections. Biology, natural history, treatment, and prevention. Ann Intern Med 1988;108(2):221–37.

30. Vichinsky EP, Neumayr LD, Earles AN, et al. Causes and outcomes of the acute chest syndrome in sickle cell disease. N Engl J Med 2000;342(25):1855–65.

31. Caboot JB, Allen JL. Pulmonary complications of sickle cell disease in children. Curr Opin Pediatr 2008;20:279–87.

32. Li MM, Klassen TP, Watters LK. Cardiovascular disorders. In: Barkin RM, Asch SM, Caputo GL, et al, editors. Pediatric emergency medicine: concepts and clinical practice. St. Louis (MO): Mosby-Year Book, Inc; 1992. p. 566–605.

33. Baren J. Breast lesions. In: Fleisher GR, Ludwig S, Henretig FM, editors. Textbook of pediatric emergency medicine. 5th edition. Philadelphia: Lippincott Williams & Wilkins; 2005. p. 193–200.

34. Tea MK, Asseryanis E, Kroiss R, et al. Surgical breast lesions in adolescent females. Pediatr Surg Int 2009;25:73–5.

35. Trupiano JK, Sebek BA, Goldfarb J, et al. Mastitis due to Mycobacterium abscessus after body piercing. Clin Infect Dis 2001;33:131–4.

36. Marks MI. Herpangina and pleurodynia associated with herpes simplex virus. Pediatrics 1971;48(2):305–7.

37. Cherry JD. Enteroviruses: polioviruses (poliomyelitis), coxsackieviruses, echoviruses, and enteroviruses. In: Feigin RD, Cherry JD, editors. Textbook of pediatric infectious disease. 2nd edition. Philadelphia: WB Saunders; 1987. p. 1729–90.

38. Santen RJ, Mansel R. Benign breast disorders. N Engl J Med 2005;353:275–85.

39. Rebhandl W, Rami B, Barcik U, et al. Neurenteric cyst mimicking pleurodynia: an unusual case of thoracic pain in a child. Pediatr Neurol 1998;18(3):272–4.

40. Layton K. Fever and worst pain ever in the chest: in one ED, out the other. Contemp Pediatr 2006;23(2):18–26.

41. Mooney DP, Shorter NA. Slipping rib syndrome in childhood. J Pediatr Surg 1997;32:1081–2.

42. Stockendahl MJ, Christensen HW. Chest pain in focal musculoskeletal disorders. Med Clin North Am 2010;94(2):259–73.

43. Kundra M, Yousaf S, Maqbool S, et al. Boerhaave syndrome—unusual cause of chest pain. Pediatr Emerg Care 2007;23(7):489–91.

Postscript

The following article is an addition to Nutritional Deficiencies, the October 2010 issue of Pediatric Clinics (Volume 56, Issue 5).

Nutritional Deficiencies in the Developing World: Current Status and Opportunities for Intervention

Yasir Khan, MD, Zulfiqar A. Bhutta, MBBS, FRCP, FRCPCH, FCPS, PhD*

KEYWORDS

- Undernutrition • Malnurtition • Micronutrients • Disease burden
- Dietary supplementation • Food Insecurity • Stunting
- Wasting

Nutritional deficiencies are widely prevalent globally, and contribute significantly to high rates of morbidity and mortality among infants, children, and mothers in developing countries. Several contributory factors such as poverty, lack of purchasing power, household food insecurity, and limited general knowledge about appropriate nutritional practices increase the risk of undernutrition in developing countries. The most recent estimates[1] indicate that 178 million children younger than 5 years are stunted, representing 32% of all children worldwide, and a further 19 million have severe acute malnutrition (SAM).

To understand better what causes undernutrition, it is necessary to systematically evaluate the causes and determinants of undernutrition at different levels. **Fig. 1** illustrates a well-recognized conceptual framework across the life span, indicating how nutrition problems may have an impact across various age groups and could potentially lead to intergenerational effects.[2] The widely used conceptual framework of proximal and distal determinants developed by UNICEF (**Fig. 2**) also illustrates these causes, and their interactions.[2] The synergistic interaction between the 2 causes (inadequate dietary intake and disease burden) leads to a vicious cycle that accounts for much of the high morbidity and mortality in developing countries. Three groups of underlying factors contribute to inadequate dietary intake and infectious disease: inadequate maternal and child care, household food insecurity, and poor health services in an unhealthy environment.

Division of Women and Child Health, Aga Khan University, Stadium Road, PO Box 3500, Karachi 74800, Pakistan
* Corresponding author.
E-mail address: zulfiqar.bhutta@aku.edu

Pediatr Clin N Am 57 (2010) 1409–1441
doi:10.1016/j.pcl.2010.09.016
0031-3955/10/$ – see front matter © 2010 Elsevier Inc. All rights reserved.

pediatric.theclinics.com

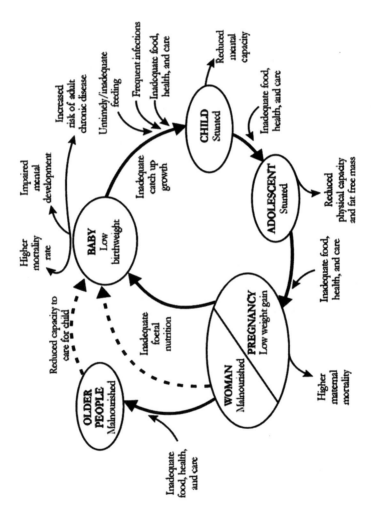

Fig. 1. Undernutrition across the life course. (*Adapted from* ACC/SCN. Fourth report on world nutrition status. Geneva: ACC/SCN in collaboration with IFPRI; 2000; with permission.)

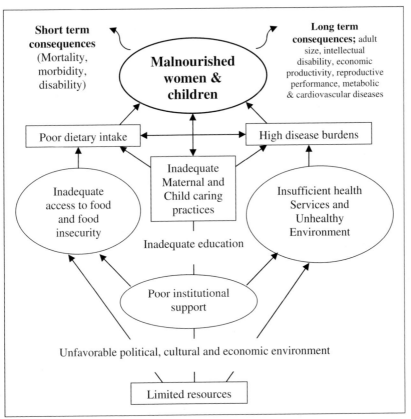

Fig. 2. Causes of maternal and newborn malnutrition. (*Data from* Strategy for Improved Nutrition of Children and Women in Developing Countries. New York: UNICEF; 1990; with permission.)

EPIDEMIOLOGY AND BURDEN OF UNDERNUTRITION

Undernutrition magnifies the effect of every disease, and children are the most visible victims of nutritional deficiencies. Poor nutrition contributes to 35% of the 9.2 million child deaths each year globally.[1] Asia, Africa, and Latin America are major contributors to the burden of disease attributable to maternal and child undernutrition, as only 1% of deaths in children younger than 5 years occurs outside these regions. The estimated proportions of deaths in which undernutrition is an underlying cause are roughly similar for diarrhea (61%), malaria (57%), pneumonia (52%), and measles (45%).[3] Micronutrient deficiencies are now recognized as important contributors to the global burden of disease, especially in developing world.

One commonly used effectiveness measure for health interventions is the disability-adjusted life year (DALY). DALYs combine years of life lost due to premature death and years of life lived with disabilities (YLD) into one indicator, allowing assessment of the total loss of health from different causes. One DALY can be regarded as roughly 1 lost year of so-called healthy life. Nutrition interventions (as general, preventive, public health measures) have an extensive estimated benefit in terms of reducing the burden of disease, as measured by DALYs. **Table 1** summarizes the estimated DALYs due to undernutrition and micronutrient deficiencies.[1]

Table 1
Global deaths and disease burden measured in disability-adjusted life-years (DALYs) in children younger than 5 years attributed to nutritional status measures and micronutrient deficiencies in 2004

	Deaths	% of Deaths in Children Younger than 5	Disease Burden (1000 DALYs)	% of DALYs in Children Younger than 5
Underweight	1957530	19.0	81358	18.7
Stunting	1491188	14.5	54912	12.6
Wasting	1505236	14.6	64566	14.8
Intrauterine growth retardation	337047	3.3	13536	3.1
Vitamin A deficiency	667771	6.5	22668	5.3
Zinc deficiency	453207	4.4	16342	3.8
Iron deficiency	20854	0.2	2156	0.5
Iodine deficiency	3619	0.03	2614	0.6

According to a recent review in the Lancet,[1] undernutrition was responsible for the largest disease burden, whereas burden with wasting is slightly less than that of stunting. Within developing countries, South Central Asia has the highest disease burden due to stunting and wasting, with India alone having 600,000 deaths annually. Undernutrition is high in Eastern, Middle, and Western Africa, with an estimated 111 million deaths in children younger than 5 years in the region. Among vitamins and minerals, vitamin A and zinc deficiencies have the largest disease burden globally, with 6% and 5% of under-5 deaths, respectively, the highest burden being in South Central Asia. On the other hand, iodine and iron deficiency contribute to a relatively small burden of disease (**Table 2**).

Maternal Undernutrition and Consequences

Maternal undernutrition remains a ubiquitous problem in developing countries, where women usually do not have equal access to food, health care, and education. The nutritional status of a woman before, during, and after pregnancy is critically important for a healthy pregnancy outcome for both mother and baby. Years of neglect causes many women to remain undernourished at birth, stunted during childhood, pregnant during adolescence, as well as underfed and overworked during pregnancy and lactation. Undernutrition undermines the woman's ability to survive childbirth and give birth to healthy children, translating into lost lives of mothers and their infants. In the developing world it impairs their productivity, income-generating capacity, and their contribution to their families, communities, and nations. Most women living in developing countries experience various biologic and social stresses that increase the risk of malnutrition throughout life. These stresses include food insecurity and inadequate diets, recurrent infections, poor health care, heavy work burdens, and gender inequities. These factors are compounded by high fertility rates, repeated pregnancies, and short intervals between pregnancies.

Low maternal body mass index
Maternal undernutrition is usually determined by body mass index (BMI; calculated as the weight in kilograms divided by height in meters squared, ie, kg/m^2) and fetal

Table 2
Burden of disease due to micronutrient deficiency

Micronutrient Deficiency	Burden of Disease
Vitamin A deficiency	Nearly 800,000 deaths among women and children worldwide can be attributed to vitamin A deficiency (VAD). 20% of maternal deaths worldwide can be attributed to VAD. South East Asia and Africa have the highest burden of VAD[2]
Iron deficiency and anemia	Iron deficiency contributes to 18.4% of total maternal deaths and 23.5% of perinatal deaths 115,000 maternal deaths and 591,000 perinatal deaths globally can be attributed to iron deficiency. 814,000 deaths globally can be attributed to iron deficiency anemia
Zinc deficiency	The estimated global prevalence of zinc deficiency is 31%. Zinc deficiency contributes to increased risk of childhood diseases, a main cause of death among children[3] It is estimated that 665,000 child deaths, or 5.5%, are related to zinc deficiency
Folic acid deficiency	Access to adequate folic acid supplementation is estimated to reduce the incidence of neural tube defects, affecting up to 5 babies per 1000 live births worldwide; 95% of cases occur from a first pregnancy

undernutrition reflected by intrauterine growth retardation (IUGR). A BMI of 17 to 18.49 is classified as underweight and a BMI of 18.5 to 24.99 is considered desirable. In adult women, a BMI of less than 18.5 is used as an indicator of chronic energy deficiency, which ranges from 10% to 19% in most countries. Almost 20% of women in sub-Saharan Africa, South Central and Southeastern Asia, and Yemen (**Fig. 3**) have a BMI of less than 18.5. In India, Bangladesh, and Eritrea, 40% of women have low BMI; this has an adverse effect on pregnancy outcomes and increases the risk of infant mortality.[1] The high proportion of women falling below the cut-off value in developing countries shows that maternal undernutrition is a staggering problem, which can lead to major consequences including increased rates of infection due to low immunity, increased risk of obstructed labor because of disproportion between the size of the baby's head and the space in the birth canal, as well as increased risk of mortality due to obstructed labor. It also increases the risk of giving birth to a low birth weight (LBW) baby, which itself is a major risk factor of neonatal and infant mortality. Studies have shown that low maternal BMI is highly associated with IUGR,[4] but at the same time it does not increase the risk of assisted delivery and pregnancy complications.[5]

Distribution of intrauterine growth retardation
Undernutrition occurs during pregnancy, childhood, and adolescence, and has a cumulative negative impact on the birth weight of future babies. IUGR represents 23.8%, or approximately 30 million newborns per year. It is estimated that at least 13.7 million infants are born every year at term with LBW (weighing <2.5 kg at birth), representing 11% of all newborns in developing countries. IUGR is most common in South Central Asia, where 20.9% of newborns are affected; this subregion accounts for about 80% of all affected newborns worldwide. LBW is also common in Middle and Western Africa, where 14.9% and 11.4% of infants are LBW at term, respectively.[6] Maternal nutritional factors account for approximately 50% of IUGR in developing countries. Studies have shown the close association of IUGR and early childhood

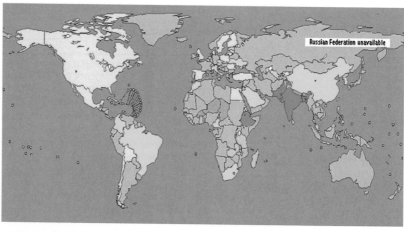

BMI Underweight Females (%), Most recent
- ≥ 40.00
- 30.00 - 40.00
- 20.00 - 30.00
- 10.00 - 20.00
- 5.00 - 10.00
- 0.00 - 5.00
- no data

Fig. 3. Global prevalence of low maternal body mass index (BMI). (*From* Black RE, Allen LH, Bhutta ZA, et al. Maternal and Child Undernutrition Study Group. Maternal and child undernutrition: global and regional exposures and health consequences. Lancet 2008;371:243–60; with permission.)

growth patterns on disease and human capital.[7] Studies from developing countries such as India, Pakistan, and Nepal shows the risk of neonatal deaths associated with IUGR[8–11] Poor fetal growth, although not the direct cause of neonatal death, increases the risk of birth asphyxia and serious infections such as sepsis, pneumonia, and diarrhea (**Table 3**).

Maternal Micronutrient Deficiencies

Malnutrition among women manifests itself at the macronutrient and/or micronutrient level. Although micronutrient deficiencies of iron, iodine, and others are highly prevalent among women in many developing countries, zinc and vitamin A deficiencies contribute to the largest disease burden among micronutrient deficiencies among women of reproductive age.

Table 3
Prevalence of IUGR-LBW by regions[1]

	Low Birth Weight % (<2500 g)	IUGR-LBW (Estimated %)	IUGR-LBW % (2000–2499 g)	IUGR-LBW % (1500–1999 g)
Africa	14.3	8.89	7.85	1.04
Asia	18.3	12.39	10.94	1.45
Latin America	10	5.29	4.67	0.62
All developing countries	16	10.81	9.55	1.26

Maternal iron deficiency

Iron deficiency and iron deficiency anemia are major public health problems, affecting an estimated 30% of the world's population, affecting mostly women of reproductive age and young children. The major clinical manifestation of iron deficiency is anemia or low blood hemoglobin concentration. Anemia affects nearly half of all pregnant women in the world, and is a risk factor for maternal morbidity and mortality. More than 90% of affected women and children live in developing countries where parasitic infections and malaria are the 2 major causes of iron deficiency. Iron deficiency, resulting in anemia, is highly prevalent in women in developing countries and increased requirements are often not met by changes in diet. During pregnancy iron requirements increase substantially, due to increased requirements by the placenta and the fetus, compounded by blood loss at delivery. Iron deficiency increases the risk of mortality among anemic women caused by hemorrhage, which remains a leading cause of maternal death in developing countries, accounting for approximately 25% of all maternal deaths.[12]

Zinc deficiency

Zinc plays a role in a large number of metabolic synthetic reactions. During periods of rapid growth and higher micronutrient requirements, such as infancy, adolescence, and late pregnancy, children and women are most susceptible to zinc deficiency. Prevalence of zinc deficiency in developing countries is probably similar to that of nutritional iron deficiency because the same dietary pattern induces both, with high prevalence in South Asia, most of sub-Saharan Africa, and parts of Central and South America.[1] A high proportion of pregnant women in developing countries are likely to be at risk of zinc deficiency because of habitually inadequate zinc intakes. Maternal zinc deficiency has negative health consequences for women and their infants. Women with low plasma zinc concentrations have 3 to 7 times higher risk of premature rupture of membranes, 2 to 9 times higher risk of prolonged second-stage labor, increased risk of preterm delivery and LBW, and increased risk of maternal and infant mortality. Studies conducted in developing countries have shown the benefits of zinc supplementation during pregnancy on the child's immune function, as well as reducing diarrhea and respiratory illnesses in infancy.[13]

Vitamin A deficiency

Vitamin A is a micronutrient that has an important influence on the health of pregnant women and the fetus. Studies have shown that vitamin A deficiency is widespread throughout the developing world. Vitamin A deficiency has long been recognized in much of South and Southeast Asia (India, Bangladesh, Indonesia, Vietnam, Thailand, and the Philippines) by the common presentation of clinical cases of xerophthalmia, mostly in the latter half of pregnancies.[14,15] In various studies, vitamin A deficiency has been associated with increased risk of morbidity and mortality from diarrhea and measles.[16–19] Breast milk is a natural source of vitamin A and is the best way to protect a newborn from vitamin A deficiency. Poor maternal vitamin A status affects its concentration in breast milk.

Folic acid deficiency

In developing countries, pregnant and lactating women are at increased risk of folic acid deficiency because their dietary folic acid intake is insufficient to meet their physiologic requirements. Maternal folic acid deficiency is associated with megaloblastic anemia because of the role of folic acid in DNA synthesis. Folic acid deficiency interferes with DNA synthesis, causing abnormal cell replication. Low folic acid levels around the time of conception may cause neural tube defects in infants. Folic acid supplementation of women during the periconceptional period reduces the incidence of neural tube defects such as anencephaly and spina bifida. Low folic acid levels during pregnancy are associated with an increased risk of LBW babies.

Riboflavin deficiency

Riboflavin deficiency is endemic in populations that exist on diets lacking dairy products and meat. The effect of energy intake on riboflavin requirement in developing countries has not been studied. Despite this lack of data, a 10% increase in riboflavin requirement is suggested to cover the increased energy use during pregnancy, and a small increase is needed to cover the inefficiencies of milk production. For lactating women an estimated 0.3 mg of riboflavin is transferred in milk daily and, because milk production is assumed to be 70% efficient, the value is adjusted upward to 0.4 mg daily.

Iodine deficiency

Some 20 million children in developing countries are affected by iodine deficiency each year, and every single case could be easily prevented with the use of iodized salt. According to World Health Organization (WHO) estimates, the number of countries where iodine deficiency is a public health problem was reduced to 54 in 2003, from 110 in 1993, showing the effectiveness of the universal salt iodization strategy. Iodine is required for the synthesis of thyroid hormones that in turn are required for the regulation of cell metabolism throughout the life cycle. This problem is most serious in pregnant women and young children. During pregnancy, iodine deficiency adversely affects fetal development. Extreme iodine deficiency may cause fetal death or severe physical and mental growth retardation, a condition known as cretinism, which affects people living in iodine-deficient areas of Africa and Asia. The potential adverse effects of mild to moderate iodine deficiency during pregnancy are unclear. It can cause a range of problems referred to as iodine deficiency disorders (IDD): fetal loss, stillbirth, goiter, congenital anomalies, and hearing impairment. The mental retardation resulting from iodine deficiency during pregnancy is irreversible. Serious iodine deficiency during pregnancy may result in stillbirths, abortions, and congenital abnormalities such as cretinism. Endemic cretinism can be prevented by the correction of iodine deficiency, especially in women before and during pregnancy.

Vitamin D deficiency

Maternal vitamin D deficiency is a widespread public health problem, especially in the developing world. Vitamin D deficiency during pregnancy has been linked with several serious short- and long-term health problems in offspring, including impaired growth, skeletal problems, type 1 diabetes, asthma, and schizophrenia.[20] Animal milk, which is the major source of vitamin D and calcium, is an expensive food in the developing world. With high prevalence of vitamin D deficiency and poor dietary calcium intake, the problem is likely to worsen during pregnancy because of the active transplacental transport of calcium to the developing fetus. Vitamin D deficiency during pregnancy has important consequences for the newborn, including fetal hypovitaminosis D, neonatal rickets and tetany, and infantile rickets. Many studies in developing countries are highlighting the high prevalence of vitamin D deficiency in certain groups, especially adolescent girls and pregnant and lactating women. A high dose of vitamin D during lactation may increase the vitamin D concentration in breast milk to levels sufficient to maintain vitamin D adequacy, and prevent rickets in the suckling infant.

Multiple micronutrient deficiencies

Many population groups in the developing world suffer from multiple nutrient deficiencies. Vitamin A, zinc, iron, and iodine have been mentioned, but there are many more significant overlaps. Given the fact that for those at certain stages of the life cycle—especially during pregnancy—changes in dietary habits are insufficient to meet micronutrients requirements, multiple micronutrient supplementations hold clear potential to address multiple nutrient deficiencies in a cost-effective manner. The breast milk of undernourished lactating women consuming a limited range of foods and with multiple micronutrient deficiencies is most likely to be low in concentrations of vitamin A (retinol), the B vitamins, iodine, and selenium. Deficiencies of vitamin B12, folate, vitamin B2 (riboflavin), and several other micronutrients can also contribute to anemia.

Child Undernutrition

The fortunes of children in the developing world have also been mixed in terms of their nutritional status. Malnutrition is one of the biggest health challenges that developing countries are facing in the twenty-first century, and the consequences for child health are enormous. The 3 main indicators of malnutrition in children are IUGR, wasting (including SAM), and stunting (low height for age). Whereas approximately 3.5% of children younger than 5 years in developing countries suffer from SAM, moderate acute malnutrition and chronic malnutrition typically affect about 10% to 30% of children younger than 5 (**Fig. 4**).[21]

Childhood stunting

Most growth failure occurs from before birth until 2 to 3 years of age. A child who is stunted at 5 years is likely to remain stunted throughout life. An estimated 32% of all children younger than 5 years are stunted in all developing countries, with Eastern and Middle Africa having the highest prevalence.[5] India has around 61 million stunted

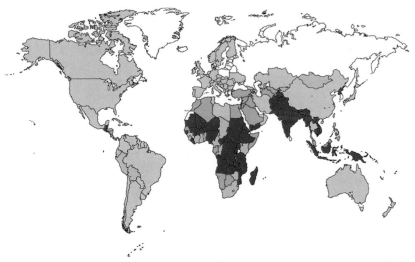

Fig. 4. Global prevalence of childhood (younger than 5 years) stunting. (*From* Haidar J, Abate G, Kogi-Makau W, et al. Risk factors for child under-nutrition with a human rights edge in rural villages of North Wollo, Ethiopia. East Afr Med J 2005;82:625–30; with permission.)

children (34% of global estimate) with a prevalence of 51%. As shown in **Table 3**, around 32% of children in all of the developing world had a height-for-age Z score of less then −2 in 2005 with the highest burden in Eastern and Middle Africa, where 50% and 42%, respectively, are stunted. Overall, with a child-stunting prevalence of 40% or more in developing countries, 23% are in Africa and 16% are in Asia. Among 52 countries where stunting prevalence is less than 20%, 17% are in Latin America, 16% are in Asia, 11% in Europe, and 4% each in Africa and Oceania (**Table 4**).[1]

Infectious diseases such as diarrhea, pneumonia, measles, and malaria are both major causes and effects of malnutrition, and can lead to growth retardation (**Fig. 5**).

Wasting and severe acute malnutrition

Wasting refers to low weight for height, whereby a child is thin for his or her height but not necessarily short. Also known as acute malnutrition, this carries an immediate increased risk of morbidity and mortality. Wasted children have a 5 to 20 times higher risk of dying from common diseases such as diarrhea or pneumonia than normally nourished children. Asia has the highest prevalence (16%) of wasting, which affects 55 million children globally.[1] South Central Asia and Middle Africa have the highest percentage of children with severe wasting (**Fig. 6**).

SAM is defined as a weight-for-height measurement of 70% or less below the median, or 3 standard deviations or more below the mean National Center for Health Statistics reference values, the presence of bilateral pitting edema of nutritional origin, or a mid-upper-arm circumference of less than 110 mm in children age 1 to 5 years. Thirteen million children younger than 5 years have SAM, and the disorder is associated with 1 to 2 million preventable child deaths each year. Severely malnourished children make up approximately 1% to 3% of the population of children younger than 5 in many African and Asian countries. About 9% of sub-Saharan African and 15% of South Asian children have moderate acute malnutrition, and about 2% of children in developing countries have SAM.[22] This figure is equivalent to approximately 1.5 million child deaths associated with severe wasting and 3.5 million child deaths associated with moderate wasting every year. These figures do not include children who die of edematous malnutrition (kwashiorkor), a form of SAM that is more common in some countries. In India alone, 2·8% of children younger than 5 years (more than 5 million children) are severely wasted[23,24] and in many poor countries, SAM is the most common reason for pediatric hospital admission.[25]

In developing countries, SAM poses a great threat to the health of infants and children. Many advanced cases of SAM are complicated by concurrent infective illness, particularly acute respiratory infection, diarrhea, and gram-negative septicemia (**Fig. 7**). Parental illiteracy is found to be associated with a higher risk of SAM. This feature is observed by many studies carried out in the developing world.[26–29] Similarly, poor family income and larger family size are other risk factors associated with SAM found in different studies.[30–32] The severity of SAM, its prognosis, and the determinants of successful treatment are primarily dependent on the lead time to presentation.

Underweight

Underweight refers to low weight for age, when a child can be either thin or short for his or her age. Underweight reflects a combination of chronic and acute malnutrition. Twenty percent of children younger than 5 year in the developing world had a weight-for-age Z score of less then −2 in 2005, with the highest burden in South Central Asia (33%) and Eastern Africa (28%).[1] The percentage of underweight children in the

Table 4
Prevalence of childhood stunting by regions[1]

	Children <5 Years in Million	% Stunted (95% CI)	Number Stunted in Millions (95% CI)	% Severely Wasted (95% CI)	Number Severely Wasted in Millions (95% CI)	Percentage Underweight (95% CI)	Number Underweight in Millions (95% CI)
Africa	141.914	40.1 (36.8–43.4)	56.9 (52.2–61.6)	3.9 (2.2–5.7)	5.6 (3.0–8.0)	21.9 (18.8–24.0)	31.1 (28.1–34.0)
Asia	356.879	31.3 (27.5–35.1)	111.6 (98.1–125.1)	3.7 (1.2–6.2)	13.3 (4.4–22.3)	22.0 (18.5–25.6)	78.6 (65.9–91.3)
Latin America	56.936	16.1 (9.4–22.8)	9.2 (5.3–13.0)	0.6 (0.2–1.0)	0.3 (0.1–0.6)	4.8 (3.1–6.4)	2.7 (1.8–3.7)
All developing countries	555.729	32.0 (29.3–34.6)	177.7 (162.9–92.5)	3.5 (1.8–5.1)	19.3 (10.0–8.6)	20.2 (17.9–22.6)	112.4 (99.3–125.5)

Abbreviation: CI, confidence interval.

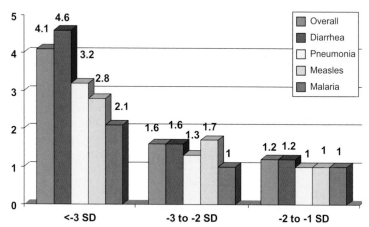

Fig. 5. Overall and cause-specific mortality risk for stunting in children younger than 5 years.

developing world, due to malnutrition, declined from 35% in 1980–1994 to 27% in 1995–2001 (**Table 5**).

Micronutrient deficiencies in children

Micronutrient deficiencies have serious repercussions for the developing fetus and for children. If iodine deficiency disorders may cause fetal brain damage or stillbirth, folate deficiency may result in neural tube or other birth defects and preterm delivery. Similarly, both iron deficiency anemia and vitamin A deficiency may have significant effects for the future infant's morbidity and mortality risk, vision, and cognitive development (**Table 6**).

Iron deficiency For children, health consequences include premature birth, LBW, infections, and elevated risk of death. Later, physical and cognitive development are impaired, resulting in lowered school performance. The major cause of iron deficiency in children of developing countries is the unavailability to the poor of food such as meat, fish, or poultry.

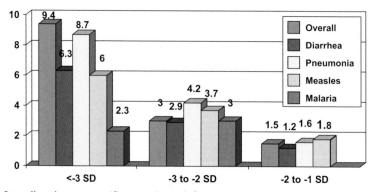

Fig. 6. Overall and cause-specific mortality risk for stunting in children younger than 5 years with severe acute malnutrition.

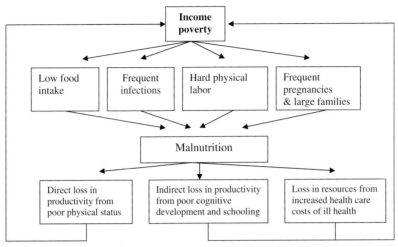

Fig. 7. Relationship between poverty and malnutrition. *(Data from* Bhagwati J, Fogel R, Frey B, et al. Ranking the opportunities. In: Lomborg B, editor. Global Crises, global Solutions. Cambridge [UK]: Cambridge University Press; 2004.)

Zinc deficiency Zinc deficiency is highly prevalent in South Asia followed by sub-Saharan Africa and South America, and the prevalence of stunting is one of the clinical manifestations of zinc deficiency. Countries where stunting prevalence is more than 20% are at higher risk for zinc deficiency. Zinc has no tissue reserves, unlike vitamin A and iron, and its turnover is rapid, especially during common gastrointestinal infections. Young children in developing countries who have a poor diet and high exposure to gastrointestinal pathogens are at greatest risk of zinc deficiency.[3] Zinc deficiency in children increases the risk of diseases such as diarrhea, pneumonia, and malaria worldwide.[33–37] The relative risk of morbidity associated with zinc deficiency is 1.09 for diarrhea, 1.25 for pneumonia, and 1.56 for malaria.[3,37] Studies from Nepal, Bangladesh, and Zanzibar have shown the relative risk estimated at around 1.29 for diarrhea, 1.18 for pneumonia, and 1.11 for malaria for mortality in infants aged 1 to 59 months.[34,36,38]

Vitamin A deficiency It is estimated that around 250 million children younger than 5 years have vitamin A deficiency. Within developing countries, Bangladesh, India, Indonesia, and the Philippines appear to be the most afflicted, but many countries

Table 5			
Trends in prevalence of underweight children younger than 5 years by region, 1980–2002 (%)			
Regions	**1980–1994**	**1990–1997**	**1995–2002**
South Asia	64	51	46
Sub-Saharan Africa	31	30	29
East Asia	23	20	17
Latin America and Caribbean	11	10	8
Middle East and North Africa	12	17	14
Developing countries	35	30	27

Data include children who are moderately or severely underweight.
Data from UNICEF 1996, 1998, 2003. Available at: http://www.unicef.org.

Table 6
Contribution of nutrition deficiencies to disease burden in developing countries: DALYs lost (%)

Factor	DALYs Lost Percentage		
	Direct effect	At risk factor	Total
General malnutrition	1.0	14.0	15.0
Micronutrient deficiencies	9.0	8.5	17.5
Total	10.0	22.5	32.5

Data from Jamison DT, Breman JG, Mesham AR, editors. Disease control priorities in developing countries, 2nd edition. New York: Oxford University Press; 2006. Table 56.1.

in Africa and some in Central and South America have the same problem. Vitamin A plays an important role in the maintenance of mucous membranes, thus enhancing local resistance to penetration of viruses and bacteria. The most vulnerable group is children from birth to 5 or 6 years of age, peaking between 2 and 3 years old. A child with vitamin A deficiency faces 25% greater risk of dying from several childhood diseases such as measles, malaria, or diarrhea. Increasing evidence now shows that improving vitamin A status among preschool children increases their chances of survival by as much as 30%. Vitamin A deficiency is the most common cause of blindness in children in many endemic areas. Xerophthalmia occurs almost entirely in children living in poverty. It has been especially prevalent in children of poor rice-eating families in South and Southeast Asia. There is a high incidence in some African countries, whereas other countries, especially in West Africa, seem to have a lower prevalence, in part because of the consumption of red palm oil, which is high in carotene. The supplementation of vitamin A reduced overall child mortality by 23%, with a 50% reduction for those infected with measles.[39] Studies have also shown the increased risk of mortality with vitamin A deficiency, with relative risk of 1.47 for diarrhea and 1.35 for measles.[1]

Riboflavin deficiency The major cause of riboflavin deficiency is inadequate dietary intake. If maternal status is poor during gestation, the infant is likely to be born riboflavin deficient. Riboflavin deficiency among schoolchildren has been documented in many developing countries where the intake of milk products and meat is limited.[40,41] It mostly occurs in combination with a deficiency of other B-complex vitamins. More advanced deficiency may result in cheilosis, angular stomatitis, dermatitis, corneal vascularization, anemia, and brain dysfunction.[42]

Iodine deficiency Relatively few child deaths are attributed to iodine deficiency, but it causes considerable loss of DALYs. According to the WHO, global iodine deficiency disorders were estimated to result in the loss of 2.5 million DALYs with 25% of this burden occurring in Africa alone. Insufficient intake of iodine can result in impaired intellectual development and physical growth. Iodine-deficient children usually experience mild mental retardation. Cretinism, caused by severe deficiency, is associated with extreme mental retardation.

Calcium and vitamin D deficiency Although fetuses are relatively protected from maternal deficiency of calcium, calcium deficiency rickets can result from low intake in young children. It is the main cause of rickets in Africa and parts of Asia, due to shrouding, inadequate exposure to sunlight, and lack of intake of a diet fortified with Vitamin D.[43] In developing countries of Asia, Africa, and Latin America, the calcium content of complementary foods provided to children during the first year of life is much less than the 50% that is suggested.[44] In India alone the daily calcium intake of children varies from 314 mg to 713 mg. Similarly, low calcium intakes have been reported from Kenya (314 mg/d), South Africa (463 mg/d girls, 528 mg/d boys), Ghana, Nigeria (214 mg/d), Malaysia, and China (374 mg/d urban, 324 mg/d rural).[45–50] Thirty-five to fifty percent of children are vitamin deficient in India, China, Lebanon, and Libya.[19] Nutritional rickets is highly prevalent in many developing countries and is relatively high in Africa, East Asia, and South Asia.[51] In fact, rickets is now said to be the most common noncommunicable childhood disease in the world.

Multiple micronutrient deficiencies Micronutrient deficiencies are more likely in children who consume diets that are poor in nutritional quality, or who have higher nutrient requirements due to high growth rates and/or the presence of bacterial infections or parasites, which are common findings in the developing world. In particular, a diet that is low in animal-source foods typically results in low intakes of iron, zinc, calcium, retinol (preformed vitamin A), vitamin B2 (riboflavin), vitamin B6, and vitamin B12. Often, poor-quality diets also lack fresh fruits and vegetables, which mean that intakes of vitamin C (ascorbic acid) and folate will also be inadequate. Improving status in one micronutrient, or even several micronutrients simultaneously in the case of multiple deficiencies, can have wider benefits to health of children in developing countries.

RISK FACTORS

Of the various risk factors recognized to affect undernutrition, the following are key.

Poverty and Food Insecurity

Extreme poverty remains an alarming problem in the world's developing regions. The causes of poverty include poor people's lack of resources, an extremely unequal income distribution in the world and within specific countries, conflict, and hunger itself. The high prevalence of undernutrition in developing countries is the result of a number of factors of which first and foremost is the presence of chronic poverty. The lack of purchasing power of people and increased population growth rates negatively affect the nutrition of the people. Poverty status had a statistically significant effect on LBW, the neonatal mortality rate, and the maternal mortality rate in developing countries (see **Fig. 7**).

Nutrition, health, and education are interrelated and mutually supporting. Inadequate nutrition in children affects long-term physical and mental development and, therefore, productivity later in life. By causing poor health, low levels of energy, and even mental impairment, hunger can lead to even greater poverty by reducing people's ability to work and learn. Education of mothers can affect the nutrition of their children, as a well-educated mother knows what food to give to her children and how to prepare it.

Household food insecurity is one of the possible underlying determinants of malnutrition.[52] A high percentage of household expenditure allocated to food is a major indicator of household food insecurity in developing countries. The best estimates of micronutrient malnutrition by the WHO indicate that the total number of people at risk of one or more of the deficiencies is around 2 billion, most of whom live in the developing countries. Persistence of malnutrition globally or increases in incidence will further imperil the socioeconomic conditions of the developing world shown by these figures, and have profound implications in today's global economic crisis.

Micronutrient deficiencies also affect displaced populations with high prevalence. For example, iron deficiency has been found with a prevalence of 23% to 75% in child refugee camps in Africa, and this deficiency contributed to the high prevalence of anemia found in many studies.[53,54] Many of the world's developing countries are locked in a tragic and vicious circle of poverty and conflicts, which have reversed development and increased global poverty levels. Children are most vulnerable to the consequences of displacement and conflicts. In many developing countries displacement and food insecurity also increase the risk of micronutrient deficiency disorders (ie, iron, iodine, and B-complex deficiencies, especially thiamine, riboflavin, and niacin), and communicable diseases are known to rapidly deplete vitamin A stores. Malnutrition contributes to physical and mental impairment in children younger than 5 years. Malnutrition undermines immune-response mechanisms and resistance to infections, thus contributing to an increase in incidence, duration, and severity of illnesses. Severely malnourished children are 8 times more likely to die from infection. Measles, diarrheal disease, acute respiratory infections (ARIs), and malaria (where malaria is endemic) with malnutrition as an underlying and aggravating factor account for 51% to 95% of all reported causes of morbidity and mortality among displaced populations (WHO and UNICEF, 2002). Malaria and ARIs, including pneumonia, are responsible for the deaths of many children. Similarly, diarrhea is another common and often deadly disease. Cholera is a constant threat, as exemplified in refugee camps in Bangladesh, Kenya, Malawi, Nepal, Somalia, Zaire, and Afghanistan.

During conflicts, mothers may experience hunger, exhaustion, and distress that can make them less able to care for their children. Breastfeeding may be endangered by the mother's loss of confidence in her ability to produce milk. The general disruption in routine can separate mothers from their children for long periods, as social structures and networks break down. Knowledge about breastfeeding is passed from one generation to the next, and this can be lost when people flee and families are broken up. Yet artificial feeding, risky at all times, is even more dangerous in unsettled circumstances.

Inadequate Feeding Practices

The first 2 years of life are a crucial window during which to break the vicious cycle of undernutrition. After birth, early and exclusive breastfeeding for 6 months followed by the introduction of complementary feeding is essential to improve the health and survival of newborns and children. Breastfeeding is important not only for the optimal growth and development, but also has a protective role in decreasing the incidence and severity of infectious diseases, and decreases the risk of morbidity and mortality in young children.[55,56] In the developing world, lack of knowledge and awareness about feeding the infant together with influences of various cultural beliefs and food taboos interfere with the feeding of infants, leading to malnutrition with a high incidence of infant morbidity and mortality. Breastfeeding provides ideal nutrition for infants and reduces the incidence and severity of infectious diseases, and also contributes to women's health. In most developing countries, women spend a large proportion of their reproductive years pregnant, lactating, or pregnant and lactating. In Asia, Africa, Latin America, and the Caribbean, only 47% to 57% of infants younger than 2 months are exclusively breastfed and for children 2 to 5 months this percentage falls to 25% to 31%.[1] The nutritional demands to support fetal growth and breast milk production during pregnancy and lactation are multiple. Breast milk completely provides the infant's nutritional and fluid needs for about the first 6 months of life. For first 6 months, infants should not receive any prelacteal feed such as water, other liquids, or ritual foods to maintain good hydration, not even in hot and dry climates (exclusive breastfeeding). In many developing countries exclusive breastfeeding is virtually nonexistent. Mothers tend to discard the first milk (colostrum), substituting prelacteal feeds such as honey, sugar water, or oil instead of the breast milk as the first feed for all newborn babies. Initiation of breastfeeding usually takes place on the third or fourth day after birth. Complementary feeding is also regarded as defective because of ignorance, lack of awareness, and influences of cultural beliefs, and consists of bulky, energy-thin feeds, with weaning occurring either too early or too late. Effective programs promoting complementary feeding could reduce deaths of children younger than 5 years in developing countries.

High Disease Burden and Inadequate Management

Undernutrition in children makes them susceptible to low immune function and confers a higher risk of developing illnesses such as diarrhea and pneumonia. It has been estimated that around 50% to 70% of the burden of diarrheal diseases, measles, malaria, and lower respiratory tract infections in childhood are attributable to undernutrition.

Globally, ARIs kill more children younger than 5 years than any other infectious disease, accounting for almost 2 million deaths a year in this age group. Ninety-nine percent of these deaths occur in developing countries. ARIs cover the spectrum of infectious illnesses of the respiratory tract, ranging from mild upper respiratory infections to serious infections of the lower respiratory tract (bronchiolitis and pneumonia). Severe ARIs are responsible for a great deal of the morbidity and mortality suffered by children in the developing world. Many risk factors have been recognized in the development of severe ARI, including age less than 1 year, malnutrition, vitamin A deficiency, LBW, lack of breastfeeding, crowding, and exposure to indoor pollutants. Without early treatment children can die very rapidly. Early recognition of ARIs is also essential for effective treatment. In malnourished children, pneumonia and ARI must be treated in a place where intravenous antibiotics can be administered.

Poor water and sanitation in developing countries is responsible for 4 billion diarrheal diseases, mostly in children younger than 5 years. In addition, diarrheal illnesses account for an estimated 12,600 deaths each day in children in developing countries in Asia, Africa, and Latin America. Diarrheal diseases lead to decreased food intake and nutrient absorption, malnutrition, reduced resistance to infection, and impaired physical growth and cognitive development. There is a bidirectional relationship between malnutrition and diarrheal diseases. There is now evidence that therapeutic use of specific nutrients early in some acute illnesses like diarrhea may reduce episode severity and duration as well as case fatality. The most effective intervention to treat diarrhea is early rehydration along with appropriate nutrition. Cases of severe dehydration need to be treated with oral rehydration therapy or intravenous fluids. However, improved diarrheal outcomes with zinc therapy, and reduced severity and duration in acute and persistent diarrhea, are now well established and may help reduce the nutritional issues associated with diarrhea.[57,58]

WHAT WORKS? EVIDENCE-BASED NUTRITION INTERVENTIONS

The sustainable solution to multiple micronutrient deficiencies must be the discovery and implementation of innovative, affordable ways to improve the diet of poor people.[59] Public health interventions to tackle the problem of malnutrition must become an area of priority for the developing world. Effective interventions exist, including promotion of breastfeeding, creating awareness about safe and proper diets for children, and provision of micronutrient supplements.

The recent *Lancet* undernutrition series published estimates on maternal and child undernutrition, giving the most up to date burden of disease as well as interventions that can implemented to decrease that burden.[60] To reduce stunting, SAM, micronutrient deficiencies, and subsequent child deaths, effective interventions are available that would reduce DALYs by about 25% in the short term if implemented on a sufficient scale. Out of many interventions available, those that focus on exclusive breastfeeding and fortification or supplementation of foods with vitamin A and zinc have the greatest potential to decrease child mortality. Improving vitamin A status reduces mortality among older infants and young children, and reduces pregnancy-related mortality; it also reduces the prevalence of severe illness and clinic attendance among children. Improving zinc status reduces morbidity from diarrheal and respiratory infections. Treatment of established infection with vitamin A is effective in measles-associated complications, but is not as useful in the majority of diarrheal or respiratory syndromes. Zinc supplements, however, have significant benefit on the clinical outcome of diarrheal and respiratory infections.

Maternal nutrition interventions to improve maternal health include supplementation of iron, folate, micronutrients such as calcium, and balanced energy and protein diets. The *Lancet* review derived data from 388 surveys from 139 countries to find preventive and therapeutic strategies to address nutritional deficiencies. These interventions include disease control measures as well as dietary diversification, supplementation, and food-fortification strategies (**Table 7** and **Fig. 8**).

According to the *Lancet* review,[60] universal coverage with general interventions could prevent 10% to 15% stunting and 1 in 8 deaths in children younger than 36 months, while universal coverage with all interventions could avert some 60 million DALYs, which is about a quarter of deaths in children younger than 36 months (**Table 8**).

Balanced Energy and Protein Supplements During Pregnancy

A review of 13 studies and a systematic review, which was weighted toward a large Gambian study that targeted women with low BMI with supplements of more than 700 kcal per day, showed that this strategy reduces the risk of a small-for-gestational age baby by 32%.[60,61]

Iron Folate or Iron Supplementation

Iron folate supplementation during pregnancy produced an increase of 12 g/L in hemoglobin at term and a 73% reduction in the risk of anemia at term.[62] Iron supplementation was seen to result in a hemoglobin concentration that was 7·4 g/L higher than in children who had no supplementation.[63] Reductions in the occurrence of anemia with iron supplementation alone ranged from 38% to 62% in nonmalarial regions and from 6% to 32% in malarial hyperendemic areas.

Vitamin A Supplementation in Mothers and Children

Some trials[64,65] of supplementation of vitamin A during pregnancy were inconsistent with respect to their effect on maternal mortality; however, in children aged 6 to 59 months, a pooled estimate showed a 24% reduction in the risk of all-cause mortality.[16,66] Vitamin A supplementation in the neonatal period in low-income countries showed a 20% reduction in mortality in babies younger than 6 months in 3 reported trials.[10,17,67]

Multiple Micronutrient Supplementation During Pregnancy

This strategy usually means providing large doses of micronutrients in the form of pills, capsules, or syrups. It has an advantage in that it provides a highly absorbable rapid way to control deficiencies in population at risk of malnutrition. In developing countries, supplementation programs have been widely used to provide iron and folic acid to pregnant women, and vitamin A to infants, children younger than 5 years,

Table 7
Interventions that may affect maternal and child undernutrition

Interventions for Which There is Sufficient Evidence for Inclusion in All Programs (Universal)	Interventions for Which There is Evidence for Inclusion in Specific Contexts (Situational)	Other Supportive Strategies
Maternal		
Iron folate supplementation[a]	Maternal balanced energy protein supplementation	Family planning interventions to promote birth spacing
Maternal iodine through iodization of salt[a]	Maternal iodine supplements	Maternal mental health interventions
Maternal multiple micronutrient supplements	Maternal deworming in pregnancy	
Maternal calcium supplementation	Intermittent preventive treatment for malaria Insecticide-treated bed nets	
Neonate		
Breastfeeding promotion strategies (individual & group counseling)	Delayed cord clamping	Baby-friendly hospital initiatives
Infant and Children		
Breastfeeding promotion strategies (individual & group counseling)	Iron fortification/ supplementation programs	Conditional cash transfer programs (with nutrition education)
Behavior change communication for improved complementary feeding	Insecticide-treated bed nets	Unconditional cash transfers & micro-credit programs
Zinc fortification/ supplementation	Provision of complementary foods	Conditional cash transfers (unspecified)
Zinc in management of diarrhea	Neonatal vitamin A supplementation	Hand washing/hygiene interventions
Vitamin A fortification/ supplementation	Multiple micronutrient supplements	Mass media strategies for breastfeeding promotion, dietary diversification, etc
Universal salt iodization	Deworming in children	Food for work programs & generalized food subsidies
Treatment of severe acute malnutrition		Dietary diversification strategies, small animal husbandry & home gardening Agricultural subsidies & land reform

[a] Includes interventions in the neonatal period of life.

and postpartum women. The evidence base for multiple micronutrient supplementation of young children and infants is weak.

A recent meta-analysis indicates a 39% reduction in maternal anemia with supplementation of multiple micronutrients when compared with placebo or with one or more micronutrients,[68] as well as reduction in LBW.[69,70] However, multiple micronutrient

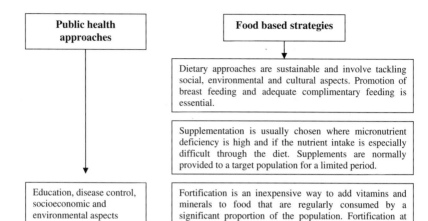

Fig. 8. Framework to address micronutrient deficiencies.

supplementations did not differ from iron and folic acid supplementation in terms of rates of LBW babies, or of those who were small for gestational age. A meta-analysis of trials of supplementation with a specific multiple micronutrient formulation for pregnant women[71] compared with iron and folic acid reported a small increase in birth weight. Two additional trials of multiple micronutrient supplements in pregnancy in India[69] and Tanzania[70] also showed that this intervention reduced the rate of LBW babies.

Zinc Supplementation in Children

Zinc supplementation in pregnancy has been shown to reduce prematurity, but its effects on IUGR have not been proven. Zinc supplementation decreases the episodes of diarrhea, persistent diarrhea, severe diarrhea, and ARI.[25,37] Adding zinc to the treatment of diarrhea reduces the duration,[72] severity, and frequency of diarrhea and infections of the lower respiratory tract by 15% to 24%. Child mortality is decreased by 9% by giving zinc supplementation.[34,38,73–76]

Supplementation with Iodine and Calcium

Calcium supplementation in women who are at greatest risk of hypertensive disorders in pregnancy and with low intake of calcium decreases the risk of preeclampsia.[77] Iodine supplementation in pregnancy is associated with reduced risk of congenital hypothyroidism at age 4 years and reduction in mortality by 29%.[78,79] It is now particularly evident that micronutrient deficiency is a major risk factor for morbidity and mortality, and that timely provision of supplements, fortified food, or a better diet is followed by a reduction in the prevalence, severity, and mortality from certain key infections among children and mothers.

Breastfeeding Promotion

The benefits of breastfeeding are extensive and well documented. For infants, ensuring a diet of breast milk is an effective way of preventing micronutrient deficiencies and, more importantly, in reducing mortality.[1,80,81] In much of the developing world, breast milk is the main source of micronutrients during the first year of life (with the exception of iron). In most of the developing world initiation of breastfeeding is not

Table 8
Effect of general and all nutrition-related interventions on mortality and stunting in 36 countries[60]

	Proportional Reduction in Deaths Before Specific Ages			Relative Reduction In Prevalence of Stunting at Specific Ages			% of DALYs Averted at 36 Months
	12 mo	24 mo	36 mo	12 mo	24 mo	36 mo	
99% coverage with balanced energy protein supplementation	3.6	3.1	2.9	1.9	0.5	0.3	2.8
99% coverage with intermittent preventive treatment	2.4	2.1	1.9	1.4	0.3	0.1	1.9
99% coverage with multiple micronutrient supplementation in pregnancy	2.0	1.7	1.6	0.9	0.3	0.1	1.5
99% coverage with breastfeeding promotion and support	11.6	9.9	0	0	0	0	8.6
99% coverage with feeding interventions (promotion of complementary feeding and other supportive strategies)	0	1.1	9.1	19.8	17.2	15.0	2.1
99% coverage with vitamin A (including neonatal in Asia)	6.9	7.1	1.5	0	0	0	6.9
99% coverage with zinc supplementation	1.3	2.8	7.2	9.1	15.5	17.0	4.2
99% coverage with hygiene interventions	0	0.1	0.2	1.9	2.4	2.4	0.2
99% coverage with all interventions	24.0	24.4	24.7	33.1	35.8	35.5	25.1
90% coverage with all interventions	22.0	22.2	22.4	31.1	32.4	32.1	22.7
70% coverage with all interventions	17.3	17.3	17.3	22.7	24.1	23.6	17.5

a problem, while exclusive breastfeeding for the first 6 months of life and continuation into the second year should be promoted.

Early cessation of breastfeeding even in the presence of human immunodeficiency virus infection leads to deficiencies of iron, zinc, and other micronutrients. Growth failure, anemia, impaired immune response, and increase in the prevalence of severe infection are all possible in the child who is not breastfed. In addition, the loss of the contraceptive benefits of breastfeeding increases the risk of early further pregnancies with associated detriment to maternal health.

In its guidelines the WHO[82] recommends exclusive breastfeeding for the first 6 months rather than the first 4 to 6 months. There are concerns that exclusive breastfeeding for this long might be difficult, particularly where maternal malnutrition is common. Multiple approaches exist to prolong exclusive breastfeeding: health education; professional support; lay support; health sector changes (eg, infant friendly hospitals); and media campaigns. Two strategies have been successful in the promotion of exclusive breastfeeding: the Baby Friendly Hospital Initiative, which increased the likelihood of exclusive breastfeeding in health facilities,[83] and the use of peer counselors in settings where most babies are delivered at home.[84,85] The second approach, based on recruitment of workers dedicated to a single intervention, is unlikely to be sustainable in health systems with few resources. Studies have shown the effect of individual as well as group counseling on the promotion of exclusive breastfeeding.[59]

Promotion of Appropriate Complementary Feeding

Complementary feeding is the process of introducing other foods and liquids into the child's diet when breast milk alone is no longer sufficient to meet nutritional requirements. Complementary feeding practices are suboptimal from several perspectives: complementary foods are introduced too early or too late, foods are served too infrequently or in insufficient amounts, or their consistency or energy density is inappropriate, the micronutrient content of foods is inadequate to meet the child's needs, or other factors in the diet impair the absorption of foods and microbial contamination may occur. In developing countries nutritional education, educational interventions, and combination of education with supplementation of food fortified with multiple micronutrients can produce major effects on reduction of stunting and achieving desired outcomes.[59] Maternal education regarding breastfeeding practices and complementary feeding has a great effect on growth and micronutrient status of infants.

Other Food Fortification Strategies

There are several benefits of fortification of food, as it requires no change in food habits, does not alter the characteristics of food, can produce desired nutritional benefits, and is a safe and cost-effective method to reach a large target population that is at risk of micronutrient deficiency. Iron fortification increases the hemoglobin level in women of child-bearing age[86,87] and pregnancy,[88] as well as achieving a 70% reduction in prevalence of anemia in school children.[89–92] Milk fortified with iron and zinc can also decrease the days of illness by 15% and incidence of ARI by 26%.[93] Water iodization reduces occurrence of goiter by 51% to 89%[94–97] whereas fortification of salt with iodine reduces this occurrence by 19% to 64%.[98–105]

Management of Severe Acute Malnutrition in Childhood in Hospitals and Community Settings

Acute malnutrition, especially SAM, is an unstable condition resulting from a relatively short duration of nutritional deficit that is often complicated by concurrent infective illness. Children with SAM have a limited ability to respond to stressful conditions and are highly vulnerable. It is thus vital to treat SAM proactively with short-duration, highly intensive treatment regimens that aim to rehabilitate the child in a few weeks.

In recent years, an increasing number of countries and international relief agencies have adopted a community-based model for the management of acute malnutrition, called community-based therapeutic care (CTC).[106,107] The CTC model consists of

4 elements: measures to mobilize the community to encourage early presentation and compliance; outpatient supplementary feeding protocols for those with moderate acute malnutrition and no serious medical complications; outpatient therapeutic protocols for those with SAM and no serious medical complications; and inpatient therapeutic protocols for those with acute malnutrition also suffering from serious medical complications.

The provision of energy- and nutrient-dense foods, including sufficient micronutrients, is a vital determinant of the successful treatment of SAM. Many studies have shown the efficacy of WHO guidelines for management of SAM in comparison with conventional treatment.[108–114] The WHO, UNICEF, and UN recommended management of SAM with ready-to-use foods in emergency settings. CTC programs have treated more than 9000 severely malnourished children in Ethiopia, Malawi, and Sudan, where case fatality rates were 4.1%, with recovery rates of 79.4% and default rates of 11.0%. Seventy-six percent of these severely malnourished children were treated solely as outpatients.[115,116] Similar positive results have recently been published from Niger, where more than 60,000 children with SAM were treated using an approach based on an outpatient treatment program (OTP) design. Approximately 70% of these children were treated solely as outpatients, and overall case fatality rates were approximately 5%.[117]

In the CTC approach, SAM is subdivided based on whether there are coexistent life-threatening complications. Children presenting with SAM complicated by life-threatening illness are admitted into "stabilization centers" where they receive inpatient care based on the WHO inpatient treatment protocols. CTC complements the existing WHO inpatient protocols, using ready-to-use therapeutic food (RUTF) to treat most children suffering from SAM solely as outpatients and reserving inpatient treatment for those with complications. RUTF is energy-dense, mineral- and vitamin-enriched food, is relatively cheap to produce and, so long as the patient has an appetite, easy to administer, making success rates high and costs per treatment low in comparison with previously used F75 and F100.

Those with SAM but without life-threatening complications (usually 80%–90% of presentations) are treated solely as outpatients through weekly or fortnightly attendance in OTPs. The OTP provides RUTF and medicines to treat simple medical conditions. Treating patients with SAM without complications solely as outpatients greatly reduces the demand for skilled staff and resources, the lack of which is itself a major problem in developing countries.

Application of WHO protocols would reduce the number of deaths by 55%, which is equivalent to 5 million deaths. Achieving the fourth millennium development goal of a two-thirds reduction in childhood mortality will not be possible if SAM is not addressed effectively. Changes must be made in funding priorities and child survival strategies if the maximum potential of CTC is to be attained.[118]

Promoting Dietary Diversity

Dietary diversification usually implies increasing both the quantity and the range of micronutrient-rich foods consumed. This strategy requires the implementation of programs, such as increasing agriculture, that improve the availability and consumption of, and access to different types of micronutrient-rich foods, but these programs have only been implemented on a small scale in poor countries and are not adequately assessed.[119–121] Increasing dietary diversity is the preferred way of improving nutrition because it increases the intake of not only important food constituents but also micronutrients, but it is not effective on a large scale.

Use of Insecticide-Treated Bed Nets

Use of insecticide-treated bed nets during pregnancy was associated with a 23% reduction in the risk of delivering LBW babies.[122,123] Few other studies have also assessed the use of these bed nets during pregnancy.[124]

Hygiene and Hand-Washing Promotion

A pooled analysis of several concurrent interventions, which included data from 7 studies in children younger than 5 years, suggested a decrease in diarrhea episodes. Three other reviews assessed the effect of hygiene interventions (eg, hand washing, water quality treatment, sanitation, and health education). Similarly pooled analysis of 6 studies of hand-washing counseling (for individuals or groups) suggested a 30% reduction in the risk of diarrhea.[125–127]

Deworming in Pregnancy and Childhood

Two studies that assessed the effect of deworming interventions during pregnancy showed that the mean decrease in hemoglobin concentration between the first and third trimesters in women who received albendazole was $6\cdot6$ g/L less than in women who received placebo.[128,129] In a systematic review of 25 studies that assessed the nutritional effect of deworming in children,[130] analysis of growth outcomes in children aged 1 to 16 years suggested that one dose was associated with an average 0.24 (95% confidence interval [CI] $0\cdot15$–$0\cdot32$) kg increase in weight. Another systematic review of deworming[131] assessed the effect on hemoglobin and anemia rates. In this study the pooled weighted mean difference of the change in hemoglobin was 1.71 (95% CI 0.70–2.73) g/L and the average estimated reduction in frequency of anemia ranged from 4.4% to 21.0% in children. In populations with high rates of intestinal helminthiasis, this can reduce the rates of anemia by 5% to 10%.

CONTROVERSIES AND UNRESOLVED ISSUES

Not everything in public health nutrition is straightforward, and there are several issues that have provoked controversy in the past such as misguided use of high protein intake supplements for malnourished children.[132] Among recent controversies, maternal multiple micronutrient supplements have been criticized for possible association with an increased risk of neonatal mortality in health systems without adequate access to skilled care.[133] Given the reported increase in malaria-associated morbidity following the use of large-scale iron supplementation in Zanzibar,[134] the entire rationale for blanket iron supplements in children has been questioned. Nutrient interactions, especially in complex formulations, are another area for research, and may underlie the apparent failure of benefits of multiple micronutrient supplements on growth in children.[135] Long-standing global programs such as growth monitoring and promotion,[136] school feeding,[137] and the Baby-Friendly Hospital Initiative[138] have been questioned because of a less than solid scientific base and evidence of impact. It is thus imperative that all nutrition interventions be based on a strong scientific foundation and are adequately monitored for impact.

SUMMARY

Maternal and child undernutrition is a global problem, largely affecting developing countries and poor populations. Stunting reflects chronic nutritional deficiency, and is a problem of greater magnitude in comparison with other forms of undernutrition. Among children younger than 5 years in the developing world, an estimated 195 million children (one-third of all children) are stunted, whereas 129 million are underweight. More than 90% of the developing world's stunted children live in Africa and Asia, and a mere 24 countries bear 80% of the burden of undernutrition as measured by stunting in the developing world.

The major risk factors for undernutrition are poverty affecting food security and dietary intake, but in many countries family behavior and feeding practices during health and disease play an equally important role. Poor environments and lack of sanitation/hygiene significantly increase the risk of diarrhea and other illnesses that deplete children of vital nutrients, which can lead to chronic undernutrition and increase the risk of death.

There is a critical window of opportunity to prevent undernutrition: during pregnancy while the fetus is growing and during a child's first 24 months of life. Evidence-based nutrition interventions can make a difference to short-term outcomes and also offer children the best opportunity for long-term growth and development. These interventions include strategies to improve maternal nutrition before and during pregnancy, early and exclusive breastfeeding, and good-quality complementary feeding for infants and young children, with appropriate micronutrient interventions. In addition to these nutrition interventions, other health promotion strategies include attention to programs to address unsafe water, inadequate sanitation, and poor hygiene.

Improving child and maternal nutrition is not only entirely feasible but also affordable and cost-effective. Nutrition interventions are among the best investments in development that countries can undertake. What is needed is the implementation of this knowledge through community participation. Large-scale programs, including the promotion, protection, and support of exclusive breastfeeding, provision of vitamins and minerals through fortified foods and supplements, and community-based treatment of SAM, have been successful in many countries. The recent global economic and food price crises have underscored the importance of preserving food and nutrition security among vulnerable populations. We now need the combined efforts of practitioners and policy makers to confine hunger and undernutrition to history.

REFERENCES

1. Black RE, Allen LH, Bhutta ZA, et al. Maternal and child undernutrition: global and regional exposures and health consequences. Lancet 2008;371:243–60.
2. United Nations ACC/SCN. Geneva (Switzerland): Fourth Report on World Nutrition Status; 2000.
3. Rice AL, West KP, Black RE. Vitamin A deficiency. In: Ezzati M, Lopez AD, Rodgers A, Murray CL, editors. Comparative quantification of health risks: global and regional burden of disease attributes to selected major risk factors. Geneva (Switzerland): World Health Organization; 2004. p. 211–56.
4. Fishman SM, Caulfield L, de Onis M, et al. Childhood and maternal underweight. In: Ezzati M, Lopez AD, Rodgers A, Murray CL, editors. Comparative quantification of health risks: global and regional burden of disease attributable to selected major risk factors. Geneva, (Switzerland): World Health Organization; 2004. p. 139–61.
5. WHO. Maternal anthropometry and pregnancy outcomes: A WHO Collaborative Study. Bull World Health Organ 1995;73(Suppl):32–7.
6. De Onis M, Blossner M, Villar J. Levels and patterns of intrauterine growth retardation in developing countries. Eur J Clin Nutr 1998;52:S5–15.
7. Victora CG, Adair L, Fall C, et al. Maternal and child undernutrition: consequences for adult health and human capital. Lancet 2008;371(9609):340–57.

8. Menezes AM, Hallal PC, Santos IS, et al. Infant mortality in pelotas, Brazil: a comparison of risk factors in two birth cohorts. Rev Panam Salud Publica 2005;18:439–46.

9. Mullany LC, Darmstadt GL, Khatry SK, et al. Topical applications of chlorhexidine to the umbilical cord for prevention of omphalitis and neonatal mortality in southern Nepal: a community-based, cluster-randomized trial. Lancet 2006; 367:910–8.

10. Rahmathullah L, Tielsch JM, Thulasiraj RD, et al. Impact of supplementing newborn infants with vitamin A on early infant mortality: community based randomized trial in southern India. BMJ 2003;327:254–60.

11. Christian P, West KP, Khatry SK, et al. Effects of maternal micronutrient supplementation on fetal loss and infant mortality: a cluster-randomized trial in Nepal. Am J Clin Nutr 2003;78:1194–202.

12. World Health Organization Comparative Quantification of Health Risks: childhood and maternal undernutrition, WHO library cataloguing-in-publication data. Available at: http://www.who.int/publications/cra/chapters/volume1/0000i-xxiv.pdf. Accessed September 15, 2010.

13. Osendarp SJ, van Raaij JM, Arifeen SE, et al. A randomized, placebo controlled trial of the effect of zinc supplementation during pregnancy on pregnancy outcomes in Bangladeshi urban poor. Am J Clin Nutr 2000;71:114–9.

14. Katz J, Khatry SK, West KP, et al. Night blindness during pregnancy and lactation in rural Nepal. J Nutr 1995;125:2122–7.

15. Christian P, West KP, Khatry SK, et al. Night blindness of pregnancy in rural Nepal—nutritional and health risks. Int J Epidemiol 1998;27:231–7.

16. Beaton GH, Martorell R, Aronson KJ, et al. Effectiveness of vitamin A supplementation in the control of young child morbidity and mortality in developing countries. Geneva, (Switzerland): United Nations Administrative Committee on Coordination/Sub-Committee on Nutrition; 1993. Report No: discussion paper No. 13. Geneva, (Switzerland): United Nations Administrative Committee on Coordination/Sub-Committee on Nutrition; 1993.

17. Humphrey JH, Agoestina T, Wu L, et al. Impact of neonatal vitamin A supplementation on infant morbidity and mortality. J Pediatr 1996;128:489–96.

18. Klemm R, Labrique A, Christian P, et al. Efficacy of newborn vitamin A supplementation in reducing infant mortality in rural Bangladesh: the JiVitA-2 trial. In: Proceedings of the Micronutrient Forum. Consequences and control of micronutrient deficiencies: science, policy, and programs—defining the issues. Istanbul (Turkey), April 16–18, 2007.

19. Holick MF. Resurrection of vitamin D deficiency and rickets. J Clin Invest 2006; 116:2062–72.

20. Pettifor JM. Vitamin D and/or calcium deficiency rickets in infants and children: a concern for developing countries? Indian Pediatr 2007;44:893–5.

21. Haidar J, Abate G, Kogi-Makau W, et al. Risk factors for child under-nutrition with a human rights edge in rural villages of North Wollo, Ethiopia. East Afr med J 2005;82:625–30.

22. Bhan MK, Bhandari N, Bhal R. Management of the severely malnourished child: perspective from developing countries. BMJ 2003;326:146–51.

23. International Institute of Population Sciences. National family health survey (NFHS2), 1998–99. Mumbai (India): International Institute of Population Sciences; 2000.

24. Manary MJ, Ndkeha MJ, Ashorn P, et al. Home based therapy for severe malnutrition with ready-to-use food. Arch Dis Child 2004;89:557–61.

25. Bhutta ZA, Black RE, Brown KH. Prevention of diarrhea and pneumonia by zinc supplementation in children in developing countries: pooled analysis of randomized controlled trials. Zinc Investigators' Collaborative Group. J Pediatr 1999; 135:689–97.
26. Appoh LY, Krekling S. Maternal nutritional knowledge and child nutritional status in the Volta region of Ghana. Matern Child Nutr 2005;1:100–10.
27. Kikafunda JK, Walker AF, Collett D, et al. Risk factors for early childhood malnutrition in Uganda. Pediatrics 1998;102:E45.
28. Sakisaka K, Wakai S, Kuroiwa C, et al. Nutritional status and associated factors in children aged 0–23 months in Granada, Nicaragua. Public Health 2006;120: 400–11.
29. Odunayo SI, Oyewole AO. Risk factors for malnutrition among rural Nigerian children. Asia Pac J Clin Nutr 2006;15:491–5.
30. Jeyaseelan L, Lakshman M. Risk factors for malnutrition in south Indian children. J Biosoc Sci 1997;29:93–100.
31. Islam MA, Rahman MM, Mahalanabis D. Maternal and socioeconomic factors and risk of severe malnutrition in a child: a case-control study. Eur J Clin Nutr 1994;48:416–24.
32. UNICEF. State of the world's children 2005. New York: UNICEF; 2005.
33. Walker CF, Black RE. Zinc and the risk for infectious disease. Annu Rev Nutr 2004;24:255–75.
34. Sazawal S, Black RE, Ramsan M, et al. Effect of zinc supplementation on mortality in children aged 1–48 months: a community-based randomized placebo-controlled trial. Lancet 2007;369:927–34.
35. Brooks WA, Yunus M, Santosham M, et al. Zinc for severe pneumonia in very young children: double-blind placebo-controlled trial. Lancet 2004;363: 1683–8.
36. Tielsch JM, Khatry SK, Stoltzfus RJ, et al. Effect of daily zinc supplementation on child mortality in southern Nepal: a community-based, cluster randomised, placebo-controlled trial. Lancet 2007;370:1230–9.
37. Aggarwal R, Sentz J, Miller MA. Role of zinc administration in prevention of childhood diarrhea and respiratory illnesses: a meta-analysis. Pediatrics 2007; 119:1120–30.
38. Brooks WA, Santosham M, Naheed A, et al. Effect of weekly zinc supplements on incidence of pneumonia and diarrhoea in children younger than 2 years in an urban, low-income population in Bangladesh: randomised controlled trial. Lancet 2005;366:999–1004.
39. Dalmiya N, Palmer A, Darnton-Hill I. Sustaining vitamin A supplementation requires a new vision. Lancet 2006;368:1052–4.
40. Powers HJ, Bates CJ, Lamb WH. Hematological response to supplements of iron and riboflavin to pregnant and lactating women in rural Gambia. Hum Nutr Clin Nutr 1985;39C:117–29.
41. Prasad PA, Bamji MS, Kakshmi AV, et al. Functional impact of riboflavin supplementation in urban schoolchildren. Nutr Res 1990;10:275–81.
42. Rivlin RS. Riboflavin. In: Bowman BA, Russel RM, editors. Present knowledge in nutrition. 8th Edition. Washington, DC: International Life Sciences Institute; 2001. p. 191–8, Chapter 18.
43. Bhutta ZA. Micronutrient needs of malnourished children. Curr Opin Clin Nutr Metab Care 2008;11:309–14.
44. Lutter CK, Rivera JA. Nutritional status of infants and young children and characteristics of their diets. J Nutr 2003;133:2941S–9S.

45. Bhatia V. Dietary calcium intake—a critical appraisal. Indian J Med Res 2008; 127:269–73.

46. Grillenberger M, Neumann CG, Murphy SP, et al. Intake of micronutrients high in animal-source foods is associated with better growth in rural Kenyan school children. Br J Nutr 2006;95:379–90.

47. Norris SA, Sheppard ZA, Griffiths PL, et al. Current socio-economic measures, and not those measured during infancy, affects bone mass in poor urban South African children. J Bone Miner Res 2008;23(9):1409–16.

48. Takyi EE. Nutritional status and nutrient intake of preschool children in northern Ghana. East Afr Med J 1999;76:510–5.

49. Norhayati M, Noor Hayati MI, Oothuman P, et al. Nutrient intake and socio-economic status among children attending a health exhibition in Malaysian rural villages. Med J Malaysia 1995;50:382–90.

50. Ma G, Li Y, Jin Y, et al. Phytate intake and molar rations of phytate to zinc, iron and calcium in the diets of people in China. Eur J Clin Nutr 2007;61:368–74.

51. Thacher TD, Fischer PR, Strand MA, et al. Nutritional rickets around the world: causes and future directions. Ann Trop Pediatr 2006;26:1–16.

52. Frongillo EA Jr, de Onis M, Hanson KM. Socioeconomic and demographic factors are associated with worldwide patterns of stunting and wasting of children. J Nutr 1997;127:2302–9.

53. Seal AJ, Creeke PI, Mirghani Z, et al. Iron and vitamin A deficiency in long-term African refugees. J Nutr 2005;135:808–13.

54. Kemmer TM, Bovill ME, Kongsomboon W, et al. Iron deficiency is unacceptably high in refugee children from Burma. J Nutr 2003;133:4143–9.

55. Arifeen S, Black RE, Antelman G, et al. Exclusive breastfeeding reduces acute respiratory infection and diarrhea deaths among infants in Dhaka slums. Pediatrics 2001;108:E67.

56. Bahl R, Frost C, Kirkwood BR, et al. Infant feeding patterns and risks of death and hospitalization in the first half of infancy: multicentre cohort study. Bull World Health Organ 2005;83:418–26.

57. Sazawal S, Black RE, Bhan MK, et al. Zinc supplementation in young children with acute diarrhea in India. N Engl J Med 1995;333:839–44.

58. Penny ME, Peerson JM, Marin RM, et al. Randomized community based trial of the effect of zinc supplementation with and without other micronutrients, on the duration of persistent childhood diarrhea in Lima, Peru. J Pediatr 1999;135:208–17.

59. Bhutta ZA, Ahmed T, Black RE, et al. What works? Interventions for maternal and child undernutrition and survival. Lancet 2008;371:417–40.

60. Kramer MS, Kakuma R. Energy and protein intake in pregnancy. Cochrane Database Syst Rev 2003;4:CD000032.

61. Ceesay SM, Prentice AM, Cole TJ, et al. Effects on birth weight and perinatal mortality of maternal dietary supplements in rural Gambia: 5 year randomised controlled trial. BMJ 1997;315:786–90.

62. Pena-Rosas JP, Viteri FE. Effects of routine oral iron supplementation with or without folic acid for women during pregnancy. Cochrane Database Syst Rev 2006;3:CD004736.

63. Gera T, Sachdev HP, Nestel P, et al. Effect of iron supplementation on hemoglobin response in children: systematic review of randomised controlled trials. J Pediatr Gastroenterol Nutr 2007;44:468–86.

64. West KP Jr, Katz J, Khatry SK, et al. Double blind, cluster randomised trial of low dose supplementation with vitamin A or beta carotene on mortality

related to pregnancy in Nepal. The NNIPS-2 Study Group. BMJ 1999;318: 570–5.

65. Christian P, West Jr K, Labrique A, et al. Effects of maternal vitamin A or beta-carotene supplementation on maternal and infant mortality in rural Bangladesh: the JiVitA-1 trial. In: Proceedings of the Micronutrient Forum. Consequences and control of micronutrient deficiencies: science, policy, and programs. April 16–18, 2007; Istanbul, Turkey. Washington, DC, USA: US Agency for International Development; 2007. 129.

66. Grotto I, Mimouni M, Gdalevich M, et al. Vitamin A supplementation and childhood morbidity from diarrhea and respiratory infections: a meta-analysis. J Pediatr 2003;142:297–304.

67. Malaba LC, Iliff PJ, Nathoo KJ, et al. Effect of postpartum maternal or neonatal vitamin A supplementation on infant mortality among infants born to HIV-negative mothers in Zimbabwe. Am J Clin Nutr 2005;81:454–60.

68. Haider BA, Bhutta ZA. Multiple-micronutrient supplementation for women during pregnancy. Cochrane Database Syst Rev 2006;4:CD004905.

69. Gupta P, Ray M, Dua T, et al. Multimicronutrient supplementation for undernourished pregnant women and the birth size of their offspring: a double-blind, randomized, placebo-controlled trial. Arch Pediatr Adolesc Med 2007;161: 58–64.

70. Fawzi WW, Msamanga GI, Urassa W, et al. Vitamins and perinatal outcomes among HIV-negative women in Tanzania. N Engl J Med 2007;356:1423–31.

71. UNICEF/WHO/UNU. Composition of a multi-micronutrient supplement to be used in pilot programmes among pregnant women in developing countries. New York: UNICEF; 1999.

72. Bhutta ZA, Bird SM, Black RE, et al. Therapeutic effects of oral zinc in acute and persistent diarrhea in children in developing countries: pooled analysis of randomized controlled trials. Am J Clin Nutr 2000;72:1516–22.

73. Tielsch JM, Khatry SK, Stoltzfus RJ, et al. Effect of routine prophylactic supplementation with iron and folic acid on preschool child mortality in southern Nepal: community-based, cluster-randomised, placebo-controlled trial. Lancet 2006; 367:144–52.

74. Bhandari N, Bahl R, Taneja S, et al. Substantial reduction in severe diarrheal morbidity by daily zinc supplementation in young north Indian children. Pediatrics 2002;109:e86.

75. Baqui AH, Black RE, El Arifeen S, et al. Effect of zinc supplementation started during diarrhoea on morbidity and mortality in Bangladeshi children: community randomised trial. BMJ 2002;325:1059.

76. Lira PI, Ashworth A, Morris SS. Effect of zinc supplementation on the morbidity, immune function, and growth of low-birth-weight, full-term infants in northeast Brazil. Am J Clin Nutr 1998;68:418–24.

77. Hofmeyr GJ, Atallah AN, Duley L. Calcium supplementation during pregnancy for preventing hypertensive disorders and related problems. Cochrane Database Syst Rev 2006;3:CD001059.

78. Thilly CH, Delange F, Lagasse R, et al. Fetal hypothyroidism and maternal thyroid status in severe endemic goiter. J Clin Endocrinol Metab 1978;47: 354–60.

79. Pharoah PO, Connolly KJ. A controlled trial of iodinated oil for the prevention of endemic cretinism: A long term follow up. Int J Epidemiol 1987;16:68–73.

80. Effect of breastfeeding on infant and child mortality due to infectious diseases in less developed countries: a pooled analysis. WHO collaborative study team on

the role of breastfeeding on the prevention of infant mortality. Lancet 2000;355: 451–5.

81. Jones G, Steketee RW, Black RE, et al. How many child deaths can we prevent this year? Lancet 2003;362:65–71.

82. World Health Organization. The optimal duration of exclusive breastfeeding: report of an expert consultation, Geneva, Switzerland, 28–30 March 2001. Document ref WHO/NHD/01.09. Geneva (Switzerland): WHO; 2002.

83. Kramer MS, Chalmers B, Hodnett ED, et al. Promotion of breastfeeding intervention trials (PROBIT): a randomised trial in the Republic of Belarus. JAMA 2001; 285:413–20.

84. Morrow AL, Guerrero ML, Shults J, et al. Efficacy of home-based peer counselling to promote exclusive breastfeeding: a randomised controlled trial. Lancet 1999;353:1226–31.

85. Haider R, Ashworth A, Kabir I, et al. Effect of community-based peer counselors on exclusive breastfeeding practices in Dhaka, Bangladesh: a randomised controlled trial. Lancet 2000;356:1643–7.

86. Ballot DE, MacPhail AP, Bothwell TH, et al. Fortification of curry powder with NaFe (111) EDTA in an iron-deficient population: report of a controlled iron-fortification trial. Am J Clin Nutr 1989;49:162–9.

87. Thuy PV, Berger J, Davidsson L, et al. Regular consumption of NaFeEDTA-fortified fish sauce improves iron status and reduces the prevalence of anemia in anemic Vietnamese women. Am J Clin Nutr 2003;78:284–90.

88. Thuy PV, Berger J, Nakanishi Y, et al. The use of NaFeEDTA-fortified fish sauce is an effective tool for controlling iron deficiency in women of childbearing age in rural Vietnam. J Nutr 2005;135:2596–601.

89. Nadiger HA, Krishnamachari KA, Naidu AN, et al. The use of common salt (sodium chloride) fortified with iron to control anaemia: results of a preliminary study. Br J Nutr 1980;43:45–51.

90. Walter T, Hertrampf E, Pizarro F, et al. Effect of bovine-hemoglobin-fortified cookies on iron status of schoolchildren: a nationwide program in Chile. Am J Clin Nutr 1993;57:190–4.

91. van Stuijvenberg ME, Smuts CM, Wolmarans P, et al. The efficacy of ferrous bisglycinate and electrolytic iron as fortified cants in bread in iron-deficient school children. Br J Nutr 2006;95:532–8.

92. Behrman J, Hoddinott J. An evaluation of the impact of PROGRESA on preschool child height, Discussion Paper No 104. Washington, DC: Food Consumption and Nutrition Division, International Food Policy Research Institute (IFPRI); 2001.

93. Sazawal S, Dhingra U, Dhingra P, et al. Effects of fortified milk on morbidity in young children in north India: community based, randomised, double masked placebo controlled trial. BMJ 2007;334:140.

94. Elnagar B, Eltom M, Karlsson FA, et al. Control of iodine deficiency using iodination of water in a goiter endemic area. Int J Food Sci Nutr 1997;48: 119–27.

95. Squatrito S, Vigneri R, Runello F, et al. Prevention and treatment of endemic iodine-deficiency goiter by iodination of a municipal water supply. J Clin Endocrinol Metab 1986;63:368–75.

96. Maberly GF, Eastman CJ, Corcoran JM. Effect of iodination of a village water-supply on goitre size and thyroid function. Lancet 1981;2:1270–2.

97. Pichard E, Soula G, Fisch A, et al. Prevention of iodine deficiency disorders in children in the rural African zone. Ann Pediatr 1992;39:71–8.

136. Ashworth A, Shrimpton R, Jamil K. Growth monitoring and promotion: review of evidence of impact. Matern Child Nutr 2008;1(Suppl 4):86–117.
137. Galloway R, Kristjansson E, Gelli A, et al. School feeding: outcomes and costs. Food Nutr Bull 2009;30:171–82.
138. Abrahams SW, Labbok MH. Exploring the impact of the Baby-Friendly Hospital Initiative on trends in exclusive breastfeeding. Int Breastfeed J 2009;4:11.

Index

Note: Page numbers of article titles are in **boldface** type.

Pediatr Clin N Am 57 (2010) 1443–1458
doi:10.1016/S0031-3955(10)00184-7
0031-3955/10/$ – see front matter © 2010 Elsevier Inc. All rights reserved.

pediatric.theclinics.com

United States Postal Service

Statement of Ownership, Management, and Circulation
(All Periodicals Publications Except Requestor Publications)

1. Publication Title	2. Publication Number	3. Filing Date
Pediatric Clinics of North America	4 2 4 - 6 6 0 0	9/15/10

4. Issue Frequency	5. Number of Issues Published Annually	6. Annual Subscription Price
Feb, Apr, Jun, Aug, Oct, Dec	6	$167.00

7. Complete Mailing Address of Known Office of Publication (Not printer) (Street, city, county, state, and ZIP+4®)

Elsevier Inc.
360 Park Avenue South
New York, NY 10010-1710

Contact Person
Stephen Bushing

Telephone (Include area code)
215-239-3688

8. Complete Mailing Address of Headquarters or General Business Office of Publisher (Not printer)

Elsevier Inc., 360 Park Avenue South, New York, NY 10010-1710

9. Full Names and Complete Mailing Addresses of Publisher, Editor, and Managing Editor (Do not leave blank)

Publisher (Name and complete mailing address)

Kim Murphy, Elsevier, Inc., 1600 John F. Kennedy Blvd. Suite 1800, Philadelphia, PA 19103-2899

Editor (Name and complete mailing address)

Carla Holloway, Elsevier, Inc., 1600 John F. Kennedy Blvd. Suite 1800, Philadelphia, PA 19103-2899

Managing Editor (Name and complete mailing address)

Catherine Bewick, Elsevier, Inc., 1600 John F. Kennedy Blvd. Suite 1800, Philadelphia, PA 19103-2899

10. Owner (Do not leave blank. If the publication is owned by a corporation, give the name and address of the corporation immediately followed by the names and addresses of all stockholders owning or holding 1 percent or more of the total amount of stock. If not owned by a corporation, give the names and addresses of the individual owners. If owned by a partnership or other unincorporated firm, give its name and address as well as those of each individual owner. If the publication is published by a nonprofit organization, give its name and address.)

Full Name	Complete Mailing Address
Wholly owned subsidiary of	4520 East-West Highway
Reed/Elsevier, US holdings	Bethesda, MD 20814

11. Known Bondholders, Mortgages, and Other Security Holders Owning or Holding 1 Percent or More of Total Amount of Bonds, Mortgages, or Other Securities. If none, check box ☑ None

Full Name	Complete Mailing Address
N/A	

12. Tax Status (For completion by nonprofit organizations authorized to mail at nonprofit rates) (Check one)
The purpose, function, and nonprofit status of this organization and the exempt status for federal income tax purposes:
☐ Has Not Changed During Preceding 12 Months
☐ Has Changed During Preceding 12 Months (Publisher must submit explanation of change with this statement)

PS Form **3526**, September 2007 (Page 1 of 3 (Instructions Page 3)) PSN 7530-01-000-9931 PRIVACY NOTICE: See our Privacy policy in www.usps.com

---

13. Publication Title	14. Issue Date for Circulation Data Below
Pediatric Clinics of North America	June 2010

15. Extent and Nature of Circulation		Average No. Copies Each Issue During Preceding 12 Months	No. Copies of Single Issue Published Nearest to Filing Date
a. Total Number of Copies (Net press run)		4501	4400
b. Paid Circulation (By Mail and Outside the Mail)	(1) Mailed Outside-County Paid Subscriptions Stated on PS Form 3541. (Include paid distribution above nominal rate, advertiser's proof copies, and exchange copies)	1928	1796
	(2) Mailed In-County Paid Subscriptions Stated on PS Form 3541 (Include paid distribution above nominal rate, advertiser's proof copies, and exchange copies)		
	(3) Paid Distribution Outside the Mails Including Sales Through Dealers and Carriers, Street Vendors, Counter Sales, and Other Paid Distribution Outside USPS®	1626	1303
	(4) Paid Distribution by Other Classes Mailed Through the USPS (e.g. First-Class Mail®)		
c. Total Paid Distribution (Sum of 15b (1), (2), (3), and (4))	►	3554	3099
d. Free or Nominal Rate Distribution (By Mail and Outside the Mail)	(1) Free or Nominal Rate Outside-County Copies Included on PS Form 3541	129	132
	(2) Free or Nominal Rate In-County Copies Included on PS Form 3541		
	(3) Free or Nominal Rate Copies Mailed at Other Classes Through the USPS (e.g. First-Class Mail)		
	(4) Free or Nominal Rate Distribution Outside the Mail (Carriers or other means)		
e. Total Free or Nominal Rate Distribution (Sum of 15d (1), (2), (3) and (4))	►	129	132
f. Total Distribution (Sum of 15c and 15e)	►	3683	3231
g. Copies not Distributed (See instructions to publishers #4 (page #3))	►	818	1169
h. Total (Sum of 15f and g)	►	4501	4400
i. Percent Paid (15c divided by 15f times 100)		96.50%	95.91%

16. Publication of Statement of Ownership

☐ If the publication is a general publication, publication of this statement is required. Will be printed in the October 2010 issue of this publication. ☐ Publication not required

17. Signature and Title of Editor, Publisher, Business Manager, or Owner		Date
Stephen R. Bushing — Fulfillment/Inventory Specialist		September 15, 2010

Stephen R. Bushing – Fulfillment/Inventory Specialist

I certify that all information furnished on this form is true and complete. I understand that anyone who furnishes false or misleading information on this form or who omits material or information requested on the form may be subject to criminal sanctions (including fines and imprisonment) and/or civil sanctions (including civil penalties).

PS Form **3526**, September 2007 (Page 2 of 3)

Moving?

Make sure your subscription moves with you!

To notify us of your new address, find your **Clinics Account Number** (located on your mailing label above your name), and contact customer service at:

Email: journalscustomerservice-usa@elsevier.com

800-654-2452 (subscribers in the U.S. & Canada)
314-447-8871 (subscribers outside of the U.S. & Canada)

Fax number: 314-447-8029

Elsevier Health Sciences Division
Subscription Customer Service
3251 Riverport Lane
Maryland Heights, MO 63043

*To ensure uninterrupted delivery of your subscription, please notify us at least 4 weeks in advance of move.